EATING DISORDERS - A PARADIGM OF THE BIOPSYCHOSOCIAL MODEL OF ILLNESS

Edited by **Ignacio Jáuregui-Lobera**

Eating Disorders - A Paradigm of the Biopsychosocial Model of Illness
http://dx.doi.org/10.5772/62610
Edited by Ignacio Jáuregui-Lobera

Contributors

Aurea Lumbau, Giovanni Spano, Nayelli Alvarado Sánchez, Fragiskos Gonidakis, Dafni-Alexandra Karapavlou, Annie Aime, Tanya Guitard, Lise Grousseaud, Abigail Natenshon, Lai Chong Ma, Maria Zaccagnino, Cristina Civilotti, Martina Cussino, Chiara Callerame, Isabel Fernandez, Michel Probst, Jolien Diedens, Martha Peaslee Levine, Francisco J. Vaz-Leal, María Cristina Álvarez Mateos, Laura Rodríguez Santos, María I Ramos Fuentes, Cicek Hocaoglu

Published by InTech
Janeza Trdine 9, 51000 Rijeka, Croatia

Publishing Process Manager Diana Olloni
Technical Editor SPi Global
Cover InTech Design team

First published February, 2017
Printed in Croatia
Legal deposit, Croatia: National and University Library in Zagreb

Additional hard copies can be obtained from orders@intechopen.com

Eating Disorders - A Paradigm of the Biopsychosocial Model of Illness, Edited by Ignacio Jáuregui-Lobera
p. cm.
Print ISBN 978-953-51-2899-1
Online ISBN 978-953-51-2900-4

For EU product safety concerns:
IN TECH d.o.o., Prolaz Marije Krucifikse Kozulić 3, 51000 Rijeka, Croatia,
info@intechopen.com or visit our website at intechopen.com.

Meet the editor

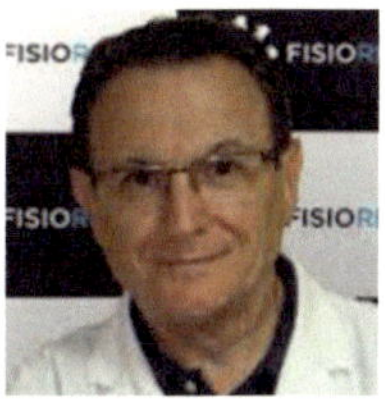

Ignacio Jáuregui-Lobera, MD, PhD, MSc, is a doctor of Medicine and Psychology. He has a Master of Science and Nutrition from the University of Barcelona, Spain and a Master of Arts in Applied Statistics from the National University of Distance Education, Spain. He is an expert in Biostatistics (UNED), Advanced Methods of Applied Statistics (UNED), and completed his post-graduate studies in Food-Drug Interactions (University of Barcelona, Spain.) He is the Director of the Behavioural Sciences Institute (Sevilla, Spain) leading the lifelong learning programme "Expert in Eating Disorders and Obesity," and an Associate Professor at the Pablo de Olavide University in Seville, Spain. He has been working in the field of eating disorders since 1993 and is a recipient of the Extraordinary PsyD Award.

Contents

Preface

Despite the relevance of eating disorders in the past years, the pure core of these mental disorders remains unknown. In this regard, it is not a surprise that the biopsychosocial model is the best way to go forward in order to understand and to improve the different approaches, biological (mainly neurobiological), psychological, and social. The integration of these various approaches have been shown to be the best way to manage eating disorders.

Eating disorders have a long history. In some Egyptian, Persian and Chinese documents it is possible to see the use of purges and disturbances to some extent similar to modern eating disorders. Later on, people who fasted due to food scarcity sometimes (or many times) continued with an extremely restrictive diet despite there being no further need for such restriction. This behaviour has also been evidenced in oral traditions from Africa where under spiritual direction some people, mainly women, have starved themselves in order to get their souls free with respect to the body - the body being a symbol of sin. Apart from these curiosities, it was in 1686 when Richard Morton described a patient ("a skeleton clad with skin") with a similar disorder to what is now known as anorexia nervosa and then, Sir William Gull and Ernest-Charles Lasegue described what is now considered "modern" anorexia nervosa. With respect to bulimia nervosa, it was medically described by Pierre Janet in 1903 ("a woman who engaged in compulsive binges in secret"), and then, Gerald Russell pointed out the first criteria of bulimia nervosa in 1979. By the 1990's binge eating disorders started to be recognised as another form of eating disorders.

Recently (2013), the DSM-5 was published including, as main eating disorders, anorexia nervosa, bulimia nervosa and binge eating disorders. Now we have clear criteria for diagnosis, notes about aetiological factors, elements with respect to the course and prognostics, etc. Nevertheless, as clinicians feel in their day-by-day practice with patients, much more must be done. This book aims to add some data in order to help doctors, psychologists and other professionals involved in the management of eating disorders.

The first section of this book focuses on the conceptualization and etiopathogenic aspects of eating disorders. The conceptualization of eating disorders has admitted different models. One of them refers to the idea of "food addiction," a concept related to a specific behavioural addiction that might be useful to understand some forms of eating disorders. In this regard, the first chapter of this book written by Francisco J. Vaz-Leal et al., states the relationship between eating disorders and substance related disorders based on animal models, epidemiological studies and neuroimaging studies.

Following with the conceptualization and etiopathogenic aspects of eating disorders, Nayelli Alvarado Sánchez and Cecilia Silva Gutiérrez bring us a chapter based on the neuropsychological functioning in anorexia and bulimia nervosas. The findings of their revision might lead to a reformulation of intervention programs. Bearing in mind the field of neuropsychology and eating disorders, Abigail H. Natenshon offers an interesting chapter with an exciting title: "Neurobiology and the Changing Face of Eating Disorder Treatment - Healing the Eating Disordered Brain." Someone wrote that we would be interested in how there is any psychopathology without brain involvement. Now, Natenshon states that in this era of the brain, through understanding more about the organ they treat, practitioners not only serve their eating disordered patients, but become instrumental in defining new directions for quantitative eating disorder research. I think this attitude is a necessity and a must-do practice.

The second section of the book refers to symptomatology and comorbidity. The section starts with a chapter by Aurea Lumbau and Giovanni Spano, which brings us a clinical reminder of some oral manifestations of eating disorders. These authors focus their chapter on dental erosions, trauma to the mucosa of the oral cavity and pharynx, dry mouth, an increased risk of caries, periodontal problems, and injuries to the soft tissues secondary to the direct actions of emesis, or indirectly because of systemically-induced effects of vomiting. Oral complications due to eating disorders are not a minor problem. Eating disorder patients usually have low self-esteem and body dissatisfaction. As the authors state, the mouth has a strong impact on interpersonal relationships as it plays a key role in facial aesthetics. They conclude that in the context of comprehensive management of eating disorders, oral manifestations should be taken into account.

With respect to the comorbidity of eating disorders, perhaps anxiety (with all types of manifestations) is the main psychopathological condition to be considered. Annie Aimé et al. point out that the role of anxiety in the onset and maintenance of disordered eating still has to be better understood. After their revision, authors concluded that anxiety symptoms and anxiety disorders are common in eating disorders. It seems that in a high proportion of patients disordered eating symptoms are preceded by symptoms of anxiety and are even considered as anxiety-driven. In this regard, anxiety disorders should be systematically assessed and addressed. Following this topic, Cicek Hocaoglu gives us a chapter about eating disorders with comorbid anxiety disorders. The comorbidity of eating disorders and anxiety disorders seems to affect the treatment and prognosis. Prof. Hocaoglu notes that there is limited evidence regarding the effectiveness of treatment options (medication and different forms of psychotherapy) used in the treatment of cases with a diagnosis of concurrent eating disorder and anxiety disorder. Therefore, this is a topic which deserves more attention in the future.

The third section of this book aims to update the field of the course and prognosis. The chapter of Fragiskos Gonidakis and Dafni-Alexandra Karapavlou is focused on the patient's perspective of the therapeutic process, something that is rarely taken into account. These authors distinguish between subjective and objective recovery. We need to consider all factors that are considered by the patients as important elements of a successful treatment. More specifically, their perception of improvement in the psychological, emotional and social domains is highly correlated with improvement in the corresponding fields in their quality of life, as well as in the overall quality of life. Most of the patients recognize recovery as a change that goes beyond eating disorder symptomatology to a more "holistic" improvement in their psychological, physical and social well being. It may be concluded that reduction of the symptomatology and nutrition restoration, normalization of body weight and absence of purging behaviours is not the end of the treatment.

The fourth section focuses on topics related to the treatment of eating disorders. The first chapter of this section by Joyce L.C. Ma, may be considered as a classical topic revisited. It contains transcultural elements about the family treatment of anorexia nervosa. Starting with two wonderful phrases "Zen is eating while eating and sleeping while sleeping," and "your everyday life is the Tao," Prof. Ma concludes that family therapists assist the family and the patient to use their resources and strengths to transcend the stifling familial context and drive away the disorder. However, similar to the learning experience of Zen, family healing is a process of self-discovery. A Zen master cannot give enlightenment to his student and so it is with the therapist. A therapist, at best, is only an observer participant in treatment and a companion on their journey to recovery.

Another chapter from Abigail H. Natenshon explains the use of the therapist's self in the treatment of eating disorders. In this chapter, Natenshon states that the practitioner's capacity to realize a full connection with his own self is a prerequisite to establish a potent connection with the patient. A very interesting part of this chapter refers to the fact of reminding that the qualities distinguishing the eating disorder specialist are found in the acronym V.I.A.B.L.E, which stands for Versatile, Integrative, Action-oriented, outcome-Based, Loving, and Educative.

Following with different facets of eating disorder treatments, Maria Zaccagnino et al. write a chapter about Eyes Movement Desensitization and Reprocessing (EMDR). The EMDR is a well-known evidence-based psychotherapy implementation. It has been firstly applied to relieve Posttraumatic Stress Disorder symptomatology and it has evolved to an integrated approach in psychotherapy. The main purpose of EMDR is to help a patient to access the unresolved memory and to metabolize it, to turn from a "frozen memory" to one integrated, neutral and healthier. The results of this study seem to confirm EMDR as an emerging scientific-validated approach that may become an effective treatment for eating disorders.

One of the main problems in eating disorder patients refers to body image and its disturbances. In this regard, Michel Probst and Jolien Diedens focus their chapter on this topic by means of a suggestive title: "The Body in Movement, a Clinical Approach." Here, the novelty is to approach the field of physiotherapy to the treatment of eating disorders. The authors state that physiotherapists have a wide array of skills, which can be applied successfully in treatment of anorexia nervosa. In addition, physiotherapeutic techniques represent a potent clinical addition to available treatments. Psychomotor therapy or body oriented therapy (BOT) can influence the distorted body experience, the hyperactivity and the fear of losing self-control.

The last section of this book aims to report some data about communication challenges within eating disorders. Martha Peaslee Levine starts her chapter with two important questions: "What is being said? And what is being heard?" She follows with a reflexion, "There are times when these two aspects are very different. For example, when a person tells another, 'You look so healthy!' Most of us would accept this as a compliment. Individuals with anorexia nervosa often hear this exact comment as 'You've gained weight.'." Prof. Levine goes on to say that, in a "world focused on a thin ideal," some media messages can "influence people's overall self-esteem and be especially triggering for individuals at risk of disordered eating." She concludes her chapter with a beautiful sentence: "We need to be aware of what we say and what those who struggle with eating disorders hear. Let's work to ensure that they are positive messages filled with compassion and care."

Eating disorders are frequent pathologies, many times severe and often devastating considering patients and their families. The biopsychosocial model is fully in force because biological, psychological, and social factors are always involved in these disorders. The specific influence of those factors and the interaction among them help us to better understand eating disorders, their expression, course and outcome as well as the different treatment modalities which should be progressively improved. This book includes different studies about the main topics of eating disorders. Professionals such as psychologists, nurses, doctors, and nutritionists, among others, may be interested in this book.

Ignacio Jáuregui-Lobera
Area of Nutrition and Food Sciences,
Department of Molecular Biology and Biochemical Engineering,
Pablo de Olavide University,
Sevilla, Spain

Behavioural Sciences Institute
Sevilla, Spain

Section 1

Conceptualization and Etiopathogenic Aspects

Chapter 1

Eating Disorders as New Forms of Addiction

Francisco J. Vaz-Leal, María I. Ramos-Fuentes,
Laura Rodríguez-Santos and
M. Cristina Álvarez-Mateos

Additional information is available at the end of the chapter

http://dx.doi.org/10.5772/65248

Abstract

Eating disorders (ED) seem to share many characteristics with substance-related disorders (SRD). As very often the two conditions run together, it has been proposed that eating dysfunctions could be understood as behavioral forms of addiction. This has lead to the concept of "food addiction," a proposed new form of addiction. This chapter reviews recent research focusing on the relationship between ED and SRD. Three specific areas are addressed: (a) animal models that suggest the association between substance dependence and compulsive overeating; (b) epidemiological studies that confirm the comorbidity between ED and SRD; and (c) neuroimaging studies that reveal the existence of modifications in the reward circuits following binge eating and other eating dysfunctions. The data from the different studies can be integrated into a model based on the consideration of "food addiction" as a specific form of behavioral addiction that could be applied at least to a group of patients suffering from eating disorders.

Keywords: eating disorder, substance-related disorder, anorexia nervosa, bulimia nervosa, binge eating disorder

1. Introduction

In the past, the study of similarities between eating disorders (ED) and substance-related disorders (SRD) has been limited to the consideration of the similarities in their clinical presentation and the existence of some common behaviors. Nevertheless, in recent years there has been growing interest in the study of the association between ED and SRD, and a significant event in this context has been the inclusion of binge eating disorder (BED) as an ED with full identity in the DSM-5. This new diagnosis has prompted the development of theories and studies that suggest the existence of a model of "food addiction," capable of explaining many observed similarities between ED and SRD, at least in some cases.

The term "food addiction" is a recent and in many ways controversial concept, proposed by Randolph in 1956 to refer to several eating patterns which were "descriptively similar to those of other addictive processes" [1]. According to the concept of "food addiction", certain foods will act as most psychoactive substances do, producing changes in brain function that would made necessary further use of the substance (or food) to restore balance in the affected areas. Although Randolph highlighted the addictive potential of foods such as wheat and corn derivatives, coffee, eggs or milk, nowadays the term is associated with the consumption of foods with high sugar and fat content.

A term related to "food addiction" is "food craving", a feature that goes beyond the simple desire to eat and the search for specific foods. It has to do in many cases with specific (negative) emotional states, in such a way that the seeking behavior can be explained in terms of emotional regulation and is not necessarily followed by increased eating [2, 3].

Several theories have been proposed to understand "food craving". Some of them link this feature with the evolution of the humans, and their tendency to overeat when food is clearly avalaible, specially after a scarcity period. Neurotransmiters (serotonin, dopamine, endogenous opiates, ghrelin, cholecystokinin, peptide YY and leptine, among others) appear to be involved in the complex control of (as well as in the loss of control over) eating [4]. Food intake is clearly influenced by metabolic activity in hypothalamic and extracerebral areas, including sensitivity of the hypothalamus to specific molecules, stomach mouvements or blood glucose levels [5], and organoleptic characteristics of some kinds of food (as for example, chocolate) seem to be element linked to the decisión to seek out for food and to start eating. Finally, from a cognitive framework, the so-called "elaborated intrusion theory" has postulated the existence of two main cognitive components in food craving: the emergence of intrusive thoughts about the craved substance via an associative process, and the emergence of supporting mental images via an elaborative process [6].

2. Food and substances

According to the American Society of Addiction Medicine, addiction is a chronic primary disease, which affects some brain circuits related to reward, memory, and motivation, producing significant changes at a biological and psychological level. Like other chronic diseases, cycles of remission and relapse are often observed. Without treatment or participation in recovery activities, addiction is progressive and can lead to disability or premature death [7].

Supporting the idea that food is "addictive" implies accepting that food contains ingredients capable of creating addiction in susceptible individuals. Except for caffeine, which has already been introduced in the DSM-5, so far there is no enough scientific evidence to support this assert. Some foods have rewarding properties, especially manipulated aliments which have been designed to maximize flavor, and can therefore participate more easily in the processes of reinforcement and reward [8]. Nevertheless, despite the fact that food and substances can act on the same brain circuits, eating habits are not only regulated by central brain structures, but also by peripheral mechanisms [9]. Another important fact is that food is necessary for survival, while recreational drugs are not. However, it seems clear that both elements, food and substances, may have similar addictive capability, as they share several elements that seem to be able to initiate and maintain their use, and have in common their high resistance to treatment [10].

Animal research has revealed how the following factors (included in the DSM-5 definition of SRD) are not only associated with substance use but also with excessive food intake, especially of food with high sugar content [10]: (a) intake/use in larger amounts or over longer periods than was intended; (b) persistent desire or unsuccessful efforts to cut down or control the intake/use; (c) great deal of time spent in activities necessary to obtain, use, or recover from its effects; (d) craving or strong desire or urge to eat/use; (e) maintenance of the pattern of intake/use despite having social or interpersonal problems caused or exacerbated by the intake/use; (f) reduction in social, occupational, or recreational activities; and (g) recurrent intake/use in situations where it is physically hazardous.

In accordance with these facts, some authors have defended the idea that overeating can be considered as an addictive behavior, especially in the cases that the individual who overeats fulfills the diagnostic criteria for BED. It is evident that some individuals are physically and psychologically dependent on foods with high fat and sugar content in a way that resembles substance dependence. It is also usual in these subjects the emergence of feelings of loss of control over consumption, as well as the maintenance of such behaviors despite the serious consequences that can have on health and social life. Another relevant element is that both drug abuse and binge eating are often accompanied by strong feelings of guilt, remorse, and anguish [11]. In short, there are reasons to support the idea that at least some ED could be conceptualized as SRD. This not only applies to BED, as the addictive nature of other eating-related behaviors, such as diet, compulsive exercise, purging, or the use of substances that promote weight loss, can also be defended. In any case, further research is needed, because tolerance and withdrawal (two key elements in addictions) have not been clearly observed in humans in relation to food [10].

Numerous investigations have attempted to isolate the elements of the neurotransmission systems that may be involved in the pathophysiology of ED and SRD [10]. Serotonin seems to be a relevant one, as it plays an important role in behavioral inhibition and impulsivity, two clinical items related to the psychopathology of ED and SRD. Norepinephrine, by its part, seems to be more related to the cognitive and emotional factors able to trigger these behaviors, but undoubtedly the star of the reward system is dopamine, the main neurotransmitter in the mesolimbic system [10]. If we feel pleasure is because dopamine (released from the neurons of the ventral tegmental area in response to a reinforcing stimulus) increases in the nucleus accumbens. Once the system has been activated, endocannabinoids and endorphins are responsible for extending the pleasant sensation; finally, the interaction of these and other neurotransmitters, such as acetylcholine, glutamate, or gamma-amino-butyric acid, supports the subjective feeling of reward [12]. In the case of restrictive eating disorders such as anorexia nervosa (AN), reward seeking seems to be associated to other elements, as drive for thinness, which is experienced as pleasurable; the maintenance of the feeling of satisfaction produced by weight lose and the immediate sense of control over hunger and eating associated with food restriction can also act as positive reinforcement elements in these cases [13].

ED and SRD overlap in many other important aspects, including clinical phenomenology, comorbidity, and response to certain types of treatment [10], but the final reasons for this association are unknown, and it is also difficult to determine which disorder occurs first, acting as a risk factor for the development of the other. What is not in doubt is the close relationship between them, as is revealed by many studies that report on the high comorbidity in people suffering from these disorders, when compared with general population.

3. Animal models: what are they teaching us?

Animal models are contributing to the understanding of the neurobiological basis of the behaviors associated with ED, bringing to light some of the mechanisms and the brain areas involved in food intake dysregulation [14].

A recent review of animal studies on compulsive overeating concludes that, under certain circumstances, overeating can produce behavioral and physiological changes similar to those observed in addictions, in such a way that addictive behaviors should not limit to substance use [15]. In fact, numerous animal studies have revealed that many of the behaviors observed in subjects with problems of drug addiction can be also associated with massive and persistent consumption of palatable food. Some of these common elements are as follows:

(a) Loss of control and compulsive consumption: In the model of sugar addiction, the animals are subjected to periods of food deprivation followed by equally long periods of free access to a sweet solution. When this routine is maintained for a time, an escalation in the daily intake of sweet solution is observed, especially in the first hour of access, with a change in eating patterns in the long term to make possible the intake of a larger amount of sugar during the period of free access [16].

(b) Use despite negative consequences: As has been already said, there are models of obesity and BED that measure the motivation of the animals to find and eat palatable foods despite potentially harmful consequences. It has been found that expanding access to palatable food of high energy density induces compulsive behavior in obese animals despite the application of a negative stimulus. It has also been found that reduction in dopamine D_2 receptors in the striatum of these animals exists, a phenomenon reported in humans addicted to drugs [17].

(c) Inflexible behavior: According to the results of some studies, animals often show an inflexible pattern of behavior, preferring limited access to appetizing food than continuous access to their usual food [18].

http://dx.doi.org/10.5772/65248

(d) Withdrawal symptoms and relapse: There are several animal studies on forced abstinence, but offer contradictory results, that in many cases depend on the type of food to be offered/restricted. According to the results of one of these studies, the excessive consumption of sugar will act similarly to opiate use both at brain and at behavioral levels, with the emergence of withdrawal symptoms following sugar restriction [19]. In animals fed with unlimited access to glucose, abstinence can be induced by the deprivation of sugar or the administration of naloxone, an opiate antagonist that increases the symptoms and somatic signs of withdrawal, such as tremors, shaking, teeth chattering, hyperphagia, and anxiety [20]. However, sugar and fat seem to have notable differences: while too much sugar can produce symptoms similar to those of opiates withdrawal and does not affect body weight, binges of fat cause weight gain but do not produce withdrawal symptoms [21]. The animals on a high-fat diet show no behavioral or somatic signs of withdrawal following the administration of naloxone [22]. According to these facts, combined diets (high sugar and fat content) could be able to produce both addictive symptoms and significant weight changes [23], with increased anxiety levels and psychomotor excitement following acute withdrawal [24].

With respect to BED, several models that highlight the etiological role of factors such as stress or food deprivation have been proposed. A recent review of the literature on animal models has evaluated the contribution of different studies to the understanding of BED [25]. The animal studies analyzed suggest that binge eating is often associated with changes in behavior similar to those observed in individuals who use/abuse substances. These behaviors are not observed in animals that, taking the same food, do not binge. This has led to the conclusion that food has no addictive qualities in itself and that the really important factor is the conditions under which food intake takes place, suggesting the replacement of the term "food addiction" by "addiction to eat" [8].

The role of stress in the genesis of binge eating has been one of the items analyzed in these studies. When animals are subjected to cycles of caloric restriction and exposed to tasty food associated (or not) with a stressor, the food intake of animals exposed to the stressor seems to be significantly higher than those who do not receive negative stimuli [25].

Another element analyzed is the propensity to binge eating. Once the animals have been classified into susceptible or resistant to binge, on the basis of their previous intake of palatable food, important behavioral differences that suggest the existence of an addictive pattern in animals prone to binge seem to exist. In this sense, whereas binge-resistant animals tend to reduce food intake following the exposure to negative stimuli, the animals prone to binge do not reduce their intake and continue eating the same amount of tasty food, enduring negative contingencies to obtain the appetizing food, not only when they are hungry, but also when they are satiated [26].

The results from another group of animal studies defend the idea that a limited and intermittent access to palatable food can be a sufficient cause for excessive intake. The intermittent access to palatable food attempts to reproduce one of the main items of the diagnostic criteria for BED, that is, the massive food intake occurring over a limited period of time. The model is based on the hypothesis that "forbidden" foods that people use to restrict when dieting are the trigger element of binge eating. This hypothesis has been supported by one study in which a group of animals with continuous access to their usual food and water were divided into two groups: animals with limited access to palatable food in the short time, but with daily access, and animals with intermittent access to tasty food on alternate days. According to the results of the study, the group of animals with intermittent access tended to present a significantly higher intake of palatable food. In addition, as the animals have no periods of caloric restriction during the experience, the statement of "overeating in the absence of hunger" is fulfilled, which corresponds to other main criteria of BED [27, 28].

Some studies have analyzed the changes in food intake after a mild and daily food restriction period which is followed by access to palatable food. In this kind of studies, and in contrast to the previously reported ones, the animals cannot have access to other types of food. The justification for this difference in the design of the study is that often people with BED are involved in periods of energy deprivation. In these studies, the animals are deprived for a period of time of several hours, and then, they are exposed to palatable food for a short time. Studies have shown that consumption in the early stages is higher in this group of animals than in the control groups, consisting of subjects with continuous access to palatable food or limited access to their usual food [29].

Combining different approaches, such as acute intermittent access or deprivation of food, another group of studies have attempted to reproduce BED in laboratory animals. The animals used in these studies had access to tasty food for short periods of time in two noncontiguous days per week. Over a long period of time prior to access, the animals were deprived of all food, while the rest of the day had continuous access to their usual food. At the end of the study period, an escalation in food intake was observed in these animals, compared with control subjects [30].

In summary, animal models seem to be able to provide valuable information for the understanding of the pathophysiology and course of eating disorders, especially for the recently identified as BED. They also reveal the existence of some addictive components of binging, being the results of vital importance for the rising of the concept of "food addiction." However, due to the undeniable influence of psychosocial factors, more research is needed before we can translate the results of basic research to the field of clinical management of the human patients.

4. Drugs and addictions: a question of comorbidity

A number of clinical studies have revealed the existence of high comorbidity between ED and SRD. These studies are usually based on population surveys or comparisons between groups and address comorbidity from different perspectives, whether looking for SRD in samples of patients with ED or investigating the presence of TCA in people with SRD. There are also some meta-analysis studies and others related to specific populations, such as adolescents, or specific subtypes of eating disorders.

A meta-analysis of studies published between 1994 and 2007 has concluded that substance use is higher in patients with ED than in healthy controls. In addition, it seems that differences between the subtypes of ED exist, being the risk of substance abuse higher in bulimia nervosa (BN), followed by BED and nonsignificant in AN [31].

One of the studies on the prevalence of SRD in AN has been developed after classifying patients according to their subtype. The findings are in accordance with the above-mentioned results. A quarter of the total sample referred history of substance use, being more common in purgative AN (about 30%). Thirteen percent of the participants in the study met criteria for substance abuse or dependence, especially the AN+BN group (32%). Restrictive AN patients had the lowest percentages for substance use (23%) and dependence (6%). Alcohol intake was detected in 20% of the sample, being more frequent in AN+BN patients (35.5%) and again less frequent in the restrictive forms of AN (14%). In addition, a statistically significant relationship between substance use and purges, but not between substance use and binge eating, was found in this study [32].

Although obesity is not considered an ED, but a chronic multifactorial disease, there is growing evidence on the coexistence of psychopathological disturbances. On the issue that is concerning us, there are a pair of publications that found a strong association between obesity and alcohol abuse [33, 34].

In order to examine comorbidities related to the new BED diagnosis, a group of patients were examined; the results demonstrated that the psychopathological associations were evident. Seventy-four percent of the patients suffer from at least one lifetime additional psychiatric disorder, being SRD present in one in four subjects, especially in male subjects. Individuals suffering from BED plus other psychiatric comorbid disorder had significantly higher body mass index (BMI) and higher levels of psychopathology [35].

Addressing comorbidity from the other side, some studies have been carried out on SRD women, revealing that at least 15% of them were at high risk of developing ED, reaching the lifetime prevalence 20%. On the other hand, the relationship of these disorders with the prognosis seems to be statistically significant, so that ED would represent an important predictor of relapse or unsuccessful treatment for patients with SRD [36]. In a similar way, other study of women in treatment for SRD has examined how "weight-related concerns" affected substance use. More than 70% of the participants admitted to be worried about gaining weight during recovery and 45% were concerned about whether weight gain could be in the future a reason for relapse. Approximately one-third of the sample admitted that weight loss had been a reason to initiate or maintain substance use and most of them admitted having used a variety of methods to change their figure, including substance use. Twenty-six percent of the subjects ate too much, and 13% skipped meals. Up to 40% of the participants admitted that their addictive behavior affected their eating patterns. Women who were concerned about weight gain had higher levels of body dissatisfaction, more eating symptoms (especially bulimic symptoms) and tended to use substances capable of modifying eating and weight [37].

Adolescents have been a target population for several epidemiological studies on the potential risk to develop psychopathological disorders. Studies in this field have stressed the influence of family and environmental factors in the process. When BMI (stratified by gender), dietary behaviors, and substance use have been examined, controlling for the influence of social and family factors, both obesity and underweight have appeared initially associated with increased substance use (20–40%), being overweight women more prone to ED and substance use more frequent in male participants. When a subset of them (people meeting criteria for overweight and substance abuse) was compared with teens who had just overweight, the first ones were characterized by an unconventional family structure, previous history of negative sexual experiences, and serious family and school problems. When, finally, the underlying psychosocial factors were controlled, the relationship between substance use and overweight disappeared [38]. In this same group of age, some studies have revealed the influence of the spectrum of compulsiveness on the emergence of ED and excessive alcohol intake. Compulsive symptoms seem to be especially associated with ED and obsessive-compulsive disorder and to a lesser extent with SRD and excessive alcohol intake. Nevertheless, in this last case the external factors seemed to be more relevant [39]. In a cohort study, aimed at determining the prevalence of ED in a university sample, the risk of developing an ED was 19.5%, being higher in women than in men. Among the isolated risk factors, excessive intake of alcohol ("binge drinking"), smoking, and/or problematic Internet use appeared as specially significant [40].

5. Does food addiction exist?

Despite the similarities between substance addiction and excessive food intake, only recently specific tools to measure "food addiction" have been developed. In 2008, the Yale Food Addiction Scale (YFAS) was proposed as an instrument for identifying signs of addiction to certain foods. The scale was based on a selection of criteria for substance dependence included in the fourth revised edition of the DSM (DSM-IV-TR), and other scales used to assess behavioral addictions, such as pathological gambling [41]. The items of the scale were adapted to evaluate excessive intake of high-calorie foods and were reviewed by experts in addictions, obesity, and ED. In 2013, a version of the YFAS for children (YFAS-C) was proposed [42]. According to the results, both YFAS for adults and YFAS for children seem to be solid psychometric tools, capable of identifying dysfunctional addictive eating patterns.

To study the association of "food addiction" with different ED, a wide group of subjects with their BMI ranging from underweight to severely obese were studied. According to YFAS, "food addiction" was found in more than a quarter of participants, being more prevalent in participants with BN than in those with BED. People with "food addiction" not only had higher BMI, greater fluctuations in body weight, and more dietary behaviors; all the variables related to ED (binge eating, dietary restrictions and concerns about weight and food) were also more prevalent in them, in such a way that the study revealed significant relationship between "food addiction" and eating psychopathology [43]. Other study analyzed the prevalence of "food addiction" in a sample of women diagnosed with different subtypes of ED, using healthy women as controls. The lowest scores on the YFAS were associated with the restrictive subtype of AN and the highest ones with the subtypes of ED associated with binge eating: purging AN (85.7%), BN (81.5%), and BED (76.9%). Higher YFAS scores were also associated with higher levels of negative affect, depressive symptoms, higher BMI, more severe eating pathology, and general psychopathology [44].

The association of BED and "food addiction" could be considered a severe form of the disorder, as shown by a study on a sample of obese patients with BED. [45]. In that sample, 41.5% of the subjects met the criteria for "food addiction" according to the YFAS. These patients had higher levels of negative affect, emotional dysregulation and eating psychopathology, and lower self-esteem. Higher scores in the YFAS were significant predictors of a higher frequency of binging and were also associated with earlier age of onset of overweight and dietary behaviors. In the same way, another study analyzed a clinical set of variables in a sample of overweight men and women who met diagnostic criteria for BED [46]. The subjects with higher scores in "food addiction" were more prone to impulsively overeat for emotional reasons, had more frequent and severe episodes of binge eating, and were more sensitive to the rewarding properties of food. In addition, they had more addictive personality traits, higher levels of impulsivity and reported more depressive symptoms. A third study tried to test the hypothesis that "food addiction" and BED were inseparable conditions [47], suggesting that overeating should be understood as a dimension that reflects different levels of severity. According to the results, the lower edge of the continuum will be represented by people who overeat passively, with little (or no) associated psychopathology; the upper edge, by its part, will be characterized by significant clinical deterioration and strong addictive behaviors and will correspond with BED. In this context, "food addiction" will represent a more severe and more psychopathologically serious form of BED.

These observations are in accordance with the results of a systematic review of the studies published from 2009 to 2014. The meta-analysis revealed that, according to the YFAS, the mean prevalence of the diagnosis of "food addiction" was almost 20%, being higher in patients suffering from BN than in cases of BED. In accordance with most of the aforementioned studies, "food addiction" was associated with higher tendency to binge eating, depressive symptoms, impulsivity, and emotional eating [48].

So far we have only considered those studies that measured "food addiction" using the YFAS, because it is the most standardized instrument. However, there are other scales and questionnaires that have been created with the same purpose. One example is a study performed on a sample of obese women in which the DSM-5 criteria for SRD were adapted, replacing "substance" by "food" [49]. The subjects fulfilled the new criteria for "food addiction," but those with BED described their binges as more "addictive," especially with regard to craving and the "use despite having persistent or recurrent physical or psychological problems." The group with BED also reported greater number and frequency of their binge episodes. Similar findings are provided by a study that applied the Goodman's criteria for SRD to the study of different subtypes of ED [50], comparing patients with restrictive AN, purgative AN, BN, SRD, and healthy controls. According to the results of the study, BN patients met the Goodman's criteria in the same proportion as the subjects with SRD (60 and 65%, respectively, compared with only 35% of patients with restrictive AN), in such a way that the concept of "food addiction" seems to be closely tied to binge and uncontrolled eating.

6. Looking at the brain: neuroimaging studies

One of the emerging fields of research in the study of the relationships between ED and SRD is neuroimaging. The literature provides us with a number of studies that shed some light on the biological basis of addictive behaviors and disordered eating. In general, neuroimaging techniques have revealed the existence of common neurotransmitter disturbances in specific anatomical regions and circuits in SRD and ED. These abnormalities mainly affect the prefrontal cortex (involved in inhibitory control), hippocampus (strongly linked to memory), and striatum (involved in reward, motivation and habit formation) [51].

Functional magnetic resonance imaging (fMRI) studies have shown specific changes in brain activity in patients with ED following the exposure to food images. Patients with AN, for example, tend to react with an increase in visual responses and prefrontal cortical activity that seem to be in accordance with their cognitive biases and excessive control over intake [52]. When patients with AN, BN, and controls are compared, each group seems to have a more or less specific pattern of response. The women with BN tend to present greater neural activity in the visual cortex, right dorsolateral prefrontal cortex, right insular cortex, and precentral gyrus. Compared to controls, the patients with BN had lower activity in the superior temporal gyrus, bilateral insula, and visual cortex. In contrast to women with AN, the patients with BN had lower activity in the posterior dorsal and parietal lobe of the cingulate cortex, but increased activity in caudate, superior temporal gyrus, right insula, and supplementary motor area [53].

When the response to the stimulation preceding the administration of food has been studied in patients with "food addiction," the results have also shown specific changes, as increased activation of anterior cingulate cortex, medial orbitofrontal cortex, and amygdala. A positive correlation between YFAS score and brain activity, with a pattern similar to that produced by drugs or alcohol, has also been found. These results reveal that specific patterns of neural activation are involved in "addictive" eating behavior and that in subjects with "food addiction," the activity of reward circuits increases in response to signals related to food [54].

There are several studies aimed at examining whether the neuronal hyperstimulation of reward pathways, typically associated with SRD, also occurs in individuals with binge episodes. The fMRI images obtained from overweight individuals who binge when they are exposed to food-related stimulus reveals that the increase in reward system activity correlates with BMI and with the number of reported binges. Caloric stimulation seems to activate the cingulate gyrus, the supplementary motor area, the thalamus and the temporal lobe, as well as the occipital areas related to visual processing and the regions involved in emotional processes, such as amygdala and hippocampus. According to these data, "food addiction" would be determined by a failure of self-regulation mechanisms [55].

Some studies of positron emission tomography (PET) have suggested that the striatal dopamine signaling process is impaired in obese people, as a consequence of the decrease in D_2 receptors, in a way similar to that observed in patients with SRD. A review of PET studies confirmed this point of view, revealing that the binding to the dopamine D_2/D_3 receptors is decreased not only in cocaine, methamphetamine, alcohol, heroin, and nicotine addicts, but

http://dx.doi.org/10.5772/65248

also in subjects with morbid obesity, compared with healthy controls [56]. PET studies have also been performed to assess the role of dopamine in the neurobiology of BED and obesity [57], through the quantification of the changes in extracellular striatal dopamine after food stimulation. The food stimuli, when administered with methylphenidate (a drug that blocks dopamine reuptake), caused changes in binge eaters, but not in the obese subjects who did not binge. In addition, increased levels of dopamine in the caudate were significantly correlated with binge eating, but not with BMI. In the same way, another study of PET imaging has detected alterations in dopamine pathways similar to those described in patients with SRD in a group of women with BN. The analysis of the data found a significant association between striatal dopamine release and the frequency of binge eating and vomiting in these patients [58].

Although the application of neuroimaging in the field of Psychiatry is still at an early stage of development, it represents a solid promise for the understanding of ED, SRD, and their relationships, in such a way that it is very possible that future research can help us to treat and prevent relapse in these patients more effectively.

Acknowledgements

Supported by grant no. GR15131 (Support to the Action Plans of Registered Research Groups). Consejería de Economía e Infraestructuras. Junta de Extremadura (Spain), and European Social Fund.

Author details

Francisco J. Vaz-Leal[1,2*], María I. Ramos-Fuentes[1], Laura Rodríguez-Santos[1] and M. Cristina Álvarez-Mateos[1]

*Address all correspondence to: fjvazleal@gmail.com

1 University of Extremadura School of Medicine, Badajoz, Spain

2 University Hospital Network, Badajoz, Spain

References

[1] Randolph TG. The descriptive features of food addiction; addictive eating and drinking. Q J Stud Alcohol 1956;17:198-224.

[2] Giuliani NR, Berkman ET. Craving is an affective state and its regulation can be understood in terms of the extended process model of emotion regulation. Psychol Inq 2015;26:48–53. DOI: 10.1080/1047840X.2015.955072

[3] Meule A, Gerhardt. Food addiction on the light of DSM-5. Nutrients 2014;6:3653–71. DOI: 10.3390/nu6093653

[4] Schwartz MW, Woods WC, Porte D, et al. Central nervous system control of food intake. Nature. 2000;404:661–71.

[5] Woods SC, Ramsay DS. Food intake, metabolism and homeostasis. Physiol Behav. 2011; 104:4–7. DOI: 10.1016/j.physbeh.2011.04.026

[6] Andrade J, Pears S, May J, Kavanagh DJ. Use of a clay modeling task to reduce chocolate craving. Appetite. 2012;58:955-63. DOI: 10.1016/j.appet.2012.02.044.

[7] American Society of Addiction Medicine (ASAM). Public policy statement: definition of addiction [Internet]. 2011. Available from: http://www.asam.org/quality-practice/definition-of-addiction [Accessed: 2016-06-27].

[8] Hebebrand J, Albayrak Ö, Adan R, Antel J, Dieguez C, de Jong J, et al. "Eating addiction", rather than "food addiction", better captures addictive-like eating behavior. Neurosci Biobehav Rev. 2014;47:295-306. doi:10.1016/j.neubiorev.2014.08.016.

[9] DiLeone RJ, Taylor JR, Picciotto MR. The drive to eat: comparisons and distinctions between mechanisms of food reward and drug addiction. Nat Neurosci. 2012;15:1330-5. DOI:10.1038/nn.3202.

[10] Brewerton T, Baker A, editors. Eating Disorders, Addictions and Substance Use Disorders: Clinical and Treatment Perspectives. New York: Springer; 2014. 664 p. DOI: 10.1007/978-3-642-45378-6.

[11] Smith DG, Robbins TW. The neurobiological underpinnings of obesity and binge eating: a rationale for adopting the food addiction model. Biol Psychiatry. 2013;73:804-10. DOI:10.1016/j.biopsych.2012.08.026.

[12] Méndez M, Ruiz AE, Prieto B, Romano A, Caynas S, Prospero O. Brain and substances: their neurobiological mechanisms. Salud Mental. 2010;33:451-56. Available from: http://www.redalyc.org/articulo.oa?id=5821079309. [Accessed: 2016-06-27].

[13] Godier LR, Park RJ. Compulsivity in anorexia nervosa: a transdiagnostic concept. Front Psychol. 2014;5:778. doi:10.3389/fpsyg.2014.00778.

[14] Avena NM, Bocarsly ME. Dysregulation of brain reward systems in eating disorders: neurochemical information from animal models of binge eating, bulimia nervosa, and anorexia nervosa. Neuropharmacology. 2012;63:87-96. doi:10.1016/j.neuropharm.2011.11.010.

[15] Di Segni M, Patrono E, Patella L, Puglisi-Allegra S, Ventura R. Animal models of compulsive eating behavior. Nutrients 2014;6:4591-609. doi:10.3390/nu6104591.

[16] Hoebel BG, Avena NM, Bocarsly ME, Rada P. Natural addiction: a behavioral and circuit model based on sugar addiction in rats. J Addict Med. 2009;3:33–41. doi:10.1097/ADM.0b013e31819aa621.

[17] Johnson PM, Kenny PJ. Addiction-like reward dysfunction and compulsive eating in obese rats: role for dopamine D_2 receptors. Nat Neurosci. 2010;13:635–41. Available from: http://www.ncbi.nlm.nih.gov/pmc/articles/PMC2947358/pdf/nihms181674.pdf [Accessed: 2016-06-27]. doi:10.1038/nn.2519.

[18] Heyne A, Kiesselbach C, Sahún I, McDonald J, Gaiffi M, Dierssen M, Wolffgramm J. An animal model of compulsive food-taking behaviour. Addict Biol. 2009;14:373-83. doi:10.1111/j.1369-1600.2009.00175.x.

[19] Avena NM, Gold MS. Food and addiction-sugars, fats and hedonic overeating. Addiction. 2011;106:1214–5. doi:10.1111/j.1360-0443.2011.03373.x.

[20] Avena NM, Rada P, Hoebel BG. Evidence for sugar addiction: behavioral and neurochemical effects of intermittent, excessive sugar intake. Neurosci Biobehav Rev. 2008;32:20–39. Available from: http://www.ncbi.nlm.nih.gov/pmc/articles/PMC2235907/[Accessed: 2016-06-27] doi:10.1016/j.neubiorev.2007.04.019.

[21] Avena NM, Rada P, Hoebel BG. Sugar and fat bingeing have notable differences in addictive-like behavior. J Nutr. 2009;139:623–8. Available from: http://www.ncbi.nlm.nih.gov/pmc/articles/PMC2714381/[Accessed: 2016-06-27]. doi: 10.3945/jn.108.097584.

[22] Bocarsly ME, Berner LA, Hoebel BG, Avena NM. Rats that binge eat fat-rich food do not show somatic signs or anxiety associated with opiate-like withdrawal: implications for nutrient-specific food addiction behaviors. Physiol Behav. 2011;104:865–72. doi: 10.1016/j.physbeh.2011.05.018.

[23] Berner LA, Avena NM, Hoebel BG. Bingeing, self-restriction, and increased body weight in rats with limited access to a sweet-fat diet. Obesity. 2008;16:1998–2002. doi: 10.1038/oby.2008.328.

[24] Teegarden SL, Bale TL. Decreases in dietary preference produce increased emotionality and risk for dietary relapse. Biol Psychiatry. 2007;61:1021–29. doi:10.1016/j.biopsych.2006.09.032.

[25] Corwin RL, Babbs RK. Rondent models of binge eating: are they models of addiction?. ILAR J. 2012;53:23-34. doi:10.1093/ilar.53.1.23.

[26] Boggiano MM, Artiga AI, Pritchett CE, Chandler-Laney PC, Smith ML, Eldridge AJ. High intake of palatable food predicts binge-eating independent of susceptibility to obesity: an animal model of lean vs obese binge-eating and obesity with and without binge-eating. Int J Obes. 2007;31:1357-67. doi:10.1038/sj.ijo.0803614.

[27] Corwin RL, Avena NM, Boggiano MM. Feeding and reward: perspectives from three rat models of binge eating. Physiol Behav. 2011;104:87–97. doi:10.1016/j.physbeh.2011.04.041.

[28] Corwin RL, Wojnicki FH. Binge eating in rats with limited access to vegetable shortening. Curr Protoc Neurosci. 2006;36:9.23B:9.23B.1–9.23B.11. doi:10.1002/0471142301.ns0923bs36.

[29] Colantuoni C, Rada P, McCarthy J, Patten C, Avena NM, Chadeayne A, Hoebel BG. Evidence that intermittent, excessive sugar intake causes endogenous opioid dependence. Obes Res. 2002;10:478–88. doi:10.1038/oby.2002.66.

[30] Bello NT, Guarda AS, Terrillion CE, Redgrave GW, Coughlin JW, Moran TH. Repeated binge access to a palatable food alters feeding behavior, hormone profile, and hindbrain c-Fos responses to a test meal in adult male rats. Am J Physiol Regul Integr Comp Physiol. 2009;297:622-63. doi:10.1152/ajpregu.00087.2009.

[31] Calero-Elvira A, Krug I, Davis K, Lopez C, Fernández-Aranda F, Treasure J. Meta-analysis on drugs in people with eating disorders. Eur Eat Disord Rev. 2009;17:243–59. doi:10.1002/erv.936.

[32] Root T, Pinheiro AP, Thornton L, Strober M, Fernández-Aranda F, Brandt H, et al. Substance use disorders in woman with anorexia nervosa. Int J Eat Disord. 2010;43:14–21. doi:10.1002/eat.20670.

[33] Petry NM, Barry D, Pietrzak RH, Wagner JA. Overweight and obesity are associated with psychiatric disorders: results from the National Epidemiologic Survey on Alcohol and Related Conditions. Psychosom Med. 2008;70:288-97. doi:10.1097/psy.0b013e3181651651.

[34] Grucza RA, Krueger RF, Racette SB, Norberg KE, Hipp PR, Bierut LJ. The emerging link between alcoholism risk and obesity in the United States. Arch Gen Psychiatry. 2010;67:1301-08. doi:10.1001/archgenpsychiatry.2010.155.

[35] Grilo CM, White MA, Masheb RM. DSM-IV psychiatric disorder comorbidity and its correlates with binge eating behavior. Int J Eat Disord. 2009;42:228–34. doi:10.1002/eat.20599.

[36] Bonfá F, Cabrini S, Avanzi M, Bettinardi O, Spotti R, Uber E. Treatment dropout in drug-addicted women: are eating disorders implicated? Eat Weight Disord. 2008;13:81-6. doi:10.1007/BF03327607.

[37] Warren CS, Lindsay AR, White EK, Claudat K, Velasquez SC. Weight-related concerns related to drug use for women in substance abuse treatment: prevalence and relationships with eating pathology. J Subst Abuse Treat. 2013;44:494-501. doi:10.1016/j.jsat.2012.08.222.

[38] Denoth F, Siciliano V, Iozzo P, Fortunato L, Molinaro S. The association between overweight and illegal drug consumption in adolescents: is there an underlying influence of the sociocultural environment? PLoS One. 2011;6(11):e27358. doi:10.1371/journal.pone.0027358.

[39] Montigny C, Castellanos-Ryan N, Whelan R, Banaschewski T, Barker GJ, Buechel C, et al. A phenotypic structure and neural correlates of compulsive behaviors in adolescents. PLoS One. 2013;8(11):e80151. doi:10.1371/journal.pone.0080151.

[40] Martínez-González L, Fernández T, Molina AJ, Ayán C, Bueno A, Capelo R, et al. Prevalence of eating disorders in college students and associated factors: Unhicos project. Nutr Hospital. 2014;30:927-34. doi:10.3305/nh.2014.30.4.7689.

[41] Gearhardt AN, Corbin WR, Brownell KD. Preliminary validation of the Yale Food Addiction Scale. Appetite. 2009;52:430-36. doi:10.1016/j.appet.2008.12.003.

[42] Gearhardt AN, Roberto CA, Seamans MJ, Corbin WR, Brownell KD. Preliminary validation of the Yale Food Addiction Scale for children. Eat Behav. 2013;14(4):508-12. doi:10.1016/j.eatbeh.2013.07.002.

[43] Gearhardt AN, Boswell RG, White MA. The association of "food addiction" with disordered eating and body mass index. Eat Behav. 2014;15:427-433. doi:10.1016/j.eatbeh.2014.05.001.

[44] Granero R, Hilker I, Agüera Z, Jiménez-Murcia S, Sauchelli S, Islam MA et al. Food addiction in a Spanish sample of eating disorders: DSM-5 diagnostic subtype differentiation and validation data. Eur Eat Disord Rev. 2014;22:389-96. doi:10.1002/erv.2311.

[45] Gearhardt AN, White MA, Masheb RM, Grilo CM. An examination of food addiction in a racially diverse sample of obese patients with binge eating disorder in primary care settings. Comp Psychiatry. 2013;54:500-5. doi:10.1016/j.comppsych.2012.12.009.

[46] Davis C. Compulsive overeating as an addictive behavior: overlap between food addiction and binge eating disorder. Curr Obes Rep. 2013;2:171-8. doi:10.1007/s13679-013-0049-8.

[47] Davis C. A narrative review of binge eating and addictive behaviors: shared associations with seasonality and personality factors. Front Psychiatry. 2013;4:183. doi:10.3389/fpsyt.2013.00183.

[48] Pursey KM, Stanwell P, Gearhardt AN, Collins CE, Burrows TL. The prevalence of food addiction as assessed by the Yale Food Addiction Scale: a systematic review. Nutrients. 2014;6:4552-4590. doi:10.3390/nu6104552.

[49] Curtis C, Davis C. A qualitative study of binge eating and obesity from an addiction perspective. Eat Disord. 2014;22:19-32. doi:10.1080/10640266.2014.857515.

[50] Speranza M, Revah-Levy A, Giquel L, Loas G, Venisse J, Jeammet P, et al. An investigation of Goodman's addictive disorder criteria in eating disorders. Eur Eat Disord Rev. 2012;20:182-9. doi:10.1002/erv.1140.

[51] Michaelides M, Thanos PK, Volkow ND, Wang GJ. Translational neuroimaging in drug addiction and obesity. ILAR J. 2012;53:59-68. doi:10.1093/ilar.53.1.59.

[52] Brooks SJ, O'Daly O, Uher R, Friederich HC, Giampietro V, Brammer M, et al. Thinking about eating food activates visual cortex with reduced bilateral cerebellar activation in

females with anorexia nervosa: an fMRI study. PLoS One. 2012;7(3):e34000. doi:10.1371/journal.pone.0034000.

[53] Brooks SJ, O'Daly OG, Uher R, et al. Differential neural responses to food images in women with bulimia versus anorexia nervosa. Tsakiris M, ed. PLoS One. 2011;6:e22259. doi:10.1371/journal.pone.0022259.

[54] Gearhardt AN, Yokum S, Orr PT, Stice E, Corbin WR, Brownell KD. Neural correlates of food addiction. Arch Gen Psychiatry. 2011;68:808-16. doi:10.1001/archgenpsychiatry.2011.32.

[55] Filbey FM, Myers US, DeWitt S. Reward circuit function in high BMI individuals with compulsive overeating: similarities with addiction. Neuroimage. 2012;63:1800-6. doi:10.1016/j.neuroimage.2012.08.073.

[56] Tomasi D, Volkow ND. Striatocortical pathway dysfunction in addiction and obesity: differences and similarities. Crit Rev Biochem Mol Biol. 2013;48:1-19. doi:10.3109/10409238.2012.735642

[57] Wang GJ, Geliebter A, Volkow ND, Telang FW, Logan J, Jayne MC, et al. Enhanced striatal dopamine release during food stimulation in binge eating disorder. Obesity. 2011;19:1601-8. doi:10.1038/oby.2011.27.

[58] Broft A, Shingleton R, Kaufman J, Liu F, Kumar D, Slifstein M, et al. Striatal dopamine in bulimia nervosa: a PET imaging study. Int J Eat Disord. 2012;4:648-56. doi:10.1002/eat.20984.

Chapter 2

Neuropsychological Functioning in Anorexia Nervosa and Bulimia Nervosa

Nayelli Alvarado Sánchez and Cecilia Silva Gutiérrez

Additional information is available at the end of the chapter

http://dx.doi.org/10.5772/65304

Abstract

Anorexia nervosa and bulimia nervosa are eating disorders in which a wide range of neuropsychological alterations are exhibited; however, the neuropsychology of bulimia nervosa has been poorly studied, and inconsistency has been found in results from different studies. Therefore, the aim of this chapter is to evaluate the differences in the neuropsychological functioning among women with anorexia nervosa and bulimia nervosa and with no eating disorders. Seventy-two women participated in this study: 18 with anorexia nervosa, 24 with bulimia nervosa and 30 without any eating disorder; all of them answered the neuropsychological version of the Wechsler Adults Intelligence Scale-III (WAIS-III), the Rey Complex Figure Test, the Tower of London Task and the Wisconsin Card Sorting Test. Overall, the results showed similar difficulties in anorexia nervosa and bulimia nervosa groups, such as in the visuoconstructive process, executive functioning (specifically in planning skills to achieve a goal, cognitive flexibility and working memory), in selective attention and in nonverbal reasoning and common sense judgment when facing complex problems. These findings open the possibility to reformulate intervention programs for management of bulimia nervosa and consider the use of cognitive remediation therapy, which is already used in anorexia nervosa with a good prognosis.

Keywords: neuropsychology, anorexia nervosa, bulimia nervosa

1. Introduction

Anorexia nervosa (AN) and bulimia nervosa (BN) are eating disorders (ED) whose prevalence is increasing [1–3]; therefore, it is important to determine the factors that could contribute to their development and maintenance in order to generate more effective and better-targeted treatment strategies.

In recent years, several studies have found a relationship between AN, BN and a wide range of neuropsychological disorders. Overall, it is reported that the affected neuropsychological functions are the visuoconstructive skills, attention, visual and working memory, learning ability and executive functions, specifically the cognitive flexibility and planning skill for solving complex problems [4–9].

From the neuropsychological point of view, AN is the most studied ED and most of the research is focused on identifying difficulties in the cognitive flexibility, planning skills and central coherence. The results are homogeneous [4] and have even allowed to test strategies for the neuropsychological rehabilitation of patients, which have been effective [8, 10, 11].

The cognitive flexibility difficulties exhibited by the patients with AN are based mainly on their inability to change thought patterns keeping a repetitive behavior in spite of the feedback provided, whereas in planning, failures are found in the anticipation, organization and integration of information to solve problems; finally, regarding the central coherence, patients have trouble integrating information, forming a global vision and putting it in a real context [12–15]. It is important to take these difficulties into consideration since they seem to have implications in the patients' daily life (e.g., accurate count of calories, excessive exercise, rigid rituals that are part of their daily routine such as grooming or going to work, and in cause-effect thoughts between noncontingent events: if I do not lose weight, I will be completely miserable).

The BN neuropsychology including the effect of its difficulties in the patients' daily life and their possible rehabilitation has been less explored. Some studies suggest that alterations in BN are different from those of AN due to the impulsivity exhibited by the people with this disease [16, 17]; however, others studies state that there are no differences in the alteration of functions, but, in any case, different combinations in failures and different degrees of severity are present probably due to the disease evolution time or malnutrition level [18–20]. In a recent research study [4], it was observed that despite the impulsive characteristics, planning and cognitive flexibility were not significantly different from the participants with AN.

The results are not entirely consistent because in some studies, patients' clinical severity or disease evolution level was not considered. It is also worth noting that the criteria used to determine the diagnosis are not always mentioned, the same test has been used to measure different neuropsychological functions, and the inclusion of control groups paired with the clinical groups has often been omitted. Finally, the total obtained scores are usually reported, but the functions involved in task solving failed are omitted [16, 20–22].

Considering the information previously described, the aim of this study was to evaluate whether there are differences in neuropsychological functioning of women with AN, BN and with no ED. The central hypothesis is that neuropsychological functioning is similar in individuals with AN or BN and different from people without these disorders.

2. Method, results and discussion

2.1. Method

2.1.1. Participants

Seventy-two women were evaluated: 18 with anorexia nervosa and 24 with bulimia nervosa who met the diagnostic criteria of the Diagnostic and Statistical Manual 5th edition (DSM-V) [23] and 30 without ED, paired according to age and educational level.

The mean age of the group without ED was 19.3 years (SD = 1.46), the mean body mass index (BMI) was 21.92 (SD = 2.31), and the mean educational level was 13.7 years (SD = 0.82). Participants with BN had a mean age of 20.12 years (SD = 2.75), a mean BMI of 23.45 (SD = 2.74) and a mean educational level of 14.24 years (SD = 0.86). In the group of participants with AN, the mean age was 18.89 years (SD = 1.4), the mean BMI was 16.88 (SD = 0.91), and the mean educational level was 13.03 years (SD = 0.62). The mean time of the ED evolution in the group was 5 years (SD = 1.23).

None of the participants showed other ED such as other nosological conditions, existence of brain lesions, alcohol or substance abuse, developmental or neurological disorders, severe malnutrition and severe anxiety or depressive states. In order to discard these conditions, some questions, taken from the DSM-V, were included to the eating disorders diagnostic interview (IDED-IV) at the time of assessment, and also, the medical records of participants with AN and BN were reviewed.

In addition to the IDED-IV, the subjective global assessment generated by the patient was also used only in the group of participants without eating disorders in order to measure nutritional status. In this test, the mean score obtained was 1.92 (SD = 1.74), that is, no problems, or risk of malnutrition was noticed. Besides, serious anxiety or depression symptoms were discarded by Beck Depression and Anxiety Inventories (scores > 30: 7.98 [SD = 4.16] and 9.52 [SD = 7.13], respectively).

2.1.2. Instruments

In order to create the study groups, IDED-IV designed to perform a differential diagnosis for ED according to the DSM-IV-TR was used; it also includes questions related to alcohol and substance abuse [24]. The version used for this research was the one translated into Spanish by [25], modified according to the DSM-V criteria and adapted for the Mexican population by the Nutrition Research Project at the National Autonomous University of Mexico (UNAM), Campus Iztacala.

The subjective global assessment generated by the patient is a method based on the original assessment of Detsky et al. [26]. This two-part assessment that evaluates the nutritional status is more specific and faster than other types of assessment such as albumin, skin sensitivity tests and anthropometric tests [27]. The first part of the assessment is a self-administered questionnaire addressed to obtain medical history data (weight differences, current dietary intake vs.

the regular intake, digestive symptoms present in the last two weeks, functional capacity and metabolic requirements), while the second part is a test performed by the health professional in order to know the physical signs (subcutaneous fat and muscle loss and the presence of edema or ascites). The rating is from zero to nine, and the higher the score, the more severe the symptoms of malnutrition.

The Beck Depression and Anxiety Inventories are self-administered questionnaires consisting of 21 multiple-choice questions, which can be used as of 13 years old. The first one has affective questions related to depressive symptoms, such as hopelessness and irritability, cognitions, such as guilt or feelings of being punished, as well as physical symptoms, such as fatigue and weight loss, while the second one is aimed to discriminate between somatic symptoms of anxiety. In Mexico, they are standardized with a reliability of 0.87 and 0.83, respectively [28, 29].

The assessment of the neuropsychological skills was carried out using the neuropsychological version of the Wechsler Adult Intelligence Scale-III (WAIS-III). This is a test of individual application that assesses the intellectual ability of people between 16 and 64 years old, it is divided into 14 subtests organized into two scales: verbal and nonverbal performance, standardized in Mexico with a reliability of 0.85 and 0.69, respectively, with an overall reliability of 0.86 [30]. The application of the neuropsychological version provides information on the most relevant aspects of cognitive functioning by performing a detailed review of the intellectual functions and allows measuring the neuropsychological functions in a global and integrative way, and it is a specific and sensitive method to neuropsychological failures [31].

The Wisconsin Card Sorting Test (WCST) is designed to measure cognitive flexibility, abstract reasoning skills and the development and maintenance of strategies to achieve a goal [32, 33]. In the Latin American population, it has been validated with a reliability of 0.82 [34]. It consists of four stimulus cards and 128 response cards; the goal is to classify the response cards with the stimulus cards according to three criteria: color, shape and number. The classification criteria are never made explicit; it is the participant who deducts them through the feedback offered by the evaluator ("right" or "wrong"). The classification criterion is changed without notice after 10 consecutive correct answers. The qualification criteria are as follows: number of applied attempts, correct answers, total number of errors, perseverative responses (when the participant insists on responding to a criterion that is not correct), perseverative errors (errors that follow the perseveration principle), nonperseverative errors (errors that do not follow the perseveration principle), number of completed categories (number of sequences of 10 consecutive correct answers), failure to maintain the attitude (an error after five or more consecutive answers but before completing the category), attempts to complete the first category and the conceptual level that reflects an understanding of the classification principles.

The Rey Complex Figure (RCF) Test assesses the visuospatial construction skills and visual memory [31, 35]. It is a paper-and-pencil test in which a complex stimulus card (5 × 7 in.) has to be copied, but it cannot be identifiable unless components are visualized and hierarchized by an analytical activity. It consists of a total of 18 perceptual units organized around a basic rectangle and divided by a horizontal and a vertical line into eight equal pieces, which in turn are intersected by two diagonal lines including a wide variety of internal and external stimuli. It is applied in two modes, copy and memory, with a time span of three minutes each. Its scoring considers rotation errors, location errors, repetition and review of the unit or its parts, distortion errors, angulation deficiencies, errors in the size of any unit or the full figure, total absence of unit and number of used colors, whose ideal is 18 (one per unit), which are essential to identify the drawing sequence. In Mexico, the test is standardized with a reliability of 0.83 for copying and 0.78 for memory [36].

The Tower of London-Drexel (TOL-DX) Task is an instrument that assesses executive functions, specifically skill planning [37] which is a process that requires the ability to conceptualize changes, generate and select alternatives, and keep attention [31, 38]. It has a reliability of 0.72 [39] and consists of two wooden bases (one for the test applicator and one for the evaluated participant) with three vertical towers and three colored beads (blue, red and green). The goal is to solve 10 problems of increasing difficulty moving the beads in the fewest possible moves to match the presented model. The test scoring criteria are as follows: number of movements (number of times that the beads are moved after surpassing the minimum necessary to solve the problems), starting, execution and overall time, the time violation at the first minute (i.e., after one minute has elapsed and the problem has not been resolved) and two rules: (I). Do not place more beads than the ones that can fit in each tower and (II). Do not move more than one bead at the same time.

2.1.3. *Procedure*

Patients from a private nutrition clinic in Mexico City were included in the AN or BN groups. The screening of participants without eating disorders was conducted in different public universities. All participants signed an informed consent (in the event of minor participants, the parents were also asked to sign an informed consent); they answered the IDED-IV in order to confirm the presence or absence of ED and exclusion criteria; medical records of participants with AN and BN were also reviewed; and all participants were weighed and measured to calculate their BMI. Later on, the RCF, the WCST and the TOL-DX were administered individually and in a different order, whereas the subscales of the WAIS-III were applied in the order proposed by Lezak [31] for the neuropsychological version: incomplete figures, vocabulary, digits and symbols keys, similarities, design with cubes, arithmetic, matrices, digit retention, information, drawing ordering, comprehension, symbol search, letter and number sequencing and object assembling.

2.1.4. *Statistical analysis*

The Shapiro-Wilk test was performed to corroborate the normal distribution of the data and its compliance with the assumptions to complete the analysis. In order to compare the neuropsychological performance among the three groups and identify statistically significant differences ($p < 0.05$), three multivariate analyses of variance (MANOVA) were carried out: one for the RCF, another for the WCST and a third one for the TOL-DX. Three ANOVAs were performed for the WAIS-III analysis in order to compare the verbal IQ, performance IQ and overall IQ, and two MANOVAS, one for the index scores and one for the 14 subtests that make up the test.

2.2. Results

A total of 72 participants were assessed: 18 with AN, 24 with BN and 30 with no ED. The mean age, BMI and educational level of the groups are shown in **Table 1**.

Group	N		Age	BMI	Edu
Without ED	30	Mean	19.3	21.92	13.7
		SD	1.46	2.31	0.82
Bulimia	24	Mean	20.12	23.45	14.24
		SD	2.75	2.74	0.86
Anorexia	18	Mean	18.89	16.88	13.03
		SD	1.4	0.91	0.62

BMI = Body Mass Index; Edu = Education.

Table 1. Age, body mass index and educational level among the groups.

In order to compare the neuropsychological performance among participants of each group and to identify whether there are statistically significant differences $p < 0.05$, four MANOVAS were conducted, one for each mode of the RCF, another for the WCST and a fourth one for the TOL-DX; three ANOVAS were performed to compare the verbal IQ, nonverbal performance IQ and overall IQ; and two more MANOVAS were carried out, one for index scores and another one for the 14 subtests of the WAIS-III.

The results of the RCF showed significant differences in both copy and memory modes, Wilk's lambda = 0.23, $F(2, 69) = 2.17$, $p < 0.05$, with an effect size of $\eta^2 = 0.52$ and Wilk's lambda = 0.23, $F(2, 69) = 1.82$, $p < 0.05$, with an effect size of $\eta^2 = 0.51$, respectively.

The univariate analyses of the copy mode showed statistically significant differences in the number of colors used, location error b (when the unit is attached to the figure, within the space that corresponds to it, but shifted) partial repetition, distortion errors a (uncoordinated trace), b (tangency error), c (closure error) and d (incomplete line), poor angulation and total score. The univariate analyses of the memory mode showed similar results to those of the copy mode; the statistically significant qualification criteria were execution time, location errors b and c (when the unit is attached to the figure, but outside its corresponding space), partial repetition (any component of the unit was drawn more than once), distortion errors a and d, omission and total score. According to Levene's statistic, the assumption of variance homogeneity was met in all cases. The means of each group and the F value for each significant variable are shown in **Tables 2** and **3**.

Rey Complex Figure—Copy							
Variable	**Group**						***F*(2, 69)**
	No ED		**Bulimia**		**Anorexia**		
	M	***SD***	**M**	***SD***	**M**	***SD***	
Colors	21.23	3.61	28.58	5.55	27.06	5.91	16.60*
Location b	1.14	0.83	1.79	1.11	1.69	1.16	3.72*
Partial repetition	0.18	0.03	1.32	0.75	0.91	0.36	4.58*
Distortion a	1.42	0.90	3.42	2.76	3.94	2.25	7.51*
Distortion b	3.73	2.42	5.87	3.16	4.00	2.60	4.49*
Distortion c	1.36	1.19	1.33	1.94	2.06	1.95	4.48*
Distortion d	1.18	0.38	1.73	1.04	1.75	1.13	3.31*
Deficient angulation	1.18	1.17	2.95	2.23	3.00	2.16	10.30*
Total score	25.44	6.13	21.10	4.53	21.81	4.53	5.64*

* $p < 0.05$.

Table 2. Univariate F means in the significant qualification criteria from the copy mode of Rey complex figure.

Rey Complex Figure—Memory							
Variable	**Group**						***F*(2, 69)**
	Without ED		**Bulimia**		**Anorexia**		
	M	***SD***	**M**	***SD***	**M**	***SD***	
Execution time	2.83	1.19	2.27	1.12	3.95	3.84	3.17*
Location b	0.93	0.86	1.79	1.41	1.78	1.47	4.70*
Location c	0.80	0.33	1.54	1.46	1.25	1.16	6.19*
Partial repetition	0.53	0.30	1.57	0.33	1.57	0.83	4.99*
Distortion a	1.45	0.88	2.63	1.83	2.91	2.39	4.26*
Distortion d	1.83	1.18	2.65	1.34	3.00	1.53	4.91*
Omission	3.80	2.09	6.46	2.02	5.00	2.40	10.20*
Total score	18.56	4.88	11.02	3.38	13.86	4.96	19.69*

* $p < 0.05$.

Table 3. Means and univariate F value in the statistically significant qualification criteria from the memory mode of Rey complex figure.

Tukey's post hoc tests showed that both AN and BN groups used a greater number of colors in the copy mode, made more location and distortion errors, had more angulation difficulties and omitted more units in the memory mode, and their scores were lower. Execution time differences were only found in participants with AN since they took longer time to complete the memory task.

The WAIS-III analyses included three ANOVAS to compare verbal IQ, performance IQ and overall IQ, and two MANOVAS, one for the four index scores (verbal comprehension, perceptual organization, working or operational memory and processing speed) and another one for the 14 subtests (picture completion, vocabulary, digit symbol- coding, similarities, block design, arithmetic, matrix reasoning, digit span, information, picture arrangement, comprehension, symbol search, letter-number sequencing, and object assembly).

The ANOVAS results showed no significant difference in verbal IQ, but they did in the performance IQ and overall IQ. Tukey's post hoc tests showed that the participants without eating disorders obtained higher scores. However, the average scores of all participants were within the expected values according to their age and educational level. The mean and coefficients are shown in **Table 4**.

IQ	Group						*F* (2, 69)
	Without ED		Bulimia		Anorexia		
	M	*SD*	M	*SD*	M	*SD*	
Verbal	101.53	5.95	100.90	7.25	101.72	1.01	2.96
Performance	106.80	4.62	101.67	4.22	101.38	5.12	11.28*
Total	102.77	4.74	100.37	5.31	101.05	5.79	8.11*

* $p < 0.05$.

Table 4. F and means of the nonverbal performance IQ and the total IQ on the WAIS-III.

The MANOVA for the index scores showed significant differences, Wilk's lambda = 0.69, F(2, 69) = 3.31, p < 0.05, with an effect size of $\eta 2 = 0.27$. According to Levene's statistic, all cases met the assumption of variance homogeneity. The univariate analyzes showed statistically significant differences in two scores: perceptual organization (picture completion, block design and matrix reasoning) and working or operational memory (arithmetic, digit span and letter-number sequencing). Tukey's post hoc tests showed that both groups, AN and BN, had more difficulties. **Table 5** shows the mean scores and the univariate F value of each index score.

	Index score						
	Group						*F*(2, 69)
	Without ED		Bulimia		Anorexia		
	M	*SD*	M	*SD*	M	*SD*	
Verbal compression	105.15	9.49	104.50	9.96	105.58	9.07	0.12
Perceptual organization	110.56	7.81	102.96	9.89	102.11	10.22	10.08*
Working memory	104.50	3.21	102.25	9.89	102.00	3.48	3.26*
Processing speed	110.46	13.61	109.83	15.66	102.72	23.92	1.74

* $p < 0.05$.

Table 5. Univariate F and means of the index score.

http://dx.doi.org/10.5772/65304

The results of the MANOVA carried out for the 14 subtests showed significant differences, Wilk's lambda = 0.45, F(2, 69) = 1.94, $p < 0.05$, with an effect size of $\eta^2 = 0.33$. According to Levene's statistic, all cases met the assumption of variance homogeneity. The univariate analyses showed statistically significant differences in picture completion, block design, picture arrangement, comprehension and symbol search. **Table 6** shows the mean scores for each group and the univariate F value in the 14 subscales. Tukey's post hoc tests showed that both groups, AN and BN, had difficulties identifying the missing parts of the figures, reproducing two-color models with cubes, rearranging the cards and telling a story, and providing solutions to everyday problems. Regarding the same stimuli found within a group of symbols, only participants with AN showed a significant difference compared with the other groups, as they had fewer trials answered.

Subscales	**Groups**						***F*(2, 69)**
	Without ED		**Bulimia**		**Anorexia**		
	M	*SD*	**M**	*SD*	**M**	*SD*	
Picture completion	22.83	0.98	21.71	1.73	20.75	1.37	4.51*
Vocabulary	36.73	7.64	35.21	5.76	36.08	6.46	0.34
Digit symbol— coding	79.93	12.15	80.95	12.32	79.97	11.79	0.18
Similarities	23.77	2.94	23.08	3.43	23.34	3.48	0.37
Block design	50.97	6.31	43.83	7.15	43.39	8.65	9.00*
Arithmetic	17.50	2.15	16.58	1.86	16.72	2.86	1.28
Matrix reasoning	22.86	2.75	21.33	2.33	21.95	2.88	2.67
Digit span	17.87	3.58	17.38	3.33	17.28	3.14	0.22
Information	22.13	3.08	22.12	2.91	22.44	2.83	0.76
Picture arrangement	20.30	2.19	16.04	3.20	16.83	3.76	15.42*
Comprehension	22.40	3.77	19.79	3.61	20.33	3.27	5.80*
Symbol search	32.36	5.04	30.08	6.72	26.63	5.65	3.84*
Letter-Number Sequencing	11.06	1.85	10.45	1.84	11.22	1.76	1.10
Object assembly	38.10	7.48	36.33	6.02	35.78	5.49	0.85

* $p < 0.05$.

Table 6. Means and univariate F in WAIS-III subtests.

In the WCST, MANOVA results showed significant differences, Wilk's lambda = 0.44, F(2, 69) = 1.70, $p < 0.05$, with an effect size of $\eta^2 = 0.42$. According to Levene's statistic, all cases met the assumption of variance homogeneity. The univariate analyses showed statistically significant differences in nine out of the 10 evaluated qualifying criteria, and the exception was the number of correct answers. **Table 7** shows the means of each group and the univariate F value of the dimensions. Tukey's post hoc tests showed that both groups, AN and BN, had a higher number of attempts and more total, perseverative and nonperseverative errors; they persisted in responding to a stimulus feature that was not correct; and they had difficulty understanding the classification principles (color, shape and number) and therefore, deducting categories (a sequence of 10 consecutive correct answers).

Wisconsin Card Sorting Test							
Dimensions	**Group**						***F* (2, 69)**
	Without ED		**Bulimia**		**Anorexia**		
	M	***SD***	**M**	***SD***	**M**	***SD***	
Number of attempts applied	82.13	9.62	103.46	20.97	111.78	21.68	18.26*
Correct answers	67.81	5.48	67.03	15.17	67.06	15.92	0.03
Total number of errors	14.57	5.29	33.88	24.01	38.61	25.45	11.31*
Perseverative responses	6.97	3.57	14.92	12.32	16.94	11.26	8.05*
Perseverative errors	6.63	3.26	13.58	10.82	15.56	10.07	8.05*
Nonperseverative errors	7.31	3.84	20.25	19.49	26.22	22.21	8.99*
Percentage of conceptual level responses	77.93	5.35	60.29	20.91	54.56	24.31	12.21*
Number of entire categories	5.94	0.31	4.87	1.75	4.22	1.81	10.51*
Attempts to complete the first category	13.13	2.54	16.67	23.87	27.33	31.99	3.91*
Failure to maintain the attitude	0.34	1.33	0.91	0.67	1.06	0.99	8.37*

* $p < 0.05$.

Table 7. Means and univariate F from the significant dimensions of the Wisconsin Card Sorting Test.

The MANOVA of the TOL-DX was statistically significant, Wilk's lambda = 0.56, $F(2, 69) = 2.18$, $p < 0.05$, with an effect size of $\eta^2 = 0.41$. According to Levene's statistic, all cases met the assumption of variance homogeneity. Regarding the number of movements exceeding the minimum necessary, the univariate analyses showed statistically significant differences in six out of the 10 problems evaluated by the instrument, as well as in the number of total movements. Tukey's post hoc tests showed that both groups, AN and BN, resorted to a greater number of moves to solve the problems. Mean and univariate F value of each of the problems and the total movements for the three groups are shown in **Table 8**.

Univariate analysis also showed significant differences in the execution time $F(2, 69) = 4.09$, $p < 0.05$ and in the violation of Rule II $F(2, 69) = 12.27$, $p < 0.05$. Tukey's post hoc tests showed that both groups, AN and BN, needed more time to solve the problems (M = 363.48 s, SD = 81.60 and M = 337.13 s, SD = 108.84 respectively) than participants without any ED (M = 193.66 s, SD = 82.60). Regarding moving more than one bead at the same time, the BN group showed a

http://dx.doi.org/10.5772/65304

difference: the number of violations of the participants with anorexia (3) was lower than those of the participants without ED (5) and the participants with bulimia (16).

Problems	Group						F (2, 69)
	No ED		Bulimia		Anorexia		
	M	SD	M	SD	M	SD	
1	2.08	1.26	3.16	2.35	2.26	1.22	2.46
2	2.83	1.06	5.87	4.33	4.89	4.74	3.13*
3	1.70	1.31	3.38	2.18	2.28	1.36	1.27
4	3.75	2.58	6.04	5.11	6.39	4.88	4.36*
5	2.70	2.11	4.67	3.68	4.17	3.24	3.61*
6	2.10	1.57	2.37	2.23	1.95	1.52	0.14
7	2.50	1.12	4.71	3.63	3.98	2.80	3.81*
8	2.26	2.11	4.33	3.66	4.00	1.41	6.72*
9	1.07	0.07	2.29	2.49	1.94	1.33	2.23
10	0.83	0.61	3.16	1.17	2.67	2.29	7.89*
Total movements	20.91	11.73	35.00	16.36	30.48	15.86	12.91*

* $p < 0.05$.

Table 8. Means and univariate F from the movement per problem and from the total of movements of the Tower of London.

2.3. Discussion

The aim of this study was to evaluate differences in the neuropsychological functioning of women with AN, BN and without ED. The main finding is that both eating disorders had similar difficulties in solving neuropsychological tests. According to the features measured by the RCF, the TOL-DX, the WCST, as well as the WAIS-III subscales of picture completion, block design, picture arrangement, comprehension and symbol search [31–33, 39, 40], failures were found in the visuoconstructive process, executive functioning, specifically in the skill planning to achieve a goal, cognitive flexibility and working memory, and in selective attention and common sense judgment when solving complex problems.

In RCF, the number of colors showed a consistent stimuli fragmentation, which implies that both groups, AN and BN, struggled to make an analysis that would allow them to visualize and prioritize the units. Therefore, at the moment of integrating the total figure, the unions of some lines were forced to coincide resulting in a disproportionate figure with errors. The participants identified the structures and organized their elements but in a fragmented way, focusing on the details and not in the stimuli globality for its construction. Organizational strategies and unit hierarchy are related to problems in the visuoconstructive process [31], whereas the detailed approach on stimuli is related to weak central coherence [41]. These results are in agreement with the results of several articles focused on AN [12, 42, 43], and they open the possibility to also consider the weak central coherence as a BN difficulty.

Regarding the memory mode, participants from both groups, AN and BN, made various omissions; nevertheless, the results of this study do not allow us to conclude about the existence of visual memory alterations, because this would require the copy to be developed without fragmenting the figure since the same fragmentation directly affects the possibility of stimulus recovery [32], and in this case, different fragmentations of origin were presented. Thus, to assess visual memory in these populations, it is worth considering one or more other tests, such as the picture set test [44] or the neuropsychological test for memory and visual learning DCS [45].

Difficulties to analyze and synthesize complex information in tasks designed to evaluate perceptual organization were also observed in the WAIS-III results. Participants at both groups, AN and BN, struggled to organize the elements that formed the stimuli and to analyze the data to conceptualize their shape and size.

In the subtest of picture completion, participants with either AN or BN focused on nonessential details and even on elements that were not present in the stimuli, concentrating more on nonrelevant details as the test difficulty increased, making the perception of globality more difficult each time. If it is considered that regardless of the task with which they are evaluated, such characteristics were observed, changes in selective attention could occur. This important finding is opposite to what some authors have mentioned about attentive difficulties being only observed when stimuli are related to food and body shape, as in the case of the Stroop Color and Word Test adapted for ED [16, 46, 47], and it also contradicts some research studies which indicate that alterations are found at the basic attention levels such as alertness and sustained attention [19, 48]. This focusing on the details also reinforces the hypothesis of the existence of weaknesses in the central coherence process.

The tendency of focusing on irrelevant details and making misinterpretations consequently was also clearly reflected in the picture arrangement subtest, which is a complex task that requires to make inferences discriminating the important information from the one that is not. Thus, the difficulties in producing a response by inhibiting others that are not relevant to solve a task together with the alterations found in the sequential thinking (i.e., the ability to identify relationships and set properties between events) make it very likely for participants with either AN or BN to struggle to pay attention to the context characteristics, which is an important skill for the implementation of goal-directed behavior [31, 32, 49], especially if we consider the difficulties in understanding concepts and social practices observed in the comprehension subtest of WAIS-III.

According to the features measured by TOL-DX and the WCST, the performance of the AN and BN participants shows neuropsychological failures in executive functioning, specifically in planning and cognitive flexibility [31–33, 39, 40]. Findings in the performance of AN participants agreed with those reported by several authors [9, 13, 16, 20, 43, 50, 51], and the difficulties exhibited by the BN participants corroborate the results of preliminary investigations [4, 14].

In the Tower of London Task, difficulties arose in delineating, organizing and integrating the sub-goals, that is, participants with either AN or BN did not follow strategies according to an overall plan of action. These difficulties are similar to those found by Alvarado and Silva [4], who considered that planning a series of sub-goals, anticipating the effects of a movement related to the ultimate goal, rejecting or accepting a move as part of the correct series and retaining the resulting sequence of correct moves for the final execution have a crucial component: the proper functioning of working memory [32]. Nevertheless, this function could suffer deterioration, which seems to have been corroborated in this investigation, not only because of the similarity in executions but also by the significant results of the WAIS-III index score (working memory).

Considering the above, it is also possible to state that there is an alteration in the prospective memory of the AN and BN participants, which is an essential element for behavioral planning as it is indispensable for the anticipation of future events for both formulating and implementing plans [49], so it would be worthwhile to conduct an investigation to asses it specifically in participants with the same characteristics and to identify whether there are difficulties affecting the solution of complex problems or not.

The results of the WCST show that the rigidity of thought is also a trait shared by the patients with either AN or BN, since both failed to make changes in response patterns and in the development and maintenance of strategies to achieve an objective despite receiving feedback [4, 14, 15], demonstrating the presence of inflexible thinking for task monitoring and plan designing.

Furthermore, considering that planning to achieve a goal focuses on the orbitofrontal area [46], that cognitive flexibility occurs in dorsolateral area [32, 33, 38, 40] and that the results suggest difficulties in sequential thinking, that is, establishing relationships between events and making common sense judgments (especially when understanding some concepts and social practices), it should be taken into consideration that people with either AN or BN have trouble with decision making, and the acquisition and use of an attribution system to interpret the intentions of others [49], especially if it is taken into account that some studies with AN patients [52, 53], designed to assess the theory of mind, have obtained similar results to those obtained in this study.

According to the results of this research, neuropsychological difficulties between AN and BN were homogeneous, and there were only differences in the execution time of the memory mode of the RCF. In the symbol search subscale of the WAIS-III for AN participants, they took longer time to deliver the figure, not only because they had not finished but also because they expected to recall other stimuli and had fewer found symbols since their answers were checked several times before continuing, and in the violation of the Rule II of the Tower of London Task in the BN group, they committed fouls when they could not solve the problem. This behavior may be attributable to their obsessive traits in the case of the AN group and to their impulsivity in the case of the BN group [18, 42, 54]. However, these characteristics did not affect their cognitive ability in the other tests.

This is consistent with the findings of some authors who observed no differences in the neuropsychological functions alteration and mentioned that the differences found in other studies may be due to the lack of consideration of the disease evolution time or severe malnutrition, especially in the case of AN [14].

It is important to note that, in patients with eating disorders, the neuropsychological difficulties may be related to certain alterations in the neural mechanisms, such as altering neurotransmitter alteration levels, decreased brain volume, blood flow and cerebral metabolism, which have been observed through neuroimaging studies [21, 55]. However, due to the huge number of variables, it is difficult to demonstrate the correlation between brain and functional changes [56]. In the case of AN, there is a preliminary study in which patients at an early stage were evaluated, and it was found that the neurobiological abnormalities may predict neuropsychological difficulties during follow-up [57]. This could be an indication that some neuropsychological disorders appear previously, so the weight of the disposition and the consequences of each type of ED should be clarified.

On this regard, there are known investigations in which executive functioning has been compared in patients with eating disorders vs. healthy relatives and similar difficulties have been found; this could be a family trait associated with an increased risk of developing these disorders [58–61]. In addition, the visuoconstructive skills, planning and flexibility of thought have been compared in participants with eating disorders associated symptoms, and it was noted that the performance is more similar to that of the participants with AN and BN than that of the participants without eating disorders; however, it should be similar to normal populations since they do not have conditions of malnutrition, dehydration or other secondary comorbidity associated with eating disorders [4, 62]. This suggests that the neuropsychological difficulties appeared prior to AN or BN and also that the degree of alteration depends on the conditions of the disease.

The simple size used in this study was limited, so studies with a larger number of participants at each study group should be conducted in order to extend and detail the data showed in this study.

In conclusion, it is possible that the impulsivity observed in participants with BN is not directly involved in the performance of neuropsychological testing as many authors have mentioned because, despite of the differences with AN, the difficulties in the neuropsychological processes were basically the same. Therefore, further research shall be conducted to reformulate BN intervention programs and to take cognitive remediation therapy into consideration, which has already been used with a good prognosis in anorexia nervosa.

Author details

Nayelli Alvarado Sánchez* and Cecilia Silva Gutiérrez

*Address all correspondence to: nayelli.alvarado.s@gmail.com

Universidad Nacional Autónoma de México [National Autonomous University of Mexico], Mexico

References

[1] Encuesta Nacional de Salud y Nutrición [National Survey on Health and Nutrition] Chapter 2: Nutrition. 2012. Retrieved from http://ensanut.insp.mx/doctos/ENSANUT2012_Sint_Ejec-24oct.pdf

[2] Smink F, Hoeken D, Hoek HW. Epidemiology of eating disorders: incidence, prevalence and mortality rates. Curr Psychiatry Rep. 2012;14(4):406–14. doi:10.1007/s11920-012-0282-y

[3] Smink F, Hoeken D, Hoek HW. Epidemiology, course, and outcome of eating disorders. Curr Opin Psychiatry. 2013;26(6):543–8. doi:10.1097/YCO.0b013e328365a24f

[4] Alvarado N, Silva C. Funciones ejecutivas y sintomatología asociada con los trastornos de la conducta alimentaria [Executive functions and symptoms associated with eating disorders]. Rev Latinoam Psicol. 2014;46(3):189–197. doi:10.1016/S0120-0534(14)70022-6

[5] Renwick B, Musiat P, Lose A, Dejong H, Broadbent H, Kenyon M, et al. Neuro- and social-cognitive clustering highlights distinct profiles in adults with anorexia nervosa. Int J Eat Disord. 2015;48(1):26–34. doi:10.1002/eat.22366

[6] Harisson A, Tchanturia K, Naumann U, Treasure J. Social emotional functioning and cognitive styles in eating disorders. Br J Clin Psychol. 2012;51(3):261–79. doi:10.1111/j.2044-8260.2011.02026.x

[7] Liao P, Uher R, Lawrence N, Treasure J, Schmidt U, Campbell I, et al. An examination of decision making in bulimia nervosa. J Clin Exp Neuropsychol. 2009;31(4):455–61. doi:10.1080/13803390802251378

[8] Pretorius N, Dimmer M, Power E, Eisler I, Simic M, Tchanturia K. Evaluation of a cognitive remediation therapy group for adolescents with anorexia nervosa: pilot study. Eur Eat Disord Rev. 2012;81(1):54–55. doi:10.1002/erv.2176

[9] Zastrow A, Kaiser S, Stippich C, Walther S, Herzog W, Tchanturia K, et al. Neural correlates of impaired cognitive-behavioral flexibility in anorexia nervosa. Am J Psychiatry. 2009;166(5):608–16. doi:10.1176/appi.ajp.2008.08050775

[10] Lang K, Treasure J, Tchanturia K. Acceptability and feasibility of self-help Cognitive Remediation Therapy for anorexia nervosa delivered in collaboration with carers: a qualitative preliminary evaluation study. Psychiatry Res. 2015;225(3):387–94. doi:10.1016/j.psychres.2014.12.008

[11] Tchanturia K, Davies H, Campbell I. Cognitive remediation therapy for patients with anorexia nervosa: preliminary findings. Ann Gen Psychiatry. 2007;6:14–20. doi:10.1186/1744-859X-6-14

[12] Lang K, Tchanturia K. A systematic review of central coherence in young people with anorexia nervosa. J Child Adolesc Behav. 2014;2:140. doi:10.4172/jcalb.1000140

[13] Marion R, Tchanturia K, Treasure J. Exploring neurocognitive inefficiencies in anorexia nervosa. J Eat Disord. 2015;3(Suppl 1):O67. doi:10.1186/2050-2974-3-S1-O67

[14] Tchanturia K, Davies H, Harrison A, Roberts M, Nakazato M, Schmidt U, et al. Poor cognitive flexibility in eating disorders: examining the evidence using the Wisconsin Card Sorting Task. PLoS One. 2012;7(1):e28331. doi:10.1371/journal.pone.0028331

[15] Westwood H, Stahl D, Mandy W, Tchanturia K. The set-shifting profiles of anorexia nervosa and autism spectrum disorder using the Wisconsin Card Sorting Test: a systematic review and meta-analysis. Psychol Med. 2016;46(9):1809–27. doi:10.1017/S0033291716000581

[16] Camacho E, Escoto M, Mancilla J. Neuropsychological evaluation in patients with eating disorders. Salud Mental. 2008;31, 441–446.

[17] Seitz J, Kahraman-Lanzerath B, Legenbauer T, Sarrar L, Herpertz S, Salbach-Andrae H, et al. The role of impulsivity, inattention and comorbid ADHD in patients with bulimia nervosa. PLoS One. 2013;8(5):e63891. doi:10.1371/journal.pone.0063891

[18] Duchesne M, Mattos P, Fontenelle L. Neuropsichology of eating disorders: a systematic review of the literature. Rev Bras Psiquiatr. 2004;26(2):107–17.

[19] Fowler L, Blackwell A, Jaffa A, Palmer R, Robbins T, Sahakian B, Dowson J. Profile of neurocognitive impairments associated with female in-patients with anorexia nervosa. Psychol Med. 2006;36:517–527. doi:10.1017/S0033291705006379

[20] Weider S1, Indredavik MS, Lydersen S, Hestad K. Neuropsychological function in patients with anorexia nervosa or bulimia nervosa. Int J Eat Disord. 2015;48(4):397–405. doi:10.1002/eat.22283

[21] Key A, O'Brien A, Gordon I, Christie D, Lask B. Assessment of neurobiology in adults with anorexia nervosa. Eur Eat Disord Rev. 2006;14:308–314. doi:10.1002/erv.696

[22] Sherman B, Savage CR, Eddy K, Blais M, Deckersbach T, Jackson SC, et al. Strategic memory in adults with anorexia nervosa: are there similarities to obsessive compulsive spectrum disorders? Int J Eat Disord. 2006;39(6):468–476. doi:10.1002/eat.20300

[23] American Psychiatric Association. Diagnostic and Statistical Manual of Mental Disorders. 5th ed. (DSM-5). Estados Unidos: Masson; 2013.

[24] Kutlesic V, Williamson A, Gleaves H, Barbin M, Murphy-Eberenz P. The Interview for the Diagnosis of Eating Disorders-IV: Application to DSMIV diagnostic criteria. Psychol Assess. 1998;10:41–48. doi:10.1037/1040-3590.10.1.41

[25] Raich R. Anorexia y bulimia: Trastornos alimentarios [Anorexia and Bulimia: Eating Disorders]. Madrid: Pirámide; 2001.

[26] Detsky A, Mc Laughlin J, Baker J, Johnson N, Whittaker S, Mendelson R, et al. What is subjective global assessment of nutritional status? J Parenter Enteral Nutr. 1987;11:8–13. doi:10.1177/014860718701100108

[27] Gómez-Candela C, Luengo L, Cos I, Martínez-Roque V, Iglesias C, Zamora P, et al. Valoración global subjetiva en el paciente neoplásico [Subjective global assessment in neoplastic patients]. Nutrición Hospitalaria. 2003;18(6):353–357.

[28] Jurado S, Villegas ME, Méndez L, Rodríguez F, Loperena V, Varela R. La estandarización del Inventario de Depresión de Beck para los residentes de la ciudad de México [The standardization of the Beck Depression Inventory for residents of Mexico City]. Salud Ment. 1998;21(3):26–31.

[29] Robles R, Varela R, Jurado S, Páez F. Versión mexicana del inventario de ansiedad de Beck: propiedades psicométricas [Mexican version of the Beck anxiety inventory: psychometric properties]. Rev Mexicana Psicol. 2001;18(2):211–218.

[30] Tulsky D, Zhu J. Escala Weschsler de Inteligencia Para Adultos – III: Manual Técnico [Wechsler Adult Intelligence Scale-III: Technical Manual]. México: Manual moderno; 2003.

[31] Lezak M. Neuropsychology Assessment. 4th ed. New York: Oxford University Press; 2004.

[32] Kenneth M, Heilman D, Valenstein E. Clinical Neuropsychology. 5th ed. New York: Oxford University Press; 2011.

[33] Parmenter A, Zivadinov R, Kerenyi L, Gavett R, Weinstock-Guttman B, Dwyer MG, et al. Validity of the Wisconsin card sorting and Delis–Kaplan executive function system (DKEFS) sorting tests in multiple sclerosis. J Clin Exp Neuropsychol. 2007;29(2):215–23. doi:10.1080/13803390600672163

[34] Heaton RK, Chelune GJ, Talley J, Kay G, Curtiss G. Manual, test de clasificación de tarjetas de Wisconsin [Wisconsin Card Sorting Test manual]. Madrid: TEA Ediciones; 2001.

[35] Salvador J, Cortés J, Galindo G. Propiedades cualitativas en la ejecución de la Figura Compleja de Rey a lo largo del desarrollo en población abierta [Qualitative properties in the execution of the Rey Complex Figure throughout development in open population]. Salud Mental. 1996;19(4):22–30.

[36] Cortés J, Galindo G, Salvador J. La figura compleja de Rey: propiedades psicométricas [Rey's Complex Figure: psychometric characteristics]. Salud Mental. 1996;19:42–48.

[37] Culbertson WC, Zillmer EA. The Tower of London – DX: a standardized approach to assessing executive functioning in children. Arch Clin Neuropsychol. 1998;13(3):285–301.

[38] Kolb B, Whishaw I. Fundamentos de neuropsicología humana [Fundamentals of Human Neuropsychology]. Barcelona: Labor; 2006.

[39] Rognoni T, Casals-Coll M, Sánchez-Benavides G, Quintana M, Manero RM, Calvo L, et al. Spanish normative studies in young adults: Norms for Stroop Color–Word Inter-

ference and Tower of London-Drexel University tests. Neurología, 2013;28(2):73–80. doi:10.1016/j.nrleng.2012.02.004

[40] Yuan P, Raz N. Prefrontal cortex and executive functions in healthy adults: A meta-analysis of structural neuroimaging studies. Neurosci Biobehav Rev. 2014;42:180–92. doi:10.1016/j.neubiorev.2014.02.005

[41] Lopez C, Tchanturia K, Stahl D, Booth R, Holliday J, Treasure J. An examination of the concept of central coherence in women with anorexia nervosa. Int J Eat Disord. 2008;41:143–152. doi:10.1002/eat.20478

[42] López B, Leekam BS. Teoría de la coherencia central: una revisión de los supuestos teóricos [Central coherence theory: a review of theoretical assumptions]. Infancia y Aprendizaje: Journal for the Study of Education and Development. 2007;30(3):439–457. doi:10.1174/021037007781787462

[43] Tapajóz F, Soneira S, Aulicino A, Martese G, Iturry M, Allegri RF. Theory of mind and central coherence in eating disorders: two sides of the same coin? Psychiatry Res. 2013;210(3):1116–1122.

[44] Tchanturia K, Anderluh M, Morris R, Rabe-Hesketh S, Collier D, Sánchez P, Treasure J. Cognitive flexibility in anorexia nervosa and bulimia nervosa. J Int Neuropsychol Soc. 2004;10(4):513–20.

[45] Lamberti G, Weidlich S. DCS: Prueba Neuropsicológica de Memoria y Aprendizaje Visual. México: Manual Moderno; 2010.

[46] Fassino S, Pieró A, Abate Daga G, Leombruni P, Mortara P, Rovera G. Attentional biases and frontal functioning in anorexia nervosa. Int J Eat Disord. 2002;31:274–283. doi: 10.1002/eat.10028

[47] Smith E, Rieger E. The effect of attentional bias toward shape- and weight-related information on body dissatisfaction. Int J Eat Disord. 2006;39(6):509–515. doi:10.1002/eat.20291

[48] Dickson H, Brooks S, Uher R, Tchanturia K, Treasure J, Campbell I. The inability to ignore: distractibility in women with restricting anorexia nervosa. Psychol Med. 2008;29:1–8. doi:10.1017/S0033291708002961

[49] Tirapu-Ustárroz J, Molina AG, Ríos-Lago M, Ardila A. Neuropsicología de la corteza prefrontal y las funciones ejecutivas [Neuropsychology of the prefrontal cortex and executive functions]. Barcelona: Viguera editores; 2012.

[50] Gillberg C, Råstam M, Wentz E, Gillberg C. Cognitive and executive functions in anorexia nervosa ten years after onset of eating disorder. J Clin Exp Neuropsychol. 2007;29(2):170–8.

[51] Lao-Kaim NP, Giampietro V, Williams SC, Simmons A, Tchanturia K. Functional MRI investigation of verbal working memory in adults with Anorexia Nervosa. Eur Psychiatry. 2013;29(4):211–218. doi:10.1016/j.eurpsy.2013.05.2003

[52] Russell TA, Schmidt U, Doherty L, Young V, Tchanturia K. Aspects of social cognition in anorexia nervosa: affective and cognitive theory of mind. Psychiatry Res. 2009;168:181–185. doi:10.1016/j.psychres.2008.10.028

[53] Schulte-Rüther M, Mainz V, Fink GR, Herpertz-Dahlmann B, Konrad K. Theory of mind and the brain in anorexia nervosa: relation to treatment outcome. J Am Acad Child Adolesc Psychiatry. 2012;51(8):832–841.e11. doi:10.1016/j.jaac.2012.06.007

[54] Lloyd S, Yiend J, Schmidt U, Tchanturia T. Perfectionism in anorexia nervosa: novel performance based evidence. PLoS One. 2014;9(10):e111697

[55] Frank GK, Shott ME, Hagman JO, Mittal VA. Alterations in brain structures related to taste reward circuitry in ill and recovered anorexia nervosa and in bulimia nervosa. Am J Psychiatry. 2013;170(10):1152–60. doi:10.1176/appi.ajp.2013.12101294

[56] Jáuregui-Lobera I. Neuropsychology of eating disorders: 1995–2012. Neuropsychiatr Dis Treat. 2013;9:415–430.

[57] Frampton I, Hutchinson A, Watkins B, Lask B. Neurobiological status at initial presentation predicts neuropsychological functioning in early onset anorexia nervosa at four-year follow up. Dev Neuropsychol. 2012;37(1):76–83. doi:10.1080/87565641.2011.583301

[58] Galimberti E, Fadda E, Cavallini MC, Martoni RM, Erzegovesi S, Bellodi L. Executive functioning in anorexia nervosa patients and their unaffected relatives. Psychiatry Res. 2013;208(3):238–44. doi:10.1016/j.psychres.2012.10.001

[59] Halmi KA, Kaye W. Susceptibility genes for anorexia and bulimia nervosa. Appetite. 2007;49:272–341. doi:10.1016/j.appet.2007.03.085

[60] Holliday J, Tchanturia K, Landau S, Collier D, Treasure J. Is impaired set-shifting an endophenotype of anorexia nervosa? Am J Psychiatry. 2005;162(12):2269–75. doi:10.1176/appi.ajp.162.12.2269

[61] Kothari R, Solmi F, Treasure J, Micali N. The neuropsychological profile of children at high risk of developing an eating disorder. Psychol Med. 2013;43(7):1543–54. doi:10.1017/S0033291712002188

[62] Alvarado-Sánchez N, Silva-Gutiérrez C, Salvador-Cruz J. Visoconstructive deficits and risk of developing eating disorders. Span J Psychol. 2009;12(2):677–85. doi:10.1017/S1138741600002043

Chapter 3

Neurobiology and the Changing Face of Eating Disorder Treatment: Healing the Eating Disordered Brain

Abigail H. Natenshon

Additional information is available at the end of the chapter

http://dx.doi.org/10.5772/66173

Abstract

By recognizing eating disorders (EDs) as disruptions in brain circuitry, neuroscience has begun to shed light on *how* people make changes in psychotherapy. The clinician who treats the eating disordered patient also treats the eating disordered brain. It is time for practitioners to become better acquainted with the organ they treat, and to apply neuroplasticity research findings to clinical practice. Eating disorders and body image disturbances signify the loss of integrity of the core self. Twenty-first century research and technology has validated the age-old notion that healthy neuronal connectivity within, and between, mind(s), brain(s), and body(s) reintegrates and defines the healthy self. The concept of the "self" as *embodied* (grounded in somatic reality) expands the scope of effective healing practices. Neurophysiological (somatosensory education and mindful psychotherapeutic attachments) interventions that support the emergence of embodied mindfulness and sensory awareness facilitate the reintegration of the eating disordered brain, and of the fragmented core self. Both lie at the heart of eating disorder recovery. Nowhere in the field of mental health are the concepts of the embedded self and embodied healing as significant as in the treatment of eating disorders and body image disturbances. This article discusses the healing impact of neurophysiological connections, intrapersonal and interpersonal, that foster recovery of the self.

Keywords: eating disorders, neurobiology, somatosensory interventions, somatic education, Feldenkrais method, neuroplasticity, neurophysiological treatment modalities, mindfulness in psychotherapy, neuronal connectivity, modern attachment theory, embodied brain, body image, self integration, neuro-cognitive retraining, trauma treatment, eating disorder recovery

"It is around the concept of the core self that psychology crosses paths with the brain and body" [1].

1. Eating disorders in the "Era of the Brain"

Eating disorders (EDs) are bio-psychosocial disorders, their origins and functional pathology based in genetics and brain structure. In the year 2006, by declaring anorexia nervosa (AN) and bulimia nervosa (BN) to be disorders of the brain, Thomas Insel, of the National Institute of Mental Health (NIMH), changed the face of ED treatment forever. "There is good reason to think that the prefrontal cortex is the brain center for some eating disorders, obsessions, addictive disorders, and alterations of body image" [2]. Studies show "substantial evidence that individuals who exhibit (ED) pathology are "wired" differently, …creating the need to define diagnosis by aberrations in brain circuitry and physiology, and then provide treatments aimed at correcting or ameliorating the aberrant circuitry" [3]. "The days of being able to talk about psychology versus biology versus neurology are fading" [2]. The NIMH initiative has not only set the stage for changes in the philosophical and clinical underpinnings of ED treatment, but also for the future of scientific research in this field. The advent of positron emission tomography (PET) scans and other neuroimaging devices capable of tracking and recording even the smallest brain changes has shed significant light on *how* people make changes in psychotherapy.

It is the functional linkage (integration) of differentiated components of a system that defines efficiency in function and well-being. "Unity within the human nervous system creates coherence, fluidity and flexibility, otherwise known as maturity. Lack of integration between spheres leads to chaos, or system rigidity" [4]. "Within psychotherapy, the focus of attention on various domains of mental, somatic, and interpersonal life creates neural firing patterns in the brain that enable new synaptic connections to be established [4]. In fact, neuronal plasticity, the changes in neural connectivity induced by experience that integrates brain function, may be the fundamental way in which psychotherapy alters the brain" [5]. Studies have shown that the more successful the (therapeutic) treatment, the greater the neuroplastic change [6]. Effective psychotherapeutic interventions "awaken" the patient's brain to attention, inviting and inspiring it to integrate learning through intrapersonal, as well as interpersonal, connections. Neuronal changes that occur over the course of an engagement between therapist and patient, when they take the form of a true "meeting of the minds," promote self-regulation [5]. The broad and integrative goals of ED recovery, which encompass emotional, physiological, neurophysiological, cognitive and social development, are best met through diverse and integrative recovery interventions, which hold the potential to facilitate a range of quantifiable changes in brain structure and function.

A brain that "marinates" in ED habits and patterns over years, and sometimes decades, will incorporate ED pathology into its structure as well as function. There is, however, a tremendous capacity for self-correction built into the human nervous system. "The brain is so plastic and changeable that alterations are not only possible, but *inevitable.* Unmasking, exposing, and strengthening secondary neural pathways are one of the main ways the plastic brain reorganizes itself" [6]. "When 'weak links in the chain' are strengthened, (through neural integration within and between regions) people gain access to skills whose development was formerly blocked. As a result, they feel enormously liberated" [6].

Quantitative neurophysiological studies across disciplines such as kinesthesiology and somatic education reveal treatment principles and interventions that support neuroplastic

http://dx.doi.org/10.5772/66173

changes at the brain level. Though relevant to ED recovery, the regrettable absence of these studies from the ED literature has made them essentially inaccessible to ED practitioners, rendering potentially beneficial outcomes lost to current mainstream ED clinical practice. Incorporating adjunctive neurophysiological treatment interventions into ED clinical practice would bridge the current research/practice chasm, facilitating brain and body integration and enhancing the healing of the ED *brain*, along with the ED patient.

2. Anorexia nervosa (AN) and bulimia nervosa (BN) are disorders of the brain

2.1. Genetic and trait-related characteristics of eating disorders

Emerging evidence suggests that both AN and BN are familial disorders, and that the clustering of these disorders in families may arise partly from genetic transmission of risk [7, 8]. A study suggests a common familial transmission of AN and obsessive-compulsive personality disorder, and the existence of a broad, genetically influenced phenotype with core features of rigid perfectionism and propensity for extreme behavioral constraint [9]. "Abnormalities in systems relevant to reward processing and the development of habit systems (in AN) have been consistently described within this population in structural and functional neuroimaging studies. Some aspects of dieting behavior are initially rewarding, but this behavior persists in individuals with AN as maladaptive behavior because it is ultimately mediated by neuronal circuits linked to habit formation" [10]. The postrecovery disturbance of such behaviors as a drive for thinness, over-concern with body shape and weight, obsessional behavior, dysphoric mood, etc., gives rise to the question of whether these elements, too, might be premorbid traits contributing to the pathogenesis of AN and BN [9].

The fact that recovered anorexic patients suffer from cognitive flexibility impairment also suggests that this is not a temporary state due to starvation, but a characteristic trait [11]. Functional MRI studies of AN demonstrate that "impaired cognitive-behavior flexibility causes behavioral rigidity which leads to maintenance of symptoms and resistance to treatment. The suppression of alternative behavior emanates from the diminished activation of a certain network pathway between the cortex and the diencephalon (that) plays a decisive role in initiating and controlling actions under rapidly changing environmental demands" [12]. Studies show that cognitive impairment in AN involves visuospatial ability, attention, memory, and cognitive flexibility [11].

A study that addresses persistent body image disturbances following ED recovery suggests an imbalance between internal and external representations of the body as a trait feature of ED, rather than just a feature of the acute state. Individuals with a lifetime history of an ED may have heightened sensitivity to visual information about the body and reduced somatosensory information processing of the body [13]. This suggests "an altered capacity of anorexic patients in processing and integration of bodily signals. Body parts are experienced as dissociated from their holistic and perceptive dimensions. Specifically, it is likely that not only perception but memory, and in particular sensorimotor/proprioceptive memory, shapes bodily experience in patients with AN" [14]. According to Norman Doidge, "because we see (perceive) with our brains and not with our eyes, the plastic brain becomes capable of reorganizing its sensory-perceptual system and with it, potentially our body image. We perceive ourselves—what we look like and feel like—with a perception that exceeds vision" [6]. It has been proposed that "restoring the balance between internal and external/visual information about the body by increasing interoceptive and/or proprioceptive awareness through sensory (neurophysiological) training should produce a less malleable and more accurate body perception. Multisensory impairment, which involves tactile and proprioceptive sensory components that may be associated with parietal cortex alterations, can best be treated through multisensory therapies" [13].

Research suggests that the altered function of neural circuitry contributes to restrictive eating in AN, and overeating in BN. "A clear link exists between AN and neural processes in the insula cortex as an integral part of ED pathology. The insula, which monitors bodily sensations and the strength of responsiveness to them, is the region where taste is sensed and integrated with reward to help determine whether an individual feels hungry or full" [15]. Identifying abnormal neural substrates could hold important implications for treatment through reformulating the basic pathology of ED and offering new targets for treatment. As an example, it may be possible to modulate the experience by enhancing insula activity in individuals with AN, or dampening the exaggerated or unstable response to food in those with BN [15]. Four separate regions within the insula cortex have been found to connect to social-emotional, sensorimotor, olfacto-gustatory, and cognitive networks of the brain. Functional systems overlapping within the insula reflect a possible linkage between them "necessary to integrate different qualities into a coherent experience of the world, setting the context for thoughts and actions" [16].

2.2. Neurological effects of ED on child and adolescent brains

The onset of AN in the developing brains of children and adolescents put young patients at risk for serious neurophysiological dysfunction. Studies show that low weight and higher cortisol levels correlate with greater structural brain abnormalities [17]. The brain's neuronal pathways multiply at a prodigious rate from birth to 6 years of age through the proliferation of gray matter, attaining 90–95% of adult brain growth. From age 6 to 12, neuronal pathways increase interneuronal connectivity, through the thickening of gray matter. Cerebral atrophy has been noted in cases of enduring AN, leading to what was initially considered to be an irreversible reduction in gray matter volume [17]. Follow up studies show that "the main brain changes seem to be reversible to some extent after adequate weight restoration, with brain changes in BN seemingly less pronounced than in AN, mainly due to chronic dietary restrictions" [18]. It is important to note, "though weight recovery may lead to the normalization of *structural* brain abnormality in ED patients, [18] weight restoration alone may be insufficient to fully rectify a nutritional insult. Adequate body composition and healthy hormonal function is also required to support optimal brain *function* in an 'all systems go' neuro-endocrine environment" [17].

The new diagnosis of 'avoidant/restrictive food intake disorder' (ARFID) has taken the place of 'feeding disorder of infancy and early childhood' in the American Psychiatric Association's Diagnostic and Statistical Manual of Mental Disorders, Fifth Edition [19]. Though not all children who experience picky eating syndrome meet the criteria for the ARFID diagnosis, one study found that, at any age, between 13 and 22 percent of children

http://dx.doi.org/10.5772/66173

were reported to be picky eaters [20]. Prevalence rates for picky eating ranges from 14 to 50 percent in preschool children and 7 to 27 percent in older children [20]. ARFID patients tend to be younger than those with AN or BN, include a higher proportion of males, and are commonly diagnosed with comorbid psychiatric and/or medical symptoms [21]. Many suffer from sensory integration disorder. Though evidence-based research has not yet proven the origins of ARFID, or of picky eating, to be in neurophysiology, tactile defensiveness and heritable factors such as variations of a specific tasting gene (dubbed TAS2R38) have shown up in "sensitive tasters, "who report that for them, vegetables take on an intolerable metallic taste. How bitter something tastes has to do with how tightly the bitter compound in foods binds with bitter receptors on the tongue" [22]. Currently, there are very few curative resources for picky eating individuals, both young and old, many of whom restrict themselves to eating no more than 5 to 15 foods. Existing solutions are based on behavioral exposure, desensitization and extinction therapy, and occupational and speech therapy, none of which have been shown to be uniformly successful. Considering the neuroplastic healing capacity of the brain, one might predict that the neurophysiological nature of this diagnosis could eventually find remediation within neurophysiological (somatosensory-based) interventions.

3. Human experience facilitates brain development

Historically, we tend to think of learning as initiated internally, within the cranial brain, but this is only partly the case. Learning also occurs externally, through the experience of movement, sensation and behavior, which create neuronal networks "from the outside, in," and from "bottom up." The nervous system's brain resides not solely in the cranium, (where learning happens "top down") but in the body. The embodied brain's sensory receptors send neuronal messages through the spinal cord to sensory receptors within the cranial-based brain. Human experience of all kinds stimulates and strengthens the formation of new and diversified neuronal pathways, guiding intelligence and instinct. "Synaptic linkages created by a combination of genes and experience shape new connections among neurons, dependent upon how genes are activated, proteins produced, and interconnections established within the neural system" [5]. The process of learning "affects which genes in our neurons are transcribed, shaping our brain's microscopic anatomy" [6]. Neuroscientist Michael Merzenich contends that practicing a new skill, under the right conditions can change hundreds of millions, and possibly billions of connections between the nerve cells in our brain maps, which develop strong connections to one another when activated at the same time. The potential for neuroplastic brain change remains viable throughout the human life span, with maps of normal body parts changing every few weeks through reorganization that occurs within and across brain sectors [6].

3.1. Awareness and attention facilitate brain integration and learning

A unified core self and feelings of well-being emerge out of a healthy integration of neurophysiological inter-relationships between moving, thinking, feeling, and sensing, and can be enhanced through mindful human connection. Any therapeutic learning experience with the capacity to move an individual towards balance, past negative habits, and closer to healing, promotes an integration and reestablishment of the once fragmented ED self. The human brain learns organically. "Organic learning is nonreductionistic, and therefore integrative, not separating the organism into its anatomical parts, but joining those parts into one continuous feedback loop [23]. The human brain's feedback loop contains the sensory domain, the motor domain, the affective domain, the cognitive, and spiritual domains, building on dimensions such as pleasure and spontaneity" [6]. Interventions that upgrade and integrate global brain function and increase neuronal connections and networks, brain weight, volume and thickness, and the number of branches among neurons, come about through focused attention, discernment, differentiation, and integration [6]. The following is an example of how the brain learns through focused attention (awareness), variation (change and novelty), differentiation (the capacity to sense and create differences,) and integration (the capacity to bring the learning to a meaningful coherence).

As an example, my 2-year-old grandson was thoroughly enjoying the attention he craved from disrupting the family dinner by kicking his shoes against his highchair. His brain sought stimulation, so I suggested that he kick the chair as loudly and as fast and hard as he possibly could. He enjoyed this experiment immensely. Then I suggested that he try to use his legs and brain differently, to kick the chair as slowly and as softly as he possibly could, seeing if he could make the sound so soft that no one else at the table would know that he was even moving his feet. In offering his brain this opportunity for attention, variation, and sensory discernment, this became not only an exercise in learning about loud and soft, fast and slow, hard and gentle, but in experiencing expansive new perspectives about how to use himself in moving towards self-regulation, self-determination, and self-satisfaction.

According to Moshe Feldenkrais, a pioneer in the field of somatic education, within the process of learning, "the more completely a person accesses and uses his entire muscular apparatus, the more the brain will become activated, with the activated regions further stimulating adjacent areas" [24]. The novelty of diverse types of therapeutic interventions stimulates different regions of the brain in facilitating connections between neurons [6].

The feedback loop of the *eating disordered* brain sustains biochemical, neuromuscular, and sensory imbalances resulting in the *dis*integration of the core self. Compensatory behavioral compulsions and dysfunctional eating rituals lead to erratic weight gain or loss, amenorrhea, bradycardia, and electrolyte imbalances. Resulting mood shifts compromise the patient's capacity for self-regulation and self-care, exacerbating behavioral pathology and physiological dysfunction. The at-risk eating disordered child who is developmentally unprepared to cope with the complexities of treatment and recovery tasks becomes most deeply vulnerable to the dire emotional, physical, and neurophysiological complications of these disorders. Diminishing cognitive, perceptual, emotional, and sensory acuity compromises a patient's capacity to benefit from psychotherapy.

3.2. Interventions that facilitate sensory connectivity promote self-integration

EDs are disorders of sensing. ED patients experience an impaired capacity to accurately sense, process and integrate bodily signals. "What emerges as the core experience of recovery is

http://dx.doi.org/10.5772/66173

the process of re-establishing a sense of self, where the word "sense" is as important as the word "self" [25]. What ED individuals *do* sense, typically, are feelings of isolation, shame, and self-loathing. ED patients experience difficulty in accurately sensing/perceiving hunger and satiety cues. For those with co-occurring mood disorders, the impulse to inflict self-harm may serve as an attempt to reconnect, through sensation, with the lost self. Sensory integration can occur through neurophysiological connections *within* the cranial brain; *between* the skull-based and body-based nervous system in the context of somatosensory, kinesthetic experience; through technological, non-invasive interventions; and through empathic and mindful psychotherapeutic attachments within psychotherapy.

The fact that "self-organization of the developing brain occurs in the context of a relationship with another being, another brain, renders psychotherapy a potentially powerful neuroplastic treatment tool" [26]. Schore defines psychotherapy as an attachment relationship that affects underlying neuronal structure and function" [26]. It is the ever-deepening sensation of connection between the therapist and patient that evokes an ever deepening sense of the patient's trust in herself. Emerging self-trust fortifies the patient to face and withstand the challenges and frustrations implicit within the ED recovery process, as well as in life itself, without the false security of the ED "crutch."

In treating eating disorders, various forms of adjunctive sensory training interventions are meant to augment, not replace more traditional mainstream approaches to ED treatment, known to promote the achievement of the "core principles" of ED recovery. The core principles of recovery include: (1) changes in the neuro-biological context, to include nutritional rehabilitation, weight normalization and stability, with no compensatory symptom substitution for the interruption of dysfunctional behaviors, (2) treating psychiatric co-morbidities to remission, (3) addressing external environmental changes, and (4) connecting to maintenance factors for recovery [17].

4. Mindfulness practice within the psychotherapeutic relationship promotes the integration of brain and self

"Healthy human attachment and mindful connectedness that results in the patient feeling "felt" through a versatile treatment relationship, creates a state of neural activation with coherence in the moment that has been shown to improve the patient's capacity for self-regulation" [5]. Within the mindful relationship, the quality of awareness and attention is broad and open, devoid of expectation, and biasing perceptual filters. The mindful quality of a treatment relationship, which has been defined as "paying attention in a particular way…on purpose, in the present moment, and non-judgmentally," [5] can be considered an intervention in itself [27]. "Two aware minds are more powerful than only one aware mind" [28]. Germer contends that mindfulness and the quality of the therapy alliance that arises from it "is more important to treatment outcomes than the particular treatment method or theory embraced by the therapist" [27]. "Empathy accounts for as much, and probably more, outcome variance than does the specific intervention. The mindful connection "may be even more influential in intervention-based treatment than in relational-based therapy" [27].

Mindfulness and empathy in psychotherapy demands the therapist's ongoing "presence" within the treatment moment, a state of "being aware, in a receptive way, of what is happening as it happens" [29]. It is the state of being present that allows a person to thrive within the experience of uncertainty [29]. Conversely, it is the *intolerance* of uncertainty that drives the patient's relentless resistance to letting go of an ED, which seductively guarantees predictability in life by providing the illusion of control over self and future. Mindful practice allows patients "to feel less resistant to, and threatened by, the vicissitudes of life experience through an acceptance of self and reality, allowing a greater capacity to choose whether to act on one's urges," [27] a concept particularly relevant to the treatment of BN and binge eating disorder (BED), which are characterized by impulsivity and self-disregulation. The fact that our intention to act is formulated in the brain *before* we become aware of it suggests that we may be able to change the brain through mindfulness practice. The individual has an opportunity to better control behavior by increasing mindful awareness of brain activity [27].

The promotion of the patient's brain integration and self-integration is a natural by-product of accepting awareness of both pleasant and unpleasant inner experience (body sensations, affects, and/or thoughts) [28]. The process of achieving mindful presence starts with a focus on bodily sensations that are connected to the issues the client brings to the therapy process, and that involve attention to body-felt experience from which other elements of subjective experience arise (emotions, cognitions, memories, etc.) [27]. It is in the state of "being present" that embodied psychotherapeutic change takes place, and where, in the end, neurons become altered, changing brain function and structure [29]. Mindfulness training has been shown to be associated with changes in gray matter concentration in brain regions involved in learning and memory processes, emotional regulation, self-referential processing, and perspective taking [30]. "Ultimately, lasting effects of psychotherapy need to harness experiences that promote the growth of new synaptic connections so that more adaptive capacities for self-regulation and well-being can be established" [5].

The mindful patient who becomes able to reject an obsessive focus in the past in order to rethink and recreate the course and flow of the present, positively affects his or her future by stimulating neurophysiological brain changes. Enabling mindfulness by creating an ongoing awareness of the patient's positive changes throughout recovery revives forgotten sensations of successful achievement, allowing the patient to *recapture* the benefits of the new circuitry that has been laid down.

Consider this example. A highly functioning woman recovering from 10 years of AN, periodically experiences herself as a failure in all her life roles, as a wife and mother, in her work, and as a recovering patient. By inviting her to join me in recalling, revisiting, and recounting the positive life experiences that she had incurred throughout her treatment, she became increasingly able to "piggy-back" on previous successes. By re-stimulating and/or simulating the previously felt sensation of confidence in anticipating novel experiences, (a process known as "faking it till you make it") she began to feel herself empowered by new neuronal pathways, having been laid down and now deepening.

Mindfulness is a revolutionary concept for psychotherapy, a profession that has traditionally seen movement and mental processes as separate processes. In offering a more unified model

http://dx.doi.org/10.5772/66173

of psychotherapy, mindfulness in clinical practice has proved to be "a teachable construct that draws clinical theory, research, and practice closer together" and that may prove to be "a tangible means for building empirically supported relationship skills" [27]. Mindfulness strategies in psychotherapy, which cultivate moment-to-moment awareness as a curative mechanism, serve most forms of psychotherapy across the board.

4.1. Clinical applications of mindfulness within ED treatment

4.1.1. Facilitating learning through mindful neurophysiological interventions in hospital settings

Though we tend to think of mindfulness as originating from the "top down" through the functioning of mind, mentality and cognition, mindful kinesthetic and bodily-based activities are also capable of evoking significant learning and healing from the "bottom up." In highlighting and addressing the ED patient's reluctance to experience herself in novel problem-solving situations, a partial hospital program assigned its adolescent patients three neurophysiologically-based tasks, designed to reinforce new sensations and learning through somatosensory movement. These included writing a sentence with one's unaccustomed hand; observing oneself in the act of walking backwards; and drawing a picture with one's eyes closed. Teaching potent lessons, these experiences challenged the patient's self-awareness and fear of the unknown, failure in the eyes of others, and the sensation of being unprepared and out of control.

When asked to discuss their responses to these tasks, the patients described feeling frightened, initially, about using themselves in unaccustomed ways. Following these experiences, they expressed surprise at how much they had improved at each task through engagement and continued practice, how helpful it had been to receive support from their peers in the process, how much they had learned from listening to each other's experiences, how acceptable it had seemed to try, and to fail, at new things, etc., all metaphors for ED recovery, and for life itself. No purely cognitive experience could have accomplished what these experiences provided these youngsters, so quickly and so potently.

Facility-based psychodrama therapy groups offer patients a liberating sense of permission to confront their "virtual" ED through community-based dramatic performances of confrontational dialogues with their disorder. Face to face with the ED and oneself, the patient's experience of expressing feelings within the context of a supportive peer and professional community tends to be a cathartic and gratifying experience among ED group populations.

Patient re-feeding becomes a pivotal soma-physiologic learning process that occurs within hospital, residential, or intensive outpatient settings. In such instances, the embodied brain comes to understand the reality that, in being required to restore weight, the body can, and will, consume goodly amounts of nutritious foods at regular intervals without becoming obese. A major concern of recovering ED patients tends to be draconian weight gain through an imagined loss of self-control upon ingesting normal amounts of food. Weight gain can be gradual and self-regulated, representing a pivotal lesson taught by the body in its wisdom.

> *A disregulated 14-year-old binging-type anorexic female who alternated binging and starvation, described her one-month experience of treatment in an outpatient treatment facility. She reported, "It wasn't till I had a chance to be fed at the program that I was finally able to understand that I can eat*

> *healthfully without getting fat ... I did it there, I know what it is like, and now I have felt what it feels like to have food in my stomach without panicking. My stomach actually became comfortable having food in it after a while, and I learned that I can choose to put it there through the decisions I make. I get hungry for meals now, without becoming frightened, and am beginning to understand what it feels like to have a normal relationship with food." This patient's bodily experience, autonomously and experientially allowed her to integrate, own, and utilize previously disintegrated cognitive and behavioral attempts to alter her eating lifestyle, this time more successfully.*

Upon release from the program, this youngster no longer engaged in binging and starving behaviors. She had become capable of eating normally and without fear, having developed new trust in her body and self. Fully prepared now to engage in the psychotherapy process, she set about to resolve the deeper emotional issues driving her disorder.

4.1.2. Mindfulness has emerged as an important focus of inpatient and outpatient treatment techniques for ED

Dialectical behavior therapy (DBT), cognitive behavioral therapy (CBT), and acceptance and commitment therapy (ACT) treatment techniques and strategies are designed to systematically ameliorate distortion in the patient's cognition, self-perception, coping. and problem-solving skills through mindfulness skills, which include emotional regulation, distress tolerance, and interpersonal effectiveness. Dialectical behavior therapy is a mindfulness-based cognitive behavioral methodology, particularly effective in the treatment of co-occurring depression, stress reduction, and borderline personality disorder. Mindfulness in DBT evokes a quality of awareness that allows one to control the mind, so the mind ceases to control the person. The roots of DBT mindfulness practice are in the benefits of "allowing," or accepting experiences, rather than suppressing or avoiding them. By reducing the anxiety that deters learning, mindfulness informs cognition, bringing the protocols of CBT into a dynamic mechanism for change" [27].

The recent advent of the inclusion of mindfulness in cognitive behavioral therapy, known as mindfulness-based cognitive therapy (MBCT) combines cognitive behavioral therapy with meditative practices and attitudes. The assignment of behavioral tasks to counteract habitual, ritualistic, and entrenched thoughts and behaviors creates new neuronal pathways in the recovering brain. ACT is a branch of cognitive therapy that acknowledges the centrality of the therapy relationship, achieving successful outcomes through mindfulness strategies coupled with commitment and behavioral change strategies. The goal of ACT is to foster emotional flexibility, emotional integration, and emotional maturity. ACT focuses on full acceptance of present experience, and mindfully letting go of obstacles, as patients identify and pursue their life goals.

4.2. The neurophysiology of effective attachment in mindful therapeutic relationships

It is through the relationship that "deficits in internal working models of the self and the world are gradually repaired" [26]. Schore's developmental model places particular emphasis upon "the experience-dependent maturation of a system in the orbital prefrontal cortex that regulates psychophysiological state and organismic energy balance. This frontolimbic system is expanded in the nonlinear right hemisphere that generates

http://dx.doi.org/10.5772/66173

stress-regulating coping strategies..." [31]. "The healing impact of the therapeutic relationship occurs through transactions where "the sensitive empathic clinician's monitoring of unconscious process, rather than content, calls for right brain attention to matching the patient's implicit affective-arousal states" [32]. By means of reverie and intuition, the therapist listens with the right brain directly to the patient's right brain [32]. Implicit right brain to right brain intersubjective transactions lie at the core of the therapeutic relationship, mediating the "moments of meeting" between patient and therapist. The right brain to right brain hemisphere connection that exists "outside our skin," gives rise to a therapy relationship so deeply ensconced in psychophysiology as to be considered sharing a common brain, "a mind being changed by a mind" [32].

Paralleling this dynamic, the infant's early emotional interactions with the primary object facilitate the neurophysiological development of the child's right brain. The attachment dynamics in psychotherapy between the therapist and patient, too, have been shown to result in learning that regulates psychobiological states of emotions. The aspects of "good parenting" that therapists offer patients become more than a metaphor, with the roots of the therapy relationship deeply ensconced in brain-related psychophysiology.

The implicit realm of communication is enhanced when the therapist is in his own enhanced state of right brain receptivity. The therapist's openness to his own bodily state is a crucial first step in establishing the interpersonal attunement and understanding that is at the heart of interpersonal integration and self-regulation. "By accessing his own neurophysiological responses to the patient's communications, the therapist's right brain connection allows him to know the patient "from inside out" [32]. "Where the therapist is sensitive to the patient's signals and also has made sense of his or her own life, the state of brain activation in the therapist serves as a vital source of resonance that can profoundly alter the ways in which the patient's brain is activated in the moment-to-moment experiences within therapy" [5]. The subconscious processing of information uses an expansive attention mechanism on the part of the therapist that includes free association, while the left brain remains more involved in the conscious processing of information, using a more restricted mode that focuses on local detail" [32]. In monitoring countertransferential responses, the clinician's right brain tracks at a preconscious level, not only the arousal rhythms and flows of the patient's affective states, but also his own interoceptive bodily-based affective responses to the patient's implicit facial, gestural, and prosodic communications" [32].

"As an interactive regulator of the patient's psychological states," [31] the therapist's emotional involvement offers a deep, fearless, and well-boundaried being. Attempting to achieve an open, receptive state of awareness of internal state changes and interpersonal signals sent by the patient, the mindful therapist who has learned to identify and disentangle his own thoughts and feelings inspires the patient to develop the same skills and insights that *he* has developed in approaching life. Sharing a common ground, therapist and client experience and discover each other from a position of equality" [27]. "Where therapists are not intimidated, and when they can feel comfortable disclosing themselves in appropriate, boundaried, and clear intentional ways, patients are offered the opportunity to bring forward more of their *own* seemingly intolerable experience. Our receptivity assures patients that they need not censor themselves, so that difficult emotions lose some of their threat. Resonance, or perceptions of another's affective expressions, may alter our own somatic and limbic states as practitioners. By accessing one's own bodily-based intuitive responses to the patient's communications, the intersubjective field between two individuals includes far more than two minds, to include two bodies" [32]. Significant to ED treatment, in light of the body image concerns of ED patients, "The right brain hemisphere contains the most comprehensive and integrated map of the body state available to the brain" [33].

4.2.1. The talking connection in psychotherapy is an embodied connection

Siegel describes the mind as relational, as well as embodied. According to him, "The mind uses the brain to create itself through the process of neuroplasticity… in turn, the functioning of the mind can actually change the structure of the brain itself" [34]. Through mindful psychotherapeutic connections, talk therapy resonates, brain to brain, as an embodied function. "When the therapist's mind and embodied self come together in relationship with those of the patient, implicit systems of the therapist interact with implicit systems of the patient, rendering psychotherapy not the "talking" cure, but the "communicating" cure" [6]. Psychiatrist Dr. Susan Vaughan has argued that the talking cure works by "talking to neurons," and that an effective psychotherapist or psychoanalyst is a "microsurgeon of the mind" who helps patients make needed alterations in neuronal networks" [6]. "The aim of talking cure… from the neurobiological point of view (is) to extend the functional sphere of influence of the prefrontal lobes" [6]. "Psychotherapy works by going deep into the brain and its neurons and changing their structure by turning on the right genes" [6].

Brain scans have shown that "talk therapy can change the brain even in a state of severe OCD brain-lock." Jeffry M. Schwartz theorized, then proved, that patients could shift the brain "manually" by paying constant effortful attention and actively focusing on something besides the worry, such as pleasurable activity, proving that what a patient *feels* is less important than what he *does*. Schwartz found that changes in the brain from mindful cognitive (talk) therapy can be similar to those from psychoactive medication" [27].

5. The ED, the brain, and the self are dynamic processes on the move

According to Albert Einstein, "Until something moves, nothing happens." The cohesion of movement and sensing plays an extensive role in how the nervous system coordinates a coherent sense of self [1]. Until the mid-twentieth century, scientists believed that the brain was "hard-wired" and unchanging, and that humans were born with a predestined potential, as well as limitations. Neuroplasticity research that began in the late 1960s and early 1970s overturned the doctrine of the unchanging brain, demonstrating that the brain changes its structure with each different activity it performs, continually perfecting its circuits so as to be better suited to any task at hand. The formation of neuronal pathways carved from deeply rutted habituated behaviors within the human brain is in some respects similar to rivers and streams carving their pathways through rock. The malleable and efficient brain develops and augments enriched networks of neuronal "tributaries, estuaries, and tide pools" through altering the direction, speed, and flow of learning. Moshe Feldenkrais contended, "Without movement there is no life [24]." He described the self as "never static… changing from action to action" [24]. Eating disorders, too, are on the move; never static, if not actively healing, they are actively securing a more profound and pernicious foothold within the patient's brain.

"Set off by a dynamic flow of electrochemical energy that creates electrical signals and patterns inside neurons, neoplastic learning and change occurs through the movement of ions in and out of brain membranes. "All experiences encompassing thought, sensation, feeling, and behavior, be it conscious or unconscious, are embedded in neurons. When movement occurs within neuropathways, the "language" of growth and change consists solely of the movement of electrical patterns along the neuropathways in the brain's cortex, as there are no visual images, sounds, smells, or feelings moving inside our neurons" [6]. Hebb proposed that "learning links neurons;" that when two neurons fire at the same time, (or when one fires causing the other to fire) chemical changes occur in both, so that the two connect more strongly. The neuroscientist Carla Shatz summarized the concept: "neurons that fire together, wire together" [6]. The more often the respective neurons "talk" to each other, "the greater the capacity for learning to become solidified" [6].

Brain-changing electrical movements originate either in externalized behaviors, through experience and behaviors, affecting the brain "from the outside in," or through thoughts, ideas, and feelings, "from the inside out" [6]. The brain changes its structure and function with each different activity it performs, continually perfecting its circuits so as to be better suited to any task at hand. According to Feldenkrais, "so smart is the human brain, that learning to do something with ease and facility once, can be sufficient to bring about change even after the brain has done that thing ineffectively a thousand times." If one "part" of the brain fails, than other parts can take over… if brain cells die, they can at times be replaced, or other parts can be recruited to take over their function [35].

5.1. Movement *with attention* facilitates learning

Where attention goes, neural firing occurs, and where neurons fire, new connections can be made. In this manner, "learning a new way to pay attention within the integration of consciousness enables the client with an open receptive mind to catalyze the integration of new combinations of previously isolated segments of his or her mental reality" [5]. "The repetition of novel, ameliorative behaviors alter neuronal pathways within the structure of the brain by "shaping" or "training," "molding new behaviors in very small steps [6]. In treating an obese individual who suffered from compulsive over-eating, Feldenkrais assigned her the daily task of slowly and mindfully counting every spoonful of cereal with milk that she puts into her mouth throughout the day. "The client's mindful self-monitored attention to the reality of the current moment cultivates an awareness of what has worked in the past, affecting what might work in the present, and what might be worth trying in the future" [27].

Rote, mindless, and undifferentiated movement, such as the mechanical repetition of an action through repetitive exercise, will not produce self-image change. Clarifying the self-image requires the reshaping of neurocircuits through self-awareness, with mindfulness of each part of the action, the patient's experience during the action, and the perception of the total body image during and following the action [36]. Attention paid to behavior has been deemed, "the specificity scalpel into the brain to recarve neurocircuits" [34].

5.2. The healthy mind, body and self weave a fabric of unified connection

Scientific evidence of the unity of mind and body in defining the healthy self has validated 2500 years of Buddhist thought and practice. Brain research points to a dynamic, experientially based notion of the healthy self as an embodied, sensory-based process grounded in kinesthetic experience [5]. The healthy "self" is a wholly integrative fabric with no one element separated from any other, the product of a neurophysiological inter-relationship between moving, thinking, feeling, and sensing. Sigmund Freud and Moshe Feldenkrais saw the unity of mind and body as an objective reality. Asserting that there is no valid distinction to be made between them, Feldenkrais observed that without a change in muscular habits of action, a person in Freudian psychoanalysis would often revert back to a habitual way of acting even when their therapeutic insights should have helped them change their behavior [6].

During 1940s, he postulated that "emotions are themselves body phenomena. We cannot be conscious of a feeling before it is expressed by a motor mobilization...They are not two states but two aspects of the same state" [37]. Toole describes body awareness as a "doorway into inner space" and an "awakening of consciousness" which "counteracts the loss of self in thinking, in emotions, or in external situations" [38]. He contends that primarily identifying with the mind to the exclusion of the body creates "an opaque screen of concepts, labels, images, words, judgments, and definitions" capable of blocking "a sense of oneness," the relationship between man and himself" [39]. In other words, the mind is embodied, built in part from roots in somatic reality" [5].

Twenty-first century magnetic resonance imaging (MRI) offers scientific evidence of the relationship between the brain's motor cortex and its visual system, language systems, memory, attention, and cognitive processes. Subsidiary neuropathways branch off from existing neuropathways through movement, sensory experience, behavior, emotions, and thinking, facilitating "patterns of gene expression which enhance factors that support the encoding and transfer of data, synaptic structure, and the activity and plasticity of neurons, facilitating learning" [40]. Implications of the brain's capacity to integrate sensing, perception and motor activity are far-reaching because the brain does not differentiate action from thought, so that the power of imagination and self-awareness can become as potent in stimulating neurological change as is the physical act of doing.

5.3. Self-image and body image are grounded in perception and kinesthetic experience

Self-image and body image, each having mental and neurophysiological components embedded in neurons, are virtually interchangeable within the neuroplastic brain [6]. "We act according to the image [self-perception] that we create of ourselves" [37]. "In order to change our mode of action, [once it becomes dysfunctional or fixed] we must change the image of ourselves that we carry within us" [37]. "When a sensory function becomes disturbed, the body part affiliated with it stops sending normal sensations from it to the brain. The brain then alters its representation of that body part. People with distorted body image report feeling unbalanced, rootless, and ungrounded – all vestibular terms" [41]. When dysfunctional habits and patterns occur over a period of years, the structure of the brain changes to incorporate these habits and patterns, so the brain does not move on or "turn the page" [41].

"The representation or image of the self is one such pattern. The brains of individuals with ED have become committed to neuronal pathways that have temporarily obliterated more adaptive pathways [41]. It is not atypical for ED individuals who have achieved significant benchmarks of recovery (full weight restoration and normal hormonal function, significantly improved mental and emotional functioning, and increasingly healthy problem-solving and attitudes about food and eating) to remain painfully and indefinitely susceptible to an obsessive, distorted perception of the embodied self and body image. A recovering anorexic patient, obsessed with a distorted body- and self-image, described herself as remaining "trapped in this body image." She was referring to her incapacity to take action in her life, to quit her job, separate from her husband, love herself, and move forward in her recovery, all due to her intolerable perception of her self.

Self-image is influenced by heritability, the socio-environment, as well as self-education [36]. Somatic education influences self-integration by providing a somatosensory, kinesthetically based, neurophysiological practice that educates and integrates the brain, creating an awareness of a sense of the inner body. By filling in gaps in body image, it redefines a more complete and accurate embodied perception of self. The repair and re-integration of perceptual-sensory dysfunction have been shown to take place through somatosensory movement. "Because the representation of the body is dominated more by external vision, and less by internal somatosensory information in healthy controls, somatosensory training increases the contribution of internal somatosensory information which could reduce or ameliorate the disturbance in the experience of the bodily self by helping to restore the balance between internal and external/visual information about the body [13]. Increasing interoceptive and/or proprioceptive awareness produces a less malleable and more accurate body perception and undistorted body representation.

"Mirror neurons reveal the fundamental integration within the brain of the perceptual and motor systems with limbic and somatic regulatory functions [5]. The "sensorimotor supremacy hypothesis" confirms that perceptual shifts draw on motor action; conscious and unconscious perception cannot be separated; and the correlations that give rise to conscious visual perception (i.e. body image distortion) can only be derived after the sensory inputs *and* their temporally trailing motor or premotor consequences" [42]. In addition, "it is likely that not only perception, but memory, and in particular sensorimotor/proprioceptive memory, shapes bodily experience in patients with AN. It has been discovered that "the relative proportion of positive to negative self-schemas (functional memory structures) available in memory may be the cognitive foundation of observed differences in global self-esteem, the affective component of the self-concept. Interventions promoting development of new positive self-schemas may be an important factor in identifying alternative sources of motivated behaviors and promoting ED recovery" [43].

6. Somatosensory interventions facilitate increased production of improved neuronal pathways and brain circuitry

The brain that drives the movement of thoughts and emotions also drives the movement of bodily feedback and sensation. Decades before the dawn of our current "era of the brain," Moshe Feldenkrais theorized that various parts and functions of the brain, when activated, can be enlisted to facilitate change and enhance function in *other* parts of the brain, creating new and improved neuropathways to take the place of damaged, nonexisting, or dysfunctional ones. In his book, "The Brain's Way of Healing: Remarkable Discoveries and Recoveries from the Frontiers of Neuroplasticity" (first edition), Doidge describes the girl named Elizabeth who was born 37 years ago, missing a third of her cerebellum [41]. At birth, confined to a rigid and painful body devoid of movement, Elizabeth's infant brain was deprived of its most potent and prolific opportunity to develop neuronal pathways that would permit learning of any kind. Her restriction of movement was so severe during her first year of life that she could not control her eyeballs, and for a time was thought to be blind. By 13 months of age, when she began treatment with Feldenkrais, the only bodily movement she had mastered was to roll over on one side. Feldenkrais worked with Elizabeth as consistently as possible during the second and third years of her life, demanding a family lifestyle of frequent intercontinental travel. Following his sudden death during her third year of life, and throughout her childhood and teen years, Elizabeth worked intensively with Anat Baniel, one of Feldenkrais' protégés.

Gently and intentionally moving her body so as to stimulate her dormant brain to awaken to life, Feldenkrais gradually triggered functionality in her cerebellum, which in turn, triggered the creation of neuronal pathways in adjacent parts of her brain to compensate for those parts that were missing and damaged. After her first four 20-min lessons, Elizabeth's once dormant brain began to engage her body in its most primal form of reptilian creeping, marking the start of what would become the full sequential development of her brain, from back to front, from the motor cortex to the pre-frontal cortex, and would lead to her body's "rebirth," and a full restoration of life quality.

Though several top pediatric neurologists offered a prognosis of profound retardation, incontinence, and institutionalization, where she would be restricted to bed and wheel chair, through on-going Feldenkrais Method treatment, Elizabeth's brain recovery would become complete, her life full and gratified. She has grown up to become a fully independent young woman today, with a rigorous education and two master's degrees, a successful and long-term marriage, and a business of her own. Feldenkrais correctly predicted that she would "dance at her wedding," which my husband and I, as her parents, were grateful and proud to provide for her.

6.1. Clinical applications of somatosensory research in eating disorder treatment

6.1.1. Somatic education/the Feldenkrais Method of Somatic Education©

Somatosensory movement techniques transmit information from the body's sensory receptors, via sensory nerves in the spinal cord, to sensory receptors in the motor cortex. "The part of the brain that processes movement is the same part of the brain that promotes learning" [40]. Most of the neural circuitry from the motor cortex is "outbound," influencing other parts of the brain involved in memory, attention, and spatial perception. Through the Feldenkrais Method of Somatic Education©, "the student learns to remain mindful and attentive to proprioceptive and exteroceptive sensations throughout the body while moving, and is taught to notice relationships and patterns of relationships between parts of the moving self" [23]. On the sensory level, communication is more direct with the unconscious, and therefore more effective and less distorted than at a verbal level [41]. Recognizing that sensory stimuli are closer to unconscious functioning than to conscious understanding, Feldenkrais' work allows patients to consciously reconnect with their unconscious sensorimotor repertoire through sensory training that expands their movement repertoire. The method enhances the kinesthetic sense, which is, as our first and basic ability to perceive, deeply connected with our self-identity [41]. It has been said that "the Feldenkrais method offers entrance to the ground floor of our sense of self," ...(taking) most adults back to infancy and mobilizing developmental processes at a fundamental level" [1]. In the end, what is recovered through somatic education in eating disorder recovery is the perception and connection to a sense of one's own authenticity.

Within the Feldenkrais Method, the concept of two brains meeting within a mindful connection takes the form of human touch in the hands-on, Functional Integration©, technique. "Through touch, two persons, the toucher and the touched, can become a new ensemble where two bodies when connected...become a new entity. These hands sense, at the same time as they direct," [44] a concept that currently resonates with the findings of Siegel and Schore vis-à-vis the dynamics of right brain to right brain resonance in psychotherapy. In Awareness through Movement© group classes, the student locates an awareness of self from within, and *inside* the teacher's awareness of him" [44].

Unique among other somatic movement alternatives, such as trauma informed yoga, Nia, Tai Chi, etc., Feldenkrais' Awareness through Movement © techniques actively and directly evoke the patient's mindful attention to sensation, thought, and feeling in the context of movement, all components required to stimulate integrative neuroplastic brain change. In facilitating the ED patient's self-awareness within mindful movement, the instructor of such somatic education techniques might inquire: "How does it feel to sustain contact with your body as you gently move and transition into the unknown?" "Is there a place inside of your body where you can go to feel fully safe...or unsafe?" "Can you sense your transition into the unknown as you move?" Filling the voids in body image and self-image through bodily movement with attention, somatosensory education fosters somatosensory reintegration and ultimately, the reintegration of the embodied self.

6.1.2. The Feldenkrais Method and ED: research outcomes

One of very few controlled studies of Feldenkrais' method as an adjunctive treatment for ED concluded that the Feldenkrais Method as a body therapy is "particularly suited for those suffering from ED in fostering an improvement of body perception and a clarification of the body image, through which the satisfaction and acceptance of the body should improve" [36].

The German study of ED inpatients found an "increasing contentment with regard to problematic zones of their body (hips, thighs, buttocks) typical for ED, and showed that through (awareness-based) physical movement, compulsive behavior can be decreased and spontaneous behavior can be increased. Outcomes indicated the development of a "felt" sense of self, self-confidence, and a general process of maturation of the whole personality" [36]. In another study of ED women averaging 34 years of age, the Feldenkrais work resulted in their ability to consciously challenge dominant social discourse by engendering concrete changes in the way they perceived themselves. They reported being able to occasionally change their daily activities and various eating habits, thus revealing transfer of learning from the Feldenkrais classes to their daily lives" [45].

As a Guild Certified Feldenkrais Practitioner, as well as a psychotherapist specializing in the treatment of ED, I have enjoyed the privilege of enhancing recovery for my own ED patients through integrating the work of brain, mind and body, using adjunctive Feldenkrais practice. This work has now become readily accessible, both individually and through classes, worldwide. Instructive DVDs and short demonstrations of Feldenkrais movements are offered free through the Internet [46], accessible to home and professional office.

6.1.3. Case example: Functional Integration©

Case study. A young woman who struggled with bulimia, co-occurring addictions, body image distortion, and physical and verbal abuse by the men she dated, during a long and trusting therapy relationship with me, came into my office one day and sank deeply into the corner of the couch, emotionally frozen. Feeling massively agitated and depressed, clutching her jacket to her chest in an act of self-protection, her speech was incoherent and perseverative. Recognizing how incapable she was of accessing her self to engage in treatment this day, as a Guild Certified practitioner of the Feldenkrais Method of Somatic Education©, I spontaneously offered her the nonverbal somatic treatment option. She chose to engage with me in a Feldenkrais Functional Integration© lesson. Through this lesson I would engage her body in sequential movements uniquely tailored to the current requirements of her musculoskeletal, and nervous systems. I moved parts of her body gently and purposefully, with the intention of differentiating, and thereby reintegrating, neuromuscular and sensory elements within her nervous system.

In discussing her experience after the lesson, she reported that as she first lay down on the treatment table, she assumed that this would be "still another new-agey, bogus healing experience." As the lesson began, she was aware of "thinking about all the things (she) needed to do once she left the session." "But when I closed my eyes," she said, "I was surprised to find myself focusing on changes that were taking place inside of me." Having been so out of touch with the sensation of her body, she was astounded to discover herself thinking, "She's touching my leg. Oh... I have a leg." "She's touching my arm. It's weird that I have an arm and that it is attached to me." The 40-minute lesson was transformational for this young woman. She left my office that day feeling whole, calmed, and at peace with herself. The jacket that had hidden her body previously, was now flung over her squared, and unconstrained shoulders as she strode out the door.

http://dx.doi.org/10.5772/66173

During the Functional Integration© lesson, the brain non-verbally integrates neurophysiological information offered by one nervous system, and accepted by another.

6.1.4. Case example: Awareness through Movement©—the group experience

After a series of Awareness through Movement© group sessions, a compulsive runner reported becoming increasingly aware of her body in motion, of the bottoms of her feet as they struck the ground, as an example. She began to experiment with alternative options for initiating (and differentiating) her movements. Her experimentation evoked novel sensations, in propelling herself forward first from her toes, then her heels, her shoulders and hips. Through an accruing sense of self-awareness and honed self-determination, she ultimately found herself becoming newly capable of altering her compulsive running behavior, including the frequency of her runs, her daily mileage, and her time spent in this activity.

Eventually, in generalizing her empowered choice-making to other life spheres, she observed, "If I can make *these* kinds of decisions now, (about running) what's to stop me from changing the way I make decisions within other parts of my life?" As she began to experience herself differently in her various life roles—as a marriage partner, parent, professional, and ED individual—her disordered behaviors began to diminish, losing their potency and purpose in her life. Some time after the group experience ended, she contacted me to report that she had recovered fully from her ED and had returned to graduate school to become a nurse, something she had wanted to do all her life.

This example of newly embodied self-sensing and self-determination demonstrates the relative immediacy of responsiveness to the Feldenkrais Method, as well as the potency of the partnership between body and brain, and its relevance to ED recovery. Part of the uniqueness of the Feldenkrais Method as an adjunct to psychotherapy is in the novelty of changing the endings of familiar internal narratives to become those that carry elements of change and limitless possibilities. In the case of ED, readiness for change is prerequisite to engaging in change.

6.2. Neuro-cognitive retraining interventions impact genetic trait characteristics and neural processing

AN research demonstrates that impairments in visuospatial ability, attention, memory and cognitive flexibility may be the result of genetically determined "trait" characteristics, rather than of a temporary state of starvation. Scientists believe that early in the course of ED, individuals may be compensating for disrupted processing during task performance by: (a) increasing the magnitude of response in neural circuits underlying attentional set-shifting and reversal learning in order to successfully complete cognitive flexibility tasks; (b) recruiting additional neural structures to offset inadequate activity in neural circuits underlying intentional set-shifting and reversal learning, or (c) both" [47]. "Cognitive retraining strategies that focus on specific processes that have relevance to particular psychiatric presentations (e.g., attention bias modification for anxiety disorders) have been shown to produce significant decreases in psychiatric symptoms when compared to control interventions. Cognitive retraining interventions have been shown to help individuals accommodate other areas of dysfunction, even if underlying deficits do not change" [47].

7. Neurophysiological interventions in the treatment of co-occurring trauma

7.1. Understanding the trauma phenomenon

Trauma phenomena, which typically include diagnoses such as posttraumatic stress disorder (PTSD,) attention-deficit/hyperactivity disorder (ADHD), mood disorders, etc., typically co-occur with ED. It is believed that 30% of individuals with an ED have been sexually abused [48]. Childhood sexual abuse survivors have been found significantly more likely to become obese (42%) in young adulthood than nonabused individuals (28%) [49]. Interestingly, the obesity in this patient population has been shown to be relatively treatment-resistant [49]. Those who have experienced traumatic events may engage in ED behaviors and other forms of self-harm in order to manage feelings and residual consequences of these events. BN's binge/purge cycle has been connected to trauma as a means of self-protection, as the cycle reduces awareness of thoughts and emotions accompanying traumatic experiences, offering a cleansing escape from the experience and opportunity to refocus [48]. The effects of malnourishment on the ED brain, in some cases, will give rise to the symptoms of ADHD. In such instances, once the ED brain has returned to its normal functioning in recovery, the ADHD diagnosis may no longer apply.

All memory begins with sensory input [50]. Trauma is stored in somatic memory and expressed as changes in the biological stress response, creating undischarged energy in the nervous system [51]. "Traumatic memory stays 'stuck' in the brain's nether regions, in the nonverbal, unconscious, subcortical regions (amygdala, thalamus, hippocampus, hypothalamus, and brain stem), where they are not accessible to the frontal lobes, the understanding, thinking, and reasoning parts of the brain [51]. " "Because traumatic memories are encoded subcortically, rather than in conscious autobiographical memory, in seeking psychic change, "interpretation is limited in effectiveness with pathologies arising from the verbal phase related to explicit memories, with no effect on the preverbal phase where implicit memories are to be found" [52]. Trauma- informed yoga, as an example, is a neurophysiological intervention that naturally regulates the overwhelmed nervous system by bringing unconscious content from trauma-related neurological and muscular patterns into consciousness.

Intense emotions at the time of the trauma initiate long-term conditioned responses to reminders of the event, associated both with chronic alterations in the physiological stress response, accompanied by the amnesias and hyperemeses characteristic of PTSD [53]. The failure of declarative memory may lead to organization of the trauma on a somatosensory level (as visual images or physical sensations) that are relatively impervious to change" [52]. "The inability of people with PTSD to integrate traumatic experiences, and their ten-

http://dx.doi.org/10.5772/66173

dency instead, to contiguously relive the past, is mirrored physiologically and hormonally in the misinterpretation of innocuous stimuli as potential threats. In instances where continued physiological hyperarousal and altered stress hormone secretion affect the ongoing evaluation of sensory stimuli, it has been shown that bottom-up neurophysiological interventions more effectively address "the repetitive, unbidden, physical sensations, movement inhibitions, and somatosensory intrusions of unresolved trauma, than do top-down interventions" [54]. In such cases, a therapeutic model that effectively integrates both top-down (where the cranial brain sends messages to the body) and bottom-up interventions (embodied sensory receptors communicate with cranial based sensory receptors) best serves recovery [55].

The attuned therapist, in revisiting traumatic memories with the patient, seeks to find meaning in the experience (through differentiation,) and to provide a new, healthy narrative for the suffering individual (through integration.) In bringing implicit and explicit memories together, patients experience the attributes of integration – flexibility, adaptability, cohesion energy, and stability [4]. As the organization of the body changes physically in term of movement, posture, and arousal level, a different, more positive sense of self emerges [52].

7.2. Trauma-Informed Yoga

Trauma-informed yoga provides an adjunctive, somatosensory treatment alternative by regulating the nervous system, bringing it from a disregulated state to a unified, centered state. Unprocessed traumatic memories stored in the brain become recycled when triggered, creating imbalanced patterns of nervous system activation. Teaching the use of breath, which evokes self-regulation, and facilitating close attention to present-moment awareness of self, yoga shifts sympathetic nervous system arousal to a balanced parasympathetic sense of calm and relaxation.

The trauma-informed yoga practitioner needs to conduct a full assessment of the patient's nervous system imbalances in order to provide postural movements that accommodate the individual's unique needs. Trauma-informed yoga has been shown to mitigate stress responses via both bottom-up (accessing the primitive brain and emotions) and top-down (psychological reappraisal) methods. Top-down cortically mediated techniques can be harnessed to observe and facilitate sensorimotor processing [56]. Controlled studies have demonstrated that certain "yoga practices decrease symptoms in PTSD, obsessive compulsive disorders, generalized anxiety disorder, panic disorder and anxiety after natural disasters…reducing the stress-induced allostatic load in the autonomic nervous system," [57] It has also been reported that in yoga practitioners, brain volume is larger in areas that: contain a mental map of the body, direct attention, control vision, reduce stress, and define the concept of self [58]. Yoga has been shown to promote affect tolerance of physical and sensory experiences associated with fear and helplessness [34]. For ED patients suffering from co-occurring substance abuse or addictions, yoga-breathing practices may be useful in counteracting various types of urges brought on by environmental triggers that could result in relapse [34].

Psychosomatic expressions of bodily experiences are typically embedded in a broad variety of psychopathological and intersubjective phenomena [52]. "In seeking control of the traumatized mind-brain arousal system, the goal of trauma recovery is integrating what happened in the past with what is happening now, bringing 'all parts of the brain online,' in creating a sense of calm and safety in the present [53]. van de Kolk believes that trauma treatment allows the patient to (1) master the limbic brain (i.e., regulating the reptilian brain rhythms through breath control in yoga, meditation, or martial arts), (2) regulate heart rate variability and fluctuations through flexibility of breathing, and (3) engage in mindfulness, where, through activation of the medial prefrontal cortex, the patient develops an awareness of his own internal organization, potentially addressing it through "parts work," that exists within the internal family systems (IFS) model of psychotherapy. In this context, patients confront and manage the dysfunctional parts of themselves (manifested in behaviors such as cutting, starving, binging and purging, substance abuse, morbid obesity, suicide attempts, etc.), which have evolved to help them "bear unbearable states, contain an unbearable internal world, and sustain them over the course of time" [50].

7.3. Eye movement desensitization and reprocessing (EMDR)

Given the correlation between ED and the trauma of physical, sexual, and verbal abuse, eye movement desensitization and reprocessing (EMDR) has been shown to be a relevant, mindfulness practice for the treatment of posttraumatic stress disorder as a co-occurring diagnosis. As an integrative psychotherapy approach involving interpersonal, experiential and body-centered therapies, EMDR processes and resolves the experience, sensations and emotions around traumatic memory that are stored in the limbic brain. The method works by essentially using bilateral stimulation, and/or stimuli (visual, auditory or tactile) that occur in a rhythmic left-right pattern. Anchoring resources may include tactile stimulation, auditory tapping, or installing stabilizing imaginal resources through guided imagery [59].

7.4. Sensorimotor psychotherapy

Sensorimotor psychotherapy is a mindful psychodynamic psychotherapy that includes the body as central in the therapeutic field of awareness. Promoting the same goals as psychotherapy, its practice blends theory and technique from cognitive and dynamic therapy with straightforward physical interventions, facilitating body awareness, sensation tracking, and empowerment. In identifying trauma reactions physically, it decreases the client's arousal level to "a window of tolerance," allowing the body itself to lead the client into a necessary resolution and calming of the physical experience [52]. "Top-down, cortically mediated techniques are harnessed to observe and facilitate sensorimotor processing. Clinically, sensorimotor practitioners observe a mitigation of autonomic dysregulation as the client becomes more adept at self-observation, raising the question of whether mindfulness serves to engage the right orbital prefrontal cortex in regulating arousal" [52].

http://dx.doi.org/10.5772/66173

8. Other neurophysiological interventions that facilitate ED recovery

8.1. Neurofeedback/ EEG biofeedback training

Neurofeedback, or EEG biofeedback training, remediates the patient's self-regulation. Biofeedback is applied to the brain directly, as a noninvasive approach to operant conditioning of the electrical activity emanating from large groupings of cortical neurons, with the purpose of normalizing deregulated EEG activity. The technique represents an effective alternative for modifying the neurophysiological activity in the brain that contributes to specific cognitive processing, and emotional and behavioral disregulation. Electrical signals can be used to present a variety of feedback stimuli that provide moment-to-moment information to an individual about the state of his or her neurophysiological functioning. Typically, sensors are placed on the scalp to measure activity, with measurements displayed using video displays or sound, which "feed back" information to the user, enabling that individual to discover how to change physiological activity to improve health and performance [60].

"Abnormalities in EEG activity are evident in people struggling with ED. These patterns of dysregulation are shown to normalize only partially with refeeding or weight gain" [60]. "According to a recent review of electroencephalography with ED, Ionacio Jauregui-Lobera notes "complementarity seems to exist between EEG and neuroimaging studies in terms of the study of overall functions, which result from an interaction among the different brain areas as well as the connections between them. ED might reflect some disturbances of a system of interconnecting pathways or circuits in the brain" [18]. These brain systems and networks are now being identified by techniques capable of refining existing operant conditioning-based therapeutic interventions for the entire spectrum of central nervous system (CNS)-mediated neuropsychiatric conditions to improve treatment outcomes [60].

It has been discovered that EEG functional abnormalities in the prefrontal, cingulate, and temporal regions respond differently to stimuli [18]. "After treatment, only those participants who had successfully normalized EEG activity in cortico-limbic/paralimbic brain regions could be considered in clinical remission for major depression. In these regions, significant correlations were found between the percentage of change of depressive symptoms and the percentage of reduction in high-beta activity [61]. These results suggest that the normalization of high-beta activity in cortico-limbic/paralimbic regions can be associated with a significant reduction of depressive symptoms" [61].

8.2. Deep transcranial magnetic stimulation (DTMS) heals co-occurring depression

Still another form of non-invasive technological brain intervention used successfully with ED patients includes deep transcranial magnetic stimulation, a high frequency repetitive transcranial magnetic stimulation applied to the left dorsolateral prefrontal cortex. This intervention sends low dose magnetic pulses to parts of the brain associated with treatment resistant depression (TRD). One study suggests "4 weeks of daily DTMS over the left dorsolateral prefrontal cortex in a patient with severe TRD is associated with clinically meaningful improvements in both depressive and anxious symptoms, as well as in subjective quality of life" [62].

9. Conclusion

Mental disorders have been discovered to be disorders of disruptions in brain circuits. Abnormal behavior and cognition have come to be understood as "late and convergent outcomes of altered brain development" [63]. These concepts render antiquated, the notion that ED are merely chemical imbalances or social constructs. Practitioners and researchers stand on the precipice of a new age of ED diagnosis and treatment. Neuroimaging has begun to yield biomarkers, patterns that predict response to treatment or possibly reflect changes in physiology prior to changes in behavior or mood [63].

Through these advances, neuroscience has begun to shed light on *how* people make changes in psychotherapy. The role of the embodied self and somatosensory, bottom up education in the etiology, maintenance, healing and possible prevention of ED enlightens our understanding of how people learn and of what constitutes healing in treatment and recovery. Nowhere in the field of mental health are the concepts of the embedded self and embodied healing as significant as in the treatment of ED and body image disturbances.

Much of what we are learning about the neural basis of mental illness, however, is unfortunately not yet ready for the clinic, as clinicians as a whole are not adequately prepared through formal professional training to take on and integrate the full import of the role of the brain in ED onset, treatment, and recovery. To keep pace with neuroscience, ED clinicians require a broader knowledge of relevant brain plasticity studies and methodologies within our own field, and *within related fields,* in order to access and apply relevant principles of brain plasticity to front-line ED practice. By understanding more about the organ they treat, practitioners not only serve their ED patients, but also become instrumental in defining new directions for quantitative ED research.

Acknowledgements

I extend my deepest appreciation to my husband Lou, and my talented daughter, Elizabeth, who edited this chapter skillfully and with love. A separate essay written by Abigail Natenshon entitled "Clinical Application of Neuroplastic Brain Research in Eating Disorder Treatment" will appear online, December 2016, through the Open Access Journal of Science and Technology (OAJoST), AgiAl Publishing House. This is to inform readers that ideas and/ or references offered in this chapter may also appear in the above-mentioned essay

http://dx.doi.org/10.5772/66173

Abbreviations

ED	Eating disorder, eating disorders, eating disordered
AN	Anorexia nervosa
BN	Bulimia nervosa
NIMH	National Institute of Mental Health
PET	Positron emission tomography
ARFID	Avoidant/restrictive food intake disorder
BED	Binge Eating Disorder
DBT	Dialectical behavior therapy
CBT	Cognitive behavioral therapy
ACT	Acceptance and Commitment therapy
MBCT	Mindfulness-based cognitive therapy
MRI	Magnetic resonance imaging
DVD	Digital video disc
PTSD	Posttraumatic stress disorder
ADHD	Attention-deficit/hyperactivity disorder
IFS	Internal family systems
EMDR	Eye movement desensitization and reprocessing
EEG	Electroencephalogram
CNS	Central Nervous System
DTMS	Deep transcranial magnetic stimulation
TRD	Treatment resistant depression

Author details

Abigail H. Natenshon

Address all correspondence to: abigailnatenshon@gmail.com

TreatingEatingDisorders.com, Highland Park, Illinois, USA

References

[1] Russell R. Movement and the Development of Sense of Self: Proceedings of the Feldenkrais Conference. August 2004; Seattle, Washington.

[2] Insel T. NIMH's Dr. Thomas Insel: Group Advocacy, More Data, Will Improve Eating Disorders Research Funding. Eating Disorders Review 2007;**8**(1) Gürze Books.

[3] Mosema S. Understanding Neurobiology and Eating Disorders. 2014. Laureate Eating Disorders Program. [http://www.eatingdisorderhope.com/treatment-for-eating-disorders/types-of-treatments/neurobiology-can-play-key-role-in-treating-eating-disorders]

[4] Siegel,DJ. The Mindful Therapist: A Clinical Guide to Mindsight and Neural Integration. New York, New York; W.W. Norton and Company; 2010.

[5] Siegel DJ. An Interpersonal Neurobiology Approach to Psychotherapy; Awareness, Mirror Neurons, and Neural Plasticity in the Development of Well-Being. Psychiatric Annals 2006;**36**(4):248–256.

[6] Doidge N. The Brain that Changes Itself: Stories of Personal Triumph from the Frontiers of Brain Science. New York: Viking; 2007.

[7] Lilenfeld LR, Kaye WH, Greeno CG, Merikangas K, Plotnicov KH, Pollice CP, Rao R, Strober M, Bulik CM, Nagy LA. Controlled Family Study of Anorexia and Bulimia Nervosa: Psychiatric and Effects of Proband Comorbidity. Archives of General Psychiatry 1998;**55**:603–610.

[8] Strober M. Family-genetic studies of eating disorders. Journal of Clinical Psychiatry 1991;**52**:9–12.

[9] Kaye W, Strober M. The Neurobiology or Eating Disorders. In: Schatzberg AF, Nemeroff CB, editors. The American Psychiatric Publishing Textbook of Psychopharmacology, 4th ed. pp.891-902; 2009.

[10] Steinglass JE, Walsh T. Neurobiological Model of the Persistence of Anorexia Nervosa. Journal of Eating Disorders 2016;**4**:19. DOI: 10.1186/s40337-016-0106-2

[11] Sato Y, Saito N, Utsumi A, Aizawa E, Shoji T, Izumiyama M, Mushiake H, Hongo M, Fukudo S. Hashimoto, Kenji, ed. Neural Basis off Impaired Cognitive Flexibility in Patients with Anorexia Nervosa. PLoS One 2013; 8(5): e61108. Published online. DOI: 10.1371/journal.pone0061108

[12] Zastrow A, Kaiser S, Stippich C, Walther S, Herzog W, Tchanturia K, Belger A, Weisbrod M, Treasure J, Friederich HC. Neural correlates of impaired cognitive-behavioral flexibility in anorexia nervosa. The American Journal of Psychiatry 2009;**166**:608–616.

[13] Eshkebari E, Rieger E, Longo M, Haggard P, Treasure J: Persistent Body Image Disturbance following Recovery from Eating Disorders. Journal of Eating Disorders 2014;**47**:400–409.

[14] Gaudio S, Brooks SJ, Riva G. Nonvisual Multisensory Impairment of Body Perception in Anorexia Nervosa: A Systematic Review of Neuropsychological Studies. PLoS One. 2014. DOI: 10.1371/journal.pone.0110087

[15] Nauert PhD, R. Anorexia, Bulimia Linked to Disturbance in Brain Region. Psych Central. 2013; http://psychcentral.com/news/2013/06/10/anorexia-bulimia-linked-to-disturbance-in-brain-region/55851.html

[16] Kurth F, Zilles K, Fox PT, Laird AR, Eickhoff SB. A Link between the Systems: Functional Differentiation and Integration within the Human Insula Revealed by Meta-Analysis. Brain Structure and Function 2010;**214**(5–6):519–534. Doi: 10.1007/s00429-010-0255-z. Epub2010 May 29.

[17] Bermudez O. Brain Rescue: The Developing Brain and the Treatment of Eating Disorders in Children and Adolescents. In: Proceedings of the Eating Recovery Center Conference; June 16, 2016.

[18] Jauregui-Lobera I. Neuroimaging in Eating Disorders. Neuropsychiatric Disease and Treatment 2011;7:577–584.

[19] American Psychiatric Association. Diagnostic and Statistical Manual of Mental Disorders. 5th ed. Arlington, VA: American Psychiatric Publishing; 2013.

[20] Mascola AJ, Bryson SW, Agras WS. Picky Eating During Childhood: A Longitudinal Study to Age 11-Years. Eating Behaviors 2010;11**(4)**:253–257. DOI: 10.1016/j.eatbeh2010.05.006.

[21] Norris ML, Spettigue WJ, Katzman DK. Update on Eating Disorders: Current Perspectives on Avoidant/Restrictive Food Intake Disorder in Children and Youth. Neuropsychiatric Disease and Treatment 2016;**12**:213–218.

[22] Eckelkamp S. Do You Have the Gene that Makes You Hate Broccoli? Prevention. November 2014. www.prevention.com/food/healthy-eating-tip-new–gene-variant-identified-makes-vegetables-taste-bitter.

[23] Cheever O, Cohen LJ. The Feldenkrais Method. In: Complementary and Alternative Medicine in Rehabilitation. Leskowitz, E, Micozzi, MS, eds. New York, Edinburgh, London, Philadelphia: Churchill Livingstone; 2003. Elsevier Science (USA): 39–50.

[24] Feldenkrais M. Awareness through Movement: Health Exercises for Personal Growth. New York: Harper and Row; 1972.

[25] Reindl S.M. Sensing the Self: Women's Recovery from Bulimia. Cambridge, MA: Harvard University Press; 2002.

[26] Schore AN. The Experience-Dependent Maturation of a Regulatory System in the Orbital Prefrontal Cortex and the Origin of Developmental Psychopathology. Development and Psychopathology 1996;**8**:59–87.

[27] Germer CK, Siegel RD, Fulton PR. Eds. Mindfulness and Psychotherapy. New York: Guilford Press; 2005.

[28] Zvelc G. Mindful Processing in Psychotherapy: Facilitating Natural Healing Process within Attuned Therapeutic Relationship. International Journal of Integrative Psychotherapy, 2012;**3**(1):15–28.

[29] Siegel DJ. The Science and Art of Presence: How Being Open and Receptive to Life Cultivates Well-being. 2016. Mindsight Digital Journal. Issue #1; Mindsight Institute, California. https://www.mindsightinstitute.com/digitaljournal?utm_source=Mindsight+Institute+Master+List&utm_campaign=3732856079-MDJ_2_2016_nonsubs&utm_medium=email&utm_term=0_562796b3c8-3732856079-292985749#previewVideo

[30] Holzel BK, Carmody J, Vangel M, Congleton C, Yerramsetti, SM, Gard T, Lazar SW. Mindfulness Practice Leads to Increases in Regional Brain Gray Matter Density. Psychiatric Research: Neuroimaging 2011;**191**:36–43.

[31] Schore AN. Early Organization of the Nonlinear Right Brain and Development of a Predisposition to Psychiatric Disorders. Development and Psychopathology 1997;**9**:(940):595–631.

[32] Schore JR, Schore AN. Modern Attachment Theory: The Central Role of Affect Regulation in Development and Treatment. Clinical Social Work Journal; 2008; **36**:9–20. DOI 10.1007/s10615-007-0111-7

[33] Schore AN. Affect Regulation and the Repair of the Self. New York, New York; W.W. Norton and Co.; 2003.

[34] Siegel DJ. Mindsight: The New Science of Personal Transformation. New York: Bantam/Random House; 2009.

[35] Feldenkrais M. Body and Mature Behavior. New York: International Universities Press; 1949.

[36] Laumer U, Bauer M, Fichter M, Milz, H. Therapeutic Effects of the Feldenkrais Method (Awareness through Movement) in Eating Disorders. IFF Academy; Feldenkrais Research Journal 1 (2004) First published in Lehrstuhl für Psychologie I., Universität Regensburg. PPmP Psychotherapie Psychsomatik Medizinische Psychologie 1997; **47**:170–180.

[37] Schechner R, Schechner H. Image, Movement, and Actor: Restoration of Potentiality; An Interview with Moshe Feldenkrais. The Tulane Drama Review. 1966;**10**(3).

[38] Tolle E. A New Earth: Awakening to Your Life's Purpose. USA: Plume, a member of the Penguin Group Inc. Previously published in a Dutton edition; 2005.

[39] Tolle E. The Power of Now: A Guide to Spiritual Enlightenment. Novato, CA; New World Library; 1999.

[40] Jensen E. Teaching with the Brain in Mind, 2nd ed. Alexandria, VA; Association for Supervision and Curriculum Development; 2005. http://www.ascd.org/publications/books/104013/chapters/Movement-and-Learning.aspx

[41] Doidge N. The Brain's Way of Healing: Remarkable Recoveries and Discoveries from the Frontiers of Neuroplasticity. New York, New York; Viking Press; 2015.

[42] Ansorge U, Neumann O, Becker SI, Kalberer H, Cruse H. Sensorimotor Supremacy: Investigating Conscious and Unconscious Vision by Masked Priming. Advances in Cognitive Psychology; 2007. **3**(1–2): 257–227.

[43] Stein KF, Nyquist L. Disturbances in the Self: A Source of Eating Disorders. Eating Disorders Review; 2001. 12:1 Gurze Books.

[44] Fried M. Elements of Psychotherapy in the Feldenkrais Method. Feldenkrais Journal Issue; 1988. p. 37.

[45] Fortin S, Vanasse C. The Feldenkrais Method and Women with Eating Disorders. Journal of Dance and Somatic Practices 2012;**3**(1–2): 127–143 (17).

[46] http://www.feldenkrais.com. [Internet]. 2016. http://www.anatbanielmethod.com. [Internet]. 2016.

[47] Wildes JE, Forbes EE, Marcus MD. Advancing Research on Cognitive Flexibility in Eating Disorders: The Importance of Distinguishing Attentional Set-Shifting and Reversal Learning. International Journal of Eating Disorders; 2014.**47**:227–230.

[48] National Eating Disorder Association (NEDA). Trauma and Eating Disorders; 2012.

[49] Faden J, Leonard D, O'Reardon J, Hanson, R. Obesity as a Defense Mechanism. International Journal of Surgery Case Reports. 2013. **4**(1): 127–129. Doi: 10.1016/j.ijscr.2012.10.011

[50] Rothschild, B. The Body Remembers: The Psychophysiology of Trauma and Trauma Treatment. New York: W.W. Norton Co. Ltd.; 2000.

[51] Burke T. How Trauma Impacts the Brain. Talking Points from Seminar for Rachel's' Vineyard Ministries. U.K. www.rachel'svineyard.org.

[52] Ogden P, Fisher J. Sensorimotor Psychotherapy: Interventions for Trauma and Attachment. New York, New York: W.W. Norton and Company; 2015.

[53] van der Kolk, B.A. The Body Keeps the Score: Memory and the Evolving Psychobiology of Post Traumatic Stress. Harvard Review of Psychiatry; Jan/Feb 1994. Doi: 10.3109/10673229409017088

[54] Andrade VM. 2005. Affect and the therapeutic action of psychoanalysis. International Journal of Psychoanalysis, **86:**677–697.

[55] Taylor AG, Goehler LE, Galper DI, Innes KE, Bourguignon C. Top-Down and Bottom-up Mechanisms in Mind-Body Medicine: Development of an Integrative Framework for Psychophysiological Research. Explore (NY) 2010;**6**(1):29. DOI: 10.1016/j.explore.2009.10.004

[56] Kinser P, Goehler, Taylor A. How Might Yoga Heal Depression? A Neurobiological Perspective. Explore (NY) 2012 Mar 1: **8**(2): 118-126 DOI: 10.1016/j.explore.2011.12.005.

[57] C.C. Streeter, P.L. Gerbarg, R.B. Saper, D.A. Ciraulo, R.P. Brown. Effects of yoga on the autonomic nervous system, gamma-aminobutyric-acid, and allostasis in epilepsy, depression, and post-traumatic stress disorder. *Medical Hypotheses*, 2012; **78**(5):571-579 DOI: 10.1016/j.mehy.2012.01.021

[58] Villemure C, Bushnell, Catherine. Yoga and the Brain. Scientific American; 2014. National Center for Complimentary and Alternative Medicine.

[59] Korn D, Leeds AM. Preliminary Evidence of Efficacy of EMDR Resource Development and Installation in the Stabilization Phase of Treatment of Complex Posttraumatic Stress Disorder. Journal of Clinical Psychology 2002;**58** (12):1465–1487.

[60] Berman MH, DiMarco C. Neurophysiological Management of Arousal: Eating Disorders and Neurofeedback Training. Perspectives: A Professional Journal of the Renfrew Fdn; Summer Perspectives; 2013; p 8–10.

[61] Paquette V, Beauregard M, Beaulieu-Prevost, D. Effect of a Psychoneurotherapy on Electromagnetic Tomography in Individual with Major Depressive Disorder. Psychiatry Research Neuroimaging 2009. DOI: http://dx.doi.org/10.1016/i.pscychresns.2009.06.002

[62] Berlim M, van den Eynde, F, Tover-Perdomo S, Chachamovich, E, Zengen, A, Turecki, G. Augmenting Antidepressants with Deep Transcranial Magnetic Stimulation (DTMS) in Treatment-Resistant Major Depression. The World Journal of Biological Psychiatry 2014. DOI: 10.3109/15622975.2014.925141.

[63] National Institute of Mental Health. (NIMH). Mental Illness Defined as Disruption in Neural Circuits. Director's blog; August 2011.

Section 2

Symptomatology and Comorbidity

Chapter 4

Oral Implications of Eating Disorders

Aurea Lumbau and Giovanni Spano

Additional information is available at the end of the chapter

http://dx.doi.org/10.5772/66185

Abstract

Eating disorders (EDs) are defined as persistent behavioural problems related to food and weight control, which significantly damage the physical and mental health with dramatic effects on the oral cavity. We briefly describe the effect on oral health and the principles of dental management.

Keywords: eating disorder, teeth, oral soft tissue, tooth erosion, mental disease

1. Introduction

Eating disorders (EDs) are classified as behavioural problems in food intake, and the main aim is body weight control. This condition is self-determined and not related to any known medical or psychiatric disease. All eating disorders bound to each other by several clinical features: the importance of body weight and body shape leading people affected to be obsessed by food checking and body checking. It is difficult to find out the true incidence of eating disorders due to the reluctance of the people affected to recognize it as a disease, thus avoiding consulting with a specialist, especially when early eating disorders are considered. There are numerous systemic manifestations caused by eating disorders; some are not pathognomonic, while others could lead the clinician to suspect the presence of a disease. Eating disorders are also characterized by intra-oral and extra-oral manifestations.

The most frequent intra-oral manifestations are dental erosion, trauma to the mucosa of the oral cavity and pharynx, dry mouth, a heightened risk of caries, periodontal problems, and lesions to the soft tissues secondary to the emesis, or effects induced indirectly by vomiting systemically [1].

2. Global view of the matter

Eating disorders (EDs) are psychiatric disorders that cause disability and chronicity. Few data are available to estimate their prevalence and correlates in the community. Current diagnostic classifications recognize main eating disorders, anorexia nervosa (AN), bulimia nervosa (BN) and binge eating disorder (BED) with symptomatic variants recorded as a global ''not otherwise specified' class [2]. They have high prevalence in women [2, 3] and a comorbidity with other psychiatric disorders such as drug abuse, personality and mood disorders, anxiety. Systematic reviews [4] and recent studies [5] point out that women fall ill from AN and BN more than men in the ratio of 10:1. In addition, EDs are not only characterized by abnormal behaviours about food but also from deficits of emotional, cognitive and social factors that frequently lead to chronicity, relapse, reduced quality of life [6–9]. Prevalence of anorexia nervosa has been reported around 0.3% in American and European studies [10, 11]. It affects roughly 3,000,000 people in Italy and is the second-leading cause of death among female adolescents after road accidents [12]. The rate of diffusion of anorexia nervosa is keeping fairly constant; as opposed to Bulimia, that is continuously increasing [13–17]. The prevalence of bulimia nervosa in the young female population has a rate of 1%. Uncontrolled feeding also better known as binge eating disorder (BED) reaches about 1% in the general population, both male and female. As for the severity of eating disorders, according to a meta-analysis [18], anorexia nervosa was the mental disorder with the highest mortality rate; data from the National Centre for Epidemiology, Surveillance and Health Promotion, and several scientific studies [19] confirm that in the USA eating disorders still constitute the leading cause of death for mental illness. Yet, data are sparse, regarding binge disorder, with an estimated prevalence of around 3.3% among women and 0.8% among men in a large-scale population-based survey, conducted with telephone interviews in Austria [20, 21], and, respectively, 3.5 and 2.0% in the USA National Comorbidity Replication study (NCS-R) [2, 6, 7].

What are the factors that induce eating disorder?

Trouble about weight may be predictive: fear of gaining weight, dieting and negative body image. A high rate of eating disorders, mood disorders and certain anxiety disorders (panic disorder, generalized anxiety disorder and obsessive compulsive disorder) is found in family members of patients with EDs.

A high rate of families with substance abuse problems is present for BN. Studies also suggest a high rate of social phobia, generalized anxiety disorder, post-traumatic stress disorder [5]. A history of childhood obesity is a factor strongly associated with BN [22]. It is evident that youth depression and anxiety disorders play a significant role in influencing the onset or persistence of eating disorder symptoms; especially for depression [5]. Due to the complexity of these disorders, doctors recommend a multidimensional approach, which is the gold standard for the treatment of these patients. The best place for these treatments is the outpatient setting. Nevertheless, a number of patients (approximately 30%) do not respond to outpatient treatment, and needs more intensive care [23]. For this reason, a higher level of care is necessary.

All structures should be able to interact with each other in an organized service network of five levels: general practitioners and paediatricians, specialist outpatient services, hospital staff or not, different types of day care services, therapeutic-rehabilitative residential, emergency [24]. Eating disorders have a high social impact but a low cost/benefit ratio.

The onset of eating disorders is often dated in adolescence or pre-adolescence. In the total population, prevalence and incidence of food disease are rare. But if we consider childhood, prevalence and incidence increase about 10 times, and in fact population aged between 12 and 16 years is considered 'at risk' [25]. So monitoring is necessary not only for treatment of overt diseases, but also for early diagnosis and prevention [24].

Eating disorders are also characterized by two complexity levels both mental and biological: we observe a frequent comorbidity with other psychiatric disorders such as anxiety, depression, obsessive-compulsive disorder, inevitable organic consequences (alterations of the cardiovascular system, bone, gastrointestinal, endocrine, gynaecological and neurological) determines from the beginning an integrated multi-professional approach. Finally, if the disease is an egosyntonic disorder (especially in case of AN), it is often difficult to start therapeutic alliance, forcing clinicians involved in care of a continuous redefinition and negotiation of therapeutic goals.

Evolution of the EDs is extremely variable

Normalization of weight, eating behaviour, absence of binge eating or compensatory behaviour is not sufficient to speak of healing. We must take into account other important aspects such as personality, family and extra-family relationships, emotional life, sexuality as well as the social and work integration [26]. The cure is possible in about 50% of cases. The other 50% have a difficult course with frequent relapses, chronic and a high risk of mortality [27–29]. Because of lack of awareness of the disease and a lack of motivation to treatment, only a small percentage of the people with anorexia and bulimia will appeal to deputies to the care services. This fact is due to a missed diagnosis general practitioners and paediatricians resulting in delayed treatment intervention and a worsening prognosis. The position of the Academy for Eating Disorders is that all eating disorders are mental illnesses and biologically determined and need the same level of treatment of other psychiatric disorders such as schizophrenia, bipolar disorder, major depression and obsessive-compulsive disorder. Despite this, eating disorders still receive little attention and insufficient treatment, compared to the high risk of complications and mortality [30].

2.1. Oral manifestation

Oral manifestations are mainly caused by nutritional deficiencies and consequent metabolic impairment, and lack of attention to personal oral hygiene and care.

Common intra-oral manifestations include erosion of dental tissues, trauma to the mucosa of the oral cavity and pharynx, dry mouth, high risk of caries, periodontal problems, and wound to the soft tissues caused to the direct actions of emesis, or indirectly because of effects induced systemically by vomiting. The extra-oral manifestations are mainly related to the pathological behavioural practice and include dysfunction and swelling of the parotid glands, TMJ disorders and cheilitis.

2.2. Dental erosion

Self-induced vomiting resulted in an increased frequency of erosion on the upper palatal, lower posterior buccal and occlusal surfaces. Some cases show erosions, both palatal and vestibular, and it is current opinion that these erosions are determined by two factors: intrinsic (gastric) acid results in palatally eroded sites and extrinsic (dietary) acids lead to labial erosion. This is known as perimolysis [31].

It may develop after frequent use of acidic sport drinks during physical activity, or from abnormal use of some caffeinated and/or carbonated drinks, to decrease the reflex hunger stimulus [32, 33] by increasing dilation of the stomach. Some patients will use vinegar and lemon juice (or slices of lemon) to eliminate/diminish the gustatory phase of the mechanism regulating hunger, which can also lead to erosion [34, 35]. Such erosion is characterized by a chemical rather than a bacterial dissolution and leads to uniform, polished and spoon-like surfaces, in contrast to abrasion, which is caused by mechanical wear [36]. Erosion can be accelerated by attrition [37, 38].

2.3. Dental caries

Whether the caries experience of eating disordered individuals is greater than that of the normal population remains unclear. Qualitative rather than quantitative differences, such as the cariogenicity of the oral flora, may occur and be dependent upon vomiting parameters. Sweetened drinks, candies or sugared chewing gum are frequently used by ED patients not only for energy, but also to reduce the sense of hunger; caries risk is high because of the frequency and the large quantity of eaten sugars, even if oral hygiene is generally acceptable in anorexic patients. Dental lesions and their complications may cause oral symptoms ranging from dental sensitivity to episodes of oral pain.

2.4. Saliva

The practice of self-induced vomiting, misuse of diuretics and laxatives may cause body dehydration with a negative impact on the salivary flow. Additionally, it may also influence salivary gland function. The saliva synthesis process (a dynamic process) also affects the blood and interstitial fluid, the metabolic state of the glands, electrolytes and protein synthesis that can be changed. Therefore, abnormalities such as alkalosis, acidosis and other general disturbances may affect the quantity and quality of the saliva. Salivary functions of buffering and lubrication are important in eating disorders. The salivary flow increases dramatically prior to vomiting because the medullary centre that controls vomiting is connected to salivary nuclei. Saliva concentration of bicarbonate and viscosity may change in patients with ED. Bicarbonate reduction and increased salivary viscosity act as a co-factor in dental erosion. The concentrations of other components like potassium, chloride, calcium, urea nitrogen and albumin can be normal. Episodic benign parotid enlargement has been described in bulimics by several workers. The swelling of the major salivary glands, parotids in particular, is a frequent manifestation of EDs and sometimes may be the presenting sign [39]. It is because of sialadenosis: a non-inflammatory enlargement of the salivary glands caused by a peripheral autonomic neuropathy, which is responsible for disordered metabolism and secretion, resulting in acinar enlargement and functional impairment. Salivary gland inflammation can also produce variable size of calculi, which can occlude the salivary ducts and cause intense pain. The parotid gland tends to change the physiognomy of the face, giving a puffy look; this phenomenon is usually reversible in a few weeks with the abstention from compensatory practices (especially vomiting). Sialadenosis may also involve minor intraoral salivary glands [40].

2.5. Periodontal disease

The evidence on periodontal status is conflicting.

Patients affected by ED may have poor oral hygiene, which may lead to gingival inflammation and potentially predisposition to periodontitis. Adequate oral care habits are impeded by binge eating and purging episodes. Nutritional deficiencies [41], especially in vitamin C [42], may also predispose one to gingivitis.

The deficiency of vitamin C causes defective collagen synthesis, which can be associated with generalized swollen gingiva, spontaneous bleeding, ulcerations, tooth mobility and increased periodontitis [43].

2.6. Soft tissue lesions

Reduction in intake of vitamins and other nutrients, induce general metabolic alterations, iron deficiency anaemia, causing generalized mucosal atrophy. In particular, a deficiency of vitamins in the B group, especially B1, B6 and B12, has been classically associated with a decrease in epithelial cell turnover.

Angular cheilitis, candidosis, glossitis and oral mucosal ulceration are effects of nutritional deficiencies. Generally, this is particularly evident on the tongue; here, in association with erythema, it produces the clinical picture of atrophic glossitis. Mucosal atrophy may also cause diffuse oral burning sensation, which can be more intense on the tongue (glossodynia). Dysgeusia (altered taste sensation) and xerostomia (dry mouth) can be independent and disconnected from oral signs being of psychogenic origin and expressing somatization of underlying disorders. Erythematous mucosal lesions, especially on the soft palate in purging-type behaviour, may be related to the direct offending action of acid during vomiting (epithelial erosion), and sometimes to repetitive frictional trauma (palatal haematoma) caused by the object used to induce vomiting. Multiple nutritional deficiencies may also constitute a predisposing factor for oral opportunistic infections both directly [44] and through impairment of immunologic system function [45].

3. Management

There are numerous systemic manifestations caused by eating disorders. Several of these induce the physician to suspect a disease like the 'sign of Russell' (lesions of the dorsum of the hands, arising from their repeated use to induce vomiting). As mentioned earlier, eating disorders are also characterized by intra-oral and extra-oral manifestations. The dentist may be the first person to become aware of the eating disorder by finding a pattern of teeth erosion due to the effects of chronic vomiting [46, 47].

On the basis of the pattern of dental erosion, dentist should discuss his findings with the patient's parents and arrange for referral to a physician for evaluation and management of a possible eating disorder. In these cases, the dentist's goal is to improve the patient's oral hygiene.

It is the duty of the dentist to teach oral hygiene concepts such as brushing technique, flossing and using fluoride toothpaste or mouthwash. The patient is instructed to use a baking soda mouth rinse after vomiting. For dentinal sensitivity is indicated a desensitizing toothpastes and fluoride varnish. Anorexia nervosa may be more difficult to find out for dentist. Patients with anorexia nervosa who also are bulimic may be identified by dental signs of bulimia.

Timing of intervention for eroded teeth is controversial. Caries and periodontal disease should be managed as usual? Dentists should wait before restoring worn surfaces?

There is no definite contraindication to restoring eroded surfaces other than the continued acid dissolution of tooth substance from around the restoration if vomit continues. Pain relief, reduced dentine sensitivity and improved aesthetic will motivate the patient.

During therapy, tooth wear should be monitored with study casts and photographs. On the other hand, dentist and patient need to be aware that frequently complex restorations may fail due to illness. In the worse cases, full coverage may be required in an attempt to save teeth with conservative tooth preparation and ceramic crowns. Patients with bulimia should not have treatment planned for permanent restorative procedures until the illness is during the active phase. Once the patient is stable and wants to have the teeth with severe erosion restored, this can be done. Endodontic and prosthetic treatment must be used for teeth with little clinical crown remaining. Patients with anorexia nervosa should regain their lost weight and be stabilized before starting complex restorative or prosthodontic treatment. The dentist can make several recommendations to the anorexic and bulimic. Tooth brushing after vomiting is generally regarded as inadvisable because the softened, demineralized surface is more susceptible to toothbrush abrasion. The treatment plan will be dependent on several parameters and it would be a discretionary decision of the dentist.

Dental restoration must be done with materials that can resist to acid attacks allowing preservation of occlusal plane. Glass ionomer cements are not indicated. Even a space of less than 1 mm is amenable to restoration with composite bonded to dentine. Any eroded and sclerosed dentine should be over etched (20–30 s) in order to enhance opening of dentinal tubules and intra-tubular formation of resin tags. Adhesive dentistry has advantages over conventional forms of treatment in that it is reversible and the latest generation of dentine bonding agents are durable. Space requirements are still minimal when using these adhesive techniques.

http://dx.doi.org/10.5772/66185

4. Conclusions

Patients whose teeth have been damaged as a consequence of an eating disorder are most likely to present first to a dentist who can assist in making the initial diagnosis and efficiently influence the progress of the medical and psychological management by providing support and dental care.

Oral manifestations of ED may appear in different stages along the disease progression. In fact, some oral manifestations may occur very early during disease onset (e.g. sialadenosis, palatal erythema, clinical unexplained oral symptoms); therefore, it can be very useful for an early diagnosis and prompt recovery. The dentist may be one of the few and the first clinicians contacted by the patient for incipient oral discomfort (i.e. dental sensitivity, oral pain and unusual oral sensations) [48].

In order to strengthen communication, the visit should be conducted confidentially using appropriate language and terminology: dentists should avoid judgement and pressure, observe the patients' body language and remain calm, reassuring and supportive.

It is well known that patients with ED have low self-esteem and dislike of their body.

Mouth is one of the main factors in the relationships, teeth and eyes are one of the most attractive parts in a face to the viewer. Being less attractive leads to a decrease in self-esteem, triggering a vicious circle in those who already have problems with the body. Therefore, the oral cavity should be further considered in both diagnosis and follow-up.

'Furthermore, the treatment of these manifestations may be important to the overall prognosis by preventing or reducing damages, which can modify eating habits and function, patient's self-image [49] and consequently self-esteem'.

4.1. How to face the problem

These pathologies involve different areas and produce malnutrition acting on the central nervous system (CNS) and the various organic districts; disorders of the body image; cognitive style; emotional style; family and interpersonal dynamics. Lines of action will move in parallel with each other and will be oriented towards the recovery of the physiological body weight, through learning behaviours of functional food and a diet adequate to the different social situations; definition of a therapeutic plan, with a combination of psychological, medical and pharmacological therapies; increased awareness of the patient's family and relapse prevention through continuous treatment.

'The integrated multi-professional approach to the EDs requires a transformation of "knowledge" and "know how" in a "know-how together". For this reason, the integrated multi-professional group is made up of different specialists working from the start in a shared project with common objectives and strategies tested by weekly team meetings and, when possible, by daily briefings. Intervention protocols should be subjected to continuous verification and monitoring, in liaison with similar experiences already. The staff also will have to be placed in a permanent training process, characterized by internal teams and external supervision. In particular, within the team is of particular importance is the division of roles and responsibilities, so as to make the process of collaboration' [23].

In particular:

1. Task of the psychiatrist will be: diagnosis of any psychiatric comorbidity, psychopharmacological treatment, individual psychotherapeutic treatment or panel and the study of the dynamics of the multidisciplinary team;

2. The nutritionist/internist will be in charge of the diagnosis and treatment of medical complications, as well as the planning of medical care of nutrition;

3. The psychologist will cure the psychopathological assessment, research (evaluation of outcome and effectiveness of the treatment), individual treatment and family treatment;

4. The dietitian will be tasked to determine, plan and control meals, follow the food psychoeducation (individual and/or group), establish weighting targets and follow the patient assisted in the meals

5. Other professions where problems occur in other districts [23].

Author details

Aurea Lumbau* and Giovanni Spano

*Address all correspondence to: alumbau@uniss.it

Surgical Microsurgical and Medical Science Department, School of Dentistry, University of Sassari, Sassari, Italy

References

[1] Lumbau A., Spano G., Meloni SM, Sanna F. Lugliè PF. Eating disorders: assessment of knowledge on a dentist's sample. Int J. Child Health Nut. 2015;4:50–3.

[2] Preti A, De Girolamo G, Vilagut G, Alonso J, De Graaf R, Bruffaearts R, Demyttenaere K, Pinto-Meza A, Haro JM, Morosini P, ESEMeD-WMH investigators. The epidemiology of eating disorders in six European countries: results of the ESEMeD-WMH project. J Psych Res. 2009;43(14):1125–32. .

[3] Swanson SA, Crow SJ, Le Grange D, Swendsen J, Merikangas KR. Prevalence and correlates of eating disorders in adolescents. Arch Gen Psych. 2011;68(7):714–23.

http://dx.doi.org/10.5772/66185

[4] Stice E, Marti CN, Durant S. Risk factors for onset of eating disorders: evidence of multiple risk pathways from an 8-year prospective study. Behav Res Ther. 2011;49(10): 622–7.

[5] Hautala L, Helenius H, Karukivi M, Maunula AM, Nieminen J, Aromaa M. The role of gender, affectivity and parenting in the course of disorder eating: a 4-year prospective case-control study among adolescents. Int J Nurs Stud. 2011;48(8):959–72.

[6] Hudson JI, Pope Jr HG, Yurgelun-Todd D, Jonas JM, Frankenburg FR. A controlled study of lifetime prevalence of affective and other psychiatric disorders in bulimic outpatients. American Journal of Psychiatry 1987;144:1283–7.

[7] Hudson JI, Hiripi E, Pope Jr HG, Kessler RC. The prevalence and correlates of eating disorders in the National Comorbidity Survey Replication. Biol Psych. 2007;61:348–58.

[8] Jordan J, Joyce PR, Carter FA, Horn J, McIntosh VVW, Luty SE, McKenzie JM, Frampton CM, Mulder RT, Bulik CM. Specific and nonspecific comorbidity in anorexia nervosa. Int J Eat Disord. 2008;41(1):47–56.

[9] Swinbourne JM, Touyz SW. The comorbidity of eating disorders and anxiety disorders: a review. Eur Eat Disord Rev. 2007;15(4):253–74.

[10] Hoek HW, van Hoeken D. Review of the prevalence and incidence of eating disorders. Int J Eat Disord. 2003;34(4):383–96.

[11] Favaro A, Ferrara S, Santonastaso P. The spectrum of eating disorders in young women: a prevalence study in a general population sample. Psychosom Med. 2004;65:701–8.

[12] Renna C, La prevenzione dei DCA. Ministero della Salute, Dipartimento della Gioventù, Istituto superiore di Sanità; 2012. pp. 251–63. Roma.

[13] Willi J, Giacometti G, Limacher B. Update on the epidemiology of anorexia nervosa in a defined region of Switzerland. Am J Psychiatry. 1990;147:1514–17.

[14] Hall A, Hay P. Eating disorder patient referrals from a population region 1977–1986. Psychol Med. 1991;21:697–701.

[15] Jorgensen J. The epidemiology of eating disorders in Fyn County Denmark, 1977–1986. Acta Psych Scand. 1992;85:30–4.

[16] Hoek H, Bartelds A, Bosveld J, et al. Impact of urbanization on detection rates of eating disorders. Am J Psychiatry. 1995; 152:1272–8.

[17] Turbull S, Ward A, et al. The demand for eating disorder care: an epidemiological study using the general practice research database. British J. Psych. 1996;169:705–12.

[18] Harris EC, Barraclough B. Excess mortality of mental disorder. Br J Psychiatry. 1998;173:11–53. Review.

[19] Birmingham CL, Su J, Hlynsky JA, Goldner EM, Gao M. The mortality rate from anorexia nervosa. Int J Eat Disord. 2005;38(2):143–6.

[20] Kinzl JF, Traweger C, Trefalt E, Mangweth B, Biebl W. Binge eating disorder in males: a population-based investigation. Eating and Weight Disorders 1999;4:169–74

[21] LaVange L, Stearns S, Lafata J, Koch G. Innovative strategies using SUDAAN or analysis of health surveys with complex samples. Stat Meth Med Res. 1996;5:311–29.

[22] Pratt CA, Stevens J, Daniels S. Childhood obesity prevention and treatment: recommendations for future research. Am J Prev Med. 2008;35(3):249–52. doi: 10.1016/j.amepre.2008.05.025. Epub 2008 Jul 10.

[23] Rapporti Istisan 13/49. 30 Ottobre 2013. ISSN 1123-3117. Roma.

[24] De Virgilio G, Coclite D, Napoletano A, Barbina D, Dalla Ragione L, Spera G, Di Fiandra T. Consensus Conference on Eating Disorders (ED) in adolescents and young adults. Istituto Superiore di Sanità; 2013 (Rapporti ISTISAN 13/6). 26 Rapporti ISTISAN 13/49 27. Roma.

[25] Jaffa T, Mcdermott B, Mansi GL Eating disorders in children and adolescents. Cortina editor. 2009. Milano.

[26] De Giacomo P, Renna C, Santoni Rugiu A. Guide on eating disorders. Franco Angeli editor. 2005. Milano.

[27] Sullivan PF. Course and outcome of anorexia and bulimia nervosa. In: Fairburn CG, Brownell KD (Ed.) 2nd ed., Eating Disorders and Obesity. New York: The Guilford Press; 2002. pp. 226–30.

[28] Steinhausen HC. The outcome of anorexia nervosa in the 20th century. Am J Psich. 2002;159(8):1284–93.

[29] Steinhausen HC, Weber S, The outcome of bulimia nervosa: finding from one quarter century of research. Am J Psich. 2009;166(12):1331–41.

[30] Klump KL, Bulik CM, Kaye WH, Treasure J, Tyson E. Academy for eating disorders position paper: eating disorders are serious mental illnesses. Int J Eat Disord. 2009;42(2): 97–103.

[31] Chadwick RG, Mitchell HL Conduct of an algorithm in quantifying simulated palatal surface tooth erosion. J Oral Rehabil. 2001;28(5):450–6.

[32] Moazzez R, Smith BG, Bartlett DW.Oral pH and drinking habit during ingestion of a carbonated drink in a group of adolescents with dental erosion. J Dent. 2000;28(6):395–7.

[33] Al-Dlaigan YH, Shaw L, Smith A. Dental erosion in a group of British 14-year-old, school children. Part I: prevalence and influence of differing socioeconomic backgrounds. Br Dent J. 2001;190(3):145–9.

[34] Järvinen V, Rytömaa I, Meurman JH. Location of dental erosion in a referred population. Caries Res. 1992;26(5):391–6.

[35] Del Signore A, Campisi B, Di Giacomo F. Characterization of balsamic vinegar by multivariate statistical analysis of trace element content. J AOAC Int. 1998;81(5):1087–95.

[36] Ibarra G, Senna G, Cobb D, Denehy G. Restoration of enamel and dentin erosion due to gastroesophageal reflux disease: a case report. Pract Proced Aesthet Dent. 2001;13(4): 297–304; quiz 306.

[37] Bartlett DW, Evans DF, Smith BG. The relationship between gastro-oesophageal reflux disease and dental erosion. J Oral Rehabil. 1996;23:289–97.

[38] Scheutzel P. Etiology of dental erosion: intrinsic factors. Eur J Oral Sci. 1996;104(pt 2): 178–90.

[39] Coleman H, Altini M, Nayler S, Richards A. Sialadenosis: a presenting sign in bulimia. Head Neck. 1998;20(8):758–62.

[40] Aframian DJ. Anorexia/bulimia-related sialadenosis of palatal minor salivary glands. J Oral Pathol Med. 2005;34(6):383.

[41] Prousky JE. Pellagra may be a rare secondary complication of anorexia nervosa: a systematic review of the literature. Altern Med Rev. 2003;8(2):180–5. Review.

[42] Christopher K, Tammaro D, Wing EJ. Early scurvy complicating anorexia nervosa. South Med J. 2002;95(9):1065–6.

[43] Touyz LZ. Oral scurvy and periodontal disease. J Can Dent Assoc. 1997;63(11):837–45. Review.

[44] Paillaud E, Merlier I, Dupeyron C, Scherman E, Poupon J, Bories PN. Oral candidiasis and nutritional deficiencies in elderly hospitalised patients. Br J Nutr. 2004;92(5):861–7.

[45] Chandra RK. Nutrition and the immune system from birth to old age. Eur J Clin Nutr. 2002;56(Suppl 3:)S73–6. Review.

[46] Milosevic A, Brodie DA, Slade PD. Dental erosion, oral hygiene, and nutrition in eating disorders. Int J Eat Disord. 1997;21:195–9;

[47] Milosevic A. Eating disorders and the dentist. Br Dent J. 1999;186:109–13.

[48] Burkhart N, Roberts M, Alexander M, Dodds A. Communicating effectively with patients suspected of having bulimia nervosa. J Am Dent Assoc. 2005;136(8):1130–7. Erratum in: J Am Dent Assoc. 2005 Nov;136(11):1517.

[49] Bonilla ED, Luna O. Oral rehabilitation of a bulimic patient: a case report. Quintessence Int. 2001;32(6):469–75.

Chapter 5

Anxiety and Eating Disorders in Adult Women

Annie Aimé, Tanya Guitard and Lise Grousseaud

Additional information is available at the end of the chapter

http://dx.doi.org/10.5772/65249

Abstract

Anxiety disorders are frequently reported by women diagnosed with eating disorders (EDs). Although this association is long established and rather frequent, the role of anxiety in the onset and maintenance of eating disorders still has to be better understood. By doing so, engagement in treatment and efficacy of the interventions used will be improved. Thus, the present book chapter aims at investigating anxiety comorbidity in women diagnosed with an ED. First, the prevalence rates of anxiety disorders (AD) in ED samples and similarities and differences between both disorders are presented. Then, the chronology of onset of both disorders and possible explanations of their mechanisms of association are discussed. Finally, treatment considerations are covered.

Keywords: anxiety, eating disorders, anxiety disorders, comorbidity, prevalence rates, chronology, treatment

1. Introduction

Comorbidity with other mental health disorders is frequently found in individuals with eating disorders (EDs), mood, and anxiety disorders (ADs) being the most commonly reported [1, 2]. In ED patients, anxiety and stress have been linked to binge and restrictive eating, as well as vomiting and laxative abuse [3, 4]. ED women report high levels of anxiety in a wide variety of eating situations and tend to resort to numerous behaviours aiming at reducing or managing anxiety [5]. Available past research interested in the relationship between anxiety and ED has mainly focused on prevalence rates of ADs in EDs [6]. However, there is still a need to better understand the nature of this frequent association [5].

Additionally, the comorbidity of AD has been shown to negatively impact ED treatment as the presence of AD accentuates the severity of the symptomatology, which can complicate treatment formulation [2], maintain ED, and represent a barrier for help-seeking, engagement, and compliance in therapy [2, 3]. For instance, as a trait present in many women with ED, anxiety has been associated with higher ED psychopathology and has shown to affect the course of the ED through a longer duration of the illness, a higher number of hospitalizations, and premature treatment termination [2, 7]. Given the potential treatment complications related to a dual diagnosis of AD and ED, treatment strategies taking this comorbidity into account and aiming to provide adequate care for women having to deal with such dual diagnoses must be underscored. Thus, this chapter first yields a review of the estimated prevalence rates of ADs in EDs and of their chronology of onset. Second, it provides insights on the nature of the association between ADs and EDs, and lastly it highlights treatment considerations.

2. Strength of the association

The link between anxiety and ED is observable in the relatively high prevalence of comorbid AD in people with ED. According to the few reviews interested in the comorbidity of both disorders [2, 8, 9], there is substantial variation in the estimated prevalence rates of anxiety in adults with EDs and these rates mostly focus on women. The variations in the strength of the association between ADs and EDs are mostly due to sampling (e.g. small number of participants, participants from the community or from specialized treatment centers) and methodological issues (e.g. use of nonstructured or standardized instruments, interviews or questionnaires, number of ADs considered, lack of statistical power, varied inclusion and exclusion criteria, no control group, and retrospective study devise) [2, 8–11]. They are also attributable to diagnostic particularities such as overlaps in symptoms between disorders and changes in the nosography from one version of the *Diagnostic and Statistical Manual of Mental Disorders* (DSMs) to the other [1]. Finally, estimates of prevalence rates are further complicated by the fact that, when medication is prescribed to reduce anxiety symptoms in patients with ED, AD may be underdiagnosed [12].

2.1. Prevalence rates of ADs in EDs

According to Swinbourne and her colleagues [9, 12], lifetime prevalence rates of at least one comorbid anxiety disorder ranges from 23 to 75% in participants with anorexia nervosa and from 25 to 75% in those with bulimia nervosa [9, 12]. Lifetime diagnoses of AD are significantly more frequent in AN and BN samples than in control groups [11]. Although less often assessed, ADs have also been reported in obese individuals who binge eat, with a prevalence rate of about 36% for both generalized anxiety disorder [13] and social anxiety disorder [14].

Available prevalence rates should be taken with caution given that they were obtained by using older versions of the DSM (e.g. DSM-III, III-R, IV, and IV-R) and that they rely on various sources of patients. Consequently, while considering prevalence comorbidity rates between ADs and EDs, one must keep in mind that (1) estimates based on the DSM-5 are still lacking; (2) they include obsessive compulsive disorders, a particularly highly correlated disorder in

http://dx.doi.org/10.5772/65249

AN, which is not considered as an AD anymore [15]; and (3) higher rates of comorbidity are usually found in samples issued from clinical settings (e.g. inpatient and outpatient eating disorders samples), in which higher psychological distress and multiple diagnoses are more prevalent [8, 12].

Among the DSM-5 AD diagnoses, social anxiety disorder (SAD) and generalized anxiety disorder (GAD) have been the most frequently and systematically associated with ED across studies, any ED type confounded [12]. In AN samples, GAD is the most frequent AD diagnosis reported, followed by SAD and agoraphobia [2, 11]. In BN patients, SAD is the most frequent AD in BN patients, and GAD follows while agoraphobia remains the third most frequently reported AD [11]. Compared to women without ED, those with AN and BN, respectively, have a 6.1 and 2.6 times greater risk of being diagnosed with GAD [8]. SAD is also significantly more frequent in women with AN and BN than in control groups and has been particularly linked to an increased risk of binge eating [2, 9, 16]. Agoraphobia for its part appears to be more likely to be reported by women with binge-purge AN and BN than by controls [9].

2.2. Similarities between ADs and EDs

Some diagnostic criteria found in the DSM-5 for ED [15] refer to anxiety. For instance, an "intense fear of gaining weight" or "of becoming fat" has to be present in patients with AN, and "a sense of lack of control over eating" has to be reported by patients with BN and binge-eating disorder [15]. This criterion resembles those of ADs, for example, "fear or anxiety of social settings" found as the primary requirement for SAD. Furthermore, as stated by Webb and colleagues [5], items referring to anxious dimensions of eating such as a fear of losing control, a fear of gaining weight and intense concerns over shape and weight are also used in well-known measures of disordered eating like the Eating Disorder Examination [5].

Additionally, it has been showed that women with BN present similar anxiety symptoms than patients with GAD, with worrying, tension pains, tiredness, restlessness, avoidance of anxiety, social withdrawal, and lack of confidence being equally frequent in both groups [4].

2.3. Differences between ADs and EDs

On the contrary, some differences have been highlighted between EDs and ADs. As an example, Steere et al. [4] showed that panic attacks, muscular and nervous tensions, as well as free-floating anxiety and anxious foreboding were significantly more prevalent in participants with GAD than in BN women.

Differences between ADs and EDs are particularly important to consider for diagnostic purposes. In fact, anxiety limited to ED-specific themes must be distinguished from non-ED-specific anxiety [17]. In many women diagnosed with EDs, the anxiety symptoms they experience are specific to their ED. In other words, their anxiety symptoms mostly focus on eating, weight, and shape concerns as well as on fear of weight gain or a feeling of being fat [4, 17]. These patients also typically fear being exposed to high-calorie foods and avoid exhibiting their body in public. When their anxiety is ED-specific and when they succeed in controlling their weight and eating, women with EDs do not experience anxiety [4] and the clinician cannot conclude in a comorbid AD. However, when a nonspecific anxiety focus is found, such as a general fear of failure or a social anxiety in any public situations, a comorbid AD must be suspected [17].

3. Chronology of onset

Various temporal sequences have been suggested for the comorbidity of AD and ED [2, 12]. First, anxiety may be a risk factor for ED. This pathway of association in which anxiety tends to appear prior to the onset of ED has received the most research support [9, 11, 12, 17–19]. According to Godart and colleagues [11], between 41.8 and 48.7% of women seeking help for AN and between 51.9 and 53.3% of those with a BN diagnosis had developed an AD prior to their ED. More recently, Swinbourne and colleagues [12] found that the larger proportion of their sample of women in inpatient treatment (65%) and in outpatient treatment (75%) for ED had had an AD before the onset of their ED. Studies that support this developmental sequence have suggested that (1) excessive fears about events or situations as well as anxiety about social evaluation reported in childhood could predispose to intense preoccupations with weight, shape, and food in late adolescence and young adulthood [12]; (2) an anxious trait, independent of nutritional state, would be underlying in ED patients [20, 21]; (3) childhood anxiety negatively influences the course and outcome of EDs [7]; and (4) anxiety symptoms tends to persist after recovery from an ED [5, 18, 20] and to be significantly higher in recovered women from ED than in healthy controls [10].

Second, anxiety may be secondary to an ED. This chronology of onset has been reported by 16% of inpatient and by 14% of outpatient ED women [12]. This pathway suggests that ED could produce or exacerbate anxiety in some women. It is mainly supported by evidences that anxiety tends to increase following starvation [2, 6] and by the findings that, in AN patients, anxiety symptomatology tends to decrease over the course of ED treatment (as they regain weight) and to be significantly lower than in acutely ill patients [11, 18].

Third, AD and ED may both result from a common aetiology or a shared vulnerability [2, 11]. In this developmental model of comorbidity, it is supposed that when one of these disorders is activated, the vulnerability to the other is increased [2]. This model is supported by findings showing that anxiety and elevated rates of ADs are present in first-degree relatives and family of origin of women who developed an ED [2, 7]. Other overlapping risk factors like early childhood experiences [2] or negative affect [3] could contribute to the high comorbidity rates between both disorders. Along that line, it has been suggested that childhood negative experiences give rise to maladaptive schemas, which negatively influence the interpretation of events and experiences and can accentuate the risk of adopting anxiety- and eating-related symptomatic behaviours [2]. With regard to negative affect, Schneider et al. suggested that anxious individuals could use eating as a means of regulating negative emotions [22].

In further support for the shared vulnerability model, Levinson and Rodebaugh [3] found that social appearance and fear of negative evaluation were associated with a higher risk of experiencing ED and SAD. While social appearance anxiety refers to a fear of being negatively evaluated because of one's appearance, fear of negative evaluation refers to the idea that one's social self is likely to be judged negatively [3]. Another possible vulnerability factor shared by both types of disorders may be intolerance to uncertainty [23]. Fear or intolerance of uncertainty implies an impression of uncontrollability and unpredictability that has been found in individuals with ADs, GAD especially [24], as well as in AN and BN patients [25]. Individuals with intolerance of uncertainty perceive uncertainty as stressful, upsetting, and unfair [24]. They attribute a negative meaning to uncertainty and believe it should be avoided [24]. In individuals with ED, this personality factor has been suggested to be linked to a need for control, cognitive avoidance, and low novelty seeking [21]. It is also linked to an increased need of predictability and a disposition to avoid new situations [21]. In those who show high levels of intolerance of uncertainty, the ED represents an attempt to gain control over interpersonal and life stressors [25]. It provides security and certainty [26].

When focusing on the chronology of onset of ADs and EDs, one must take into account the natural course of both disorders as well as the fact that the sequence of onset varies according to the AD diagnosis [2]. First, with regard to the course of these disorders, it must be considered that (1) AN typically develops at a younger age than BN [15], (2) SAD is more likely to begin in childhood, and (3) GAD usually develops in adolescence or early adulthood [8]. Therefore, the associations found between AD and ED and their chronology of appearance may not represent a higher risk for AD patients to develop an ED later in life but it could instead reflect the natural course of both disorders, with ADs, in most cases, appearing earlier than EDs. Second, the sequence of onset seems to differ depending on the type of AD: while SAD and specific phobia usually occur prior to ED, GAD has been found to occur simultaneously or after the onset of ED [11, 2]. Moreover, agoraphobia and panic disorder appear more likely to develop after the ED [10].

4. Deepening the association between ADs and EDs

ED patients experience high levels of anxiety in a wide variety of eating situations. Among the eating situations that elicit anxiety in over 50% of patients with ED, Webb et al. [5] identified the following: eating more than what they had planned, eating when they had not planned to, binge eating, eating in front of others who are thinner, eating when self-conscious of what they are wearing, eating in new situations, eating in front of strangers, and eating in restaurants. In the same study, the strategies used to manage anxiety by ED patients when confronted with anxiety-provoking eating situations were avoiding thinking of calories and fat contained in food, eating in a particular way or in a particular order, and using distractions when eating [5]. Findings from this study highlight a tendency to resort to safety behaviours and cognitive avoidance strategies to manage the anxiety rising from eating situations [2, 5]. They can be understood in light of the cognitive model of anxiety disorders put forward by Beck and colleagues [27, 28] and in which anxiety occurs when a situation is perceived as dangerous [2]. According to this model, anxiety requires an excessive threat meaning to innocuous situations and an underestimation of personal coping resources [2]. Threat meaning and lack of personal coping resources are found in ED women. They perceive eating situations as menacing, as they evoke strong emotional reactions such as fear and disgust. They also tend to believe they may not have the appropriated resources for dealing with these situations and tend to avoid them.

4.1. Attentional bias towards threat and coping resources

In the field of anxiety, it has been suggested that an attentional bias towards threat contributes to the development and maintenance of ADs [29]. In ED women, attention biases are centred on threat stimuli relating to food, weight, and shape [21]. A processing priority is given to fear of weight gain as women with ED tend to focus on information that confirms rather than invalidates this fear [2]. According to Nelson and her colleagues [29], state anxiety further increases the attention bias by maintaining the attention on the threat stimuli. Consequently, women with ED who have a comorbid AD are likely to experience state anxiety more often than those without AD when confronted to their feared eating- and weigh-related stimuli, and such attention bias can exacerbate their anxiety and even precipitate binge eating [21, 29]. Thus, while trait anxiety is likely to predispose to and precede AD and ED onset, state anxiety would play an active role is the maintenance of both disorders through an attentional bias towards threat.

When encountering stressful situations, individuals with ED also tend to doubt their ability to deal with and solve these situations [30], which can anchor deeper the belief they must keep fearing eating- and weight-related threat stimuli. Such negative problem orientation has also been found in individuals with ADs [24]. In fact, negative problem orientation implies a catastrophic appraisal of stressful situations and of their consequences [24]. It has been related to poor performance on problem solving and decision making [24]. Along that line, research shows that women with ED are more susceptible than women without ED to assess stressful situations in a catastrophic way, perceive themselves as being under great amount of stress, and rely on dysfunctional coping strategies such as avoidance-oriented or emotion-oriented strategies [31]. Moreover, their active and repetitive use of behaviours such as restrictions and binge eating leads them to think this is an effective way of avoiding and getting rid of negative affect, and particularly of anxiety. It can even negatively impact their likelihood of resorting to active confrontive and more functional coping strategies [30].

4.2. Safety behaviours

In anxious individuals, safety-seeking behaviours are used as a means of gaining control over feared situations, preventing a possible catastrophe, and avoiding situations leading to worrisome thinking [2, 24]. They reduce the anxiety level in the short term but maintain it in the long term. Ritualistic and slow eating, restricting oneself to only certain foods, which are considered safe foods, eating foods in a particular order, and body checking are examples of safety behaviours in women with ED. Safety behaviours also include behaviours related to body avoidance such as refusing to be weighted, avoiding mirrors, and wearing baggy clothes [2]. While body checking involves scrutinizing one's body repeatedly, body avoidance implies not wanting to learn information from the body or to see one's body [32]. As suggested by Pallister and Waller [2], these rigid behaviours are used in an attempt to get control over eating, weight, and shape and to prevent the catastrophe of gaining weight. They provide a form of

http://dx.doi.org/10.5772/65249

reassurance that unfortunately maintains the ED and, as long as they don't try to disconfirm their fears, the anxiety is also maintained in the long term [2]. Furthermore, when eating restrictions are involved, safety behaviours can lead to a loss of control over eating through an increased risk of binge eating [33].

Safety behaviours can be related to the sense of uncontrollability and unpredictability over certain dimensions of their environment that individuals with a comorbid AD and ED experience [25]. Women with ED aim to control their eating so they may not be confronted with a perceived lack of control over the interpersonal and stressful life events they encounter [25]. That way, they manage an internal sense of certainty and diminish their negative perception of being unable to handle the stressful situation [25]. The ED therefore fulfils their need for security and certainty [23].

4.3. Cognitive avoidance strategies

Cognitive avoidance strategies for their part rely on mechanisms like cognitive narrowing, blocking, and dissociation [2]. The anxiety literature suggests that these strategies involve a form of worrisome thoughts substitution and suppression, which allows for diminished unpleasant emotional arousal [24]. They can maintain ADs by impairing the opportunity for a given individual to learn he can handle the feeling of being anxious as well as the stressful situation [24]. Pallister and Waller [2] regard cognitive narrowing as a strategy that brings the attention towards an immediate and present stimulus and requires concrete and low-level thinking. While using cognitive narrowing, a person could for example try to substitute worries by neutral or positive thoughts or use distraction. ED women who rely on cognitive narrowing can focus on and monitor their eating, which reduces their likelihood of experiencing emotional distress and anxiety. Cognitive narrowing also allows for less binge eating in the short run. However, given the food restrictions implicated, an increased risk of binge eating occurs later on [33].

The cognitive avoidance strategy of blocking is used to reduce aversive self-awareness and emotional distress [2]. In ED women, blocking mainly involves binge eating, which is used in order to block or anaesthetize negative emotional states arising from stressful and painful interpersonal situations [2]. Instead of directing their attention on trying to resolve the situation and diminish their emotional arousal, they focus on food. The affect regulation model [34] appears closely related to cognitive avoidance strategies since it posits that women with ED overeat in response to emotional arousal or stress [35]. Thus, as anxiety increases, disordered eating behaviours like binge eating and vomiting may occur more frequently in order to regulate emotions and reduce an emotional void associated with boredom or loneliness [2, 16]. Sadly, instead of alleviating the emotional distress of the women who adopt these behaviours, they can elicit undesirable emotions like shame and reinforce body dissatisfaction, which in turn further increase social anxiety when one has to expose her body to the scrutiny of others [16]. Social evaluation concerns may thereafter accentuate the need to resort to binge eating [3], creating a vicious circle for women with comorbid AD and ED.

Dissociation acts as another cognitive avoidance strategy since it blocks out painful emotions and excludes information from consciousness [2]. According to Pallister and Waller, a high proportion of BN patients report some depersonalization and derealization when they binge [2]. In restrictive AN patients, it has also been found that those who report higher social anxiety display higher dissociation [2, 36].

In sum, eating behaviours like dieting, fasting, vomiting, and exercising excessively can be used as ways of reducing and in some instances eliminating anxiety, albeit temporarily, in individuals with AN, BN, and binge-eating disorder [19, 37]. This pattern of association is highlighted in Fairburn's transdiagnostic model of ED, in which anxiety-triggering situations encountered lead to a need to resort to disordered eating behaviours as a way to modulate and reduce anxiety [33].

5. Treatment considerations

ED patients with comorbid ADs are more likely to experience persisting ED symptoms, poor functioning, and higher psychosocial impairment and mortality risk than those without such comorbidity [1]. Thus, as suggested by Hughes and colleagues, comorbidity can be seen as a marker of illness' severity. Furthermore, through fear of negative evaluation and cognitive avoidance, anxiety can complicate treatment or even negatively affect engagement in treatment [1]. Such considerations highlight the need to consider and implement anxiety-focused interventions in the treatment of EDs. Additionally, when ADs and EDs co-occur in a given patient, it appears essential to opt for interventions that have the potential to address both ED and AD [12, 17]. Doing so will assure better treatment outcomes for both disorders. However, as indicated by Steiger and Israel [17], ED cannot be treated with an approach that would exclusively focus on the management of anxiety symptoms. It therefore justifies the need for a better understanding of what unifies ED and AD in a particular individual, as well as what differentiates the two in order to obtain optimal treatment effects.

The concepts of phobias and fears may be particularly relevant to use in the treatment of ED patients in order to explain their reluctance to gain weight and their bodily concerns [17]. As suggested in the cognitive behavioural treatment approach, psychoeducation about the relationships between thoughts, emotions, and behaviours could be given to ED patients with AD [24]. Additionally, psychoeducation about anxiety as a negative effect and the inefficacity of disordered eating in dealing with distress in the long term should be provided to women seeking help for ED [38]. Relevant concepts explaining GAD, such as intolerance of uncertainty, positive beliefs about worries, negative problem orientation, and cognitive avoidance, could also be covered through psychoeducation.

Cognitive behavioural strategies used for managing and reducing anxiety can wisely be applied for treating ED women who experience high anxiety levels and ADs [5]. **Table 1** presents some ED and AD treatment focus, as well as different type of interventions considered appropriate to address these focus. Treatment of ED should involve reflecting about threat-related cognitions [2], developing coping skills through problem-solving training, as well as developing behavioural experiments aiming at softening rigid cognitive and behavioural eating patterns [3]. More realistic estimates and evaluations of feared eating- and weight-

http://dx.doi.org/10.5772/65249

related stimuli need to be developed by women with ED, and negative problem orientation could be worked on by identifying the consequences of such negative orientation and developing a perception of threats and problems as opportunities and normal parts of life [24].

Treatment focus	Types of intervention
Intolerance of uncertainty and excessive worry	• Challenging positive beliefs about worry • Recognizing that certainty cannot be attained • Identifying manifestations of intolerance of uncertainty • In vivo exposure to uncertainty
Attentional bias towards threat and negative problem orientation	• Reflecting about threat-related cognitions • Discussing the emotional, cognitive, and behavioural consequences of a negative problem orientation • Cognitive restructuring: problems and stressful situations as a normal part of life and an opportunity rather than a threat
Coping skills	• Problem-solving training • Mindfulness and relaxation techniques • Behavioural activation and decision making
Behavioural avoidance (e.g. Ritualistic eating, body checking, and body avoidance)	• Exposure to fearful situations • Mirror exposure • Graded body image exposure • Exposure plus response prevention
Cognitive avoidance (e.g. cognitive narrowing, blocking, and dissociation)	• Exploring of the relationship between emotions, cognitions and behaviours • Tolerance of emotional distress • Emotional processing • Imaginal exposure

Table 1. AD- and ED-related focus of treatment and appropriate types of intervention.

Selected interventions, encompassing ADs and EDs, should focus on reducing safety behaviours such as eating only certain foods perceived as less risky and fattening, eating in a particular way, and using body checking to maintain control over weight and eating [2, 5]. By using behavioural experiments, ED women with a comorbid AD can test out whether or not their fears and dysfunctional beliefs regarding the non-use of their safety behaviours prove to be true [2]. As suggested by Levinson and Rodebaugh [3], some behavioural experiments could be centred on social appearance anxiety. For example, ED patients could be instructed to talk about a certain aspect of their appearance with others in order to disconfirm their belief that others mainly focus on that aspect of their physical anatomy and that they may reject them based on their perceived physical flaws [3].

To deal with behavioural avoidance, exposure to anxiety-provoking eating situations also seems essential to use as an intervention strategy. As for behavioural experiments, exposure allows for disconfirming the ED patients' fears of catastrophe and improving their beliefs that they have the internal resources to cope with the situations they avoid. In an exposure plus response prevention intervention strategy, patients with ED are encouraged to eat forbidden foods (exposure) and to keep themselves from vomiting (response prevention) [39]. Past research has shown that body checking and body avoidance, which can be conceptualized as behavioural manifestations of an overvaluation of weight and shape, can be effectively addressed through exposure [32]. In fact, interventions strategies like mirror exposure and graded body image exposure are promising for ED women [32]. Mirror exposure allows for habituation to and a reduction of the distressing thoughts and feelings experienced towards the body. It has been shown to significantly increase body satisfaction and decrease of body avoidance [32]. For its part, graded body image exposure uses psychoeducation about body avoidance and the overvaluation of weight and shape as well as a hierarchy of anxiety-provoking situations that are avoided with the goal of helping women with ED learning that their fears with regard to their weight and shape are harmful to them and unlikely to happen [32].

Treatment also has to consider cognitive avoidance strategies that are used to either escape from or reduce aversive self-awareness and negative affect [2]. Cognitive narrowing and blocking can be targeted by focusing on the underlying emotions and distress that ED women are anaesthetizing through restrictive and binge eating. As suggested by Haynos and colleagues [40], treatment involves increasing the patient's capacity to tolerate distress as well as identifying how cognitions and emotions are associated. Considering that intolerance of uncertainty may represent a shared vulnerability between ADs and EDs [23], developing a tolerance to uncertainty and unpredictability may also be relevant for treatment. While doing so, manifestations of intolerance of uncertainty should be identified and addressed through exposure [24]. Finally, interventions addressing cognitive narrowing and blocking should investigate and test the ED patients' beliefs about negative emotions, and particularly about anxiety [40].

6. Conclusion

Anxiety symptoms and ADs are frequently reported in women with ED. In fact, comorbid ADs are prevalent across the full spectrum of ED and particularly likely to be observed in clinical inpatient and outpatient samples. Although the understanding of the nature of the link between anxiety and ED still has to be explored and deepened, most available research focusing on the AD-ED comorbidity suggests that, in an high proportion of ED women, disordered eating symptoms are preceded by symptoms of anxiety and even considered as anxiety driven. Therefore, AD should be systematically assessed and addressed in women with ED. ADs play a maintaining role in the symptomatology of ED and thus must be recognized and treated as soon as possible [18]. Moreover, different mechanisms involved in both ADs and EDs need to be considered as treatment-appropriate focus. Among them, intolerance of uncertainty, attentional bias towards threat, negative problem orientation, and behavioural and cognitive avoidance appear particularly relevant.

In sum,

- Up to 75% of women with AN and BN present an AD.
- GAD and SAD are the most frequently AD diagnoses in women with ED.
- Three temporal sequences of the onset of AD and ED have been suggested, with the one in which AD precedes ED disposing of the most empirical support.
- ED and AD present a shared vulnerability through adverse childhood experiences, negative affect, fear of negative evaluation, and intolerance of uncertainty.
- Attentional bias, coping resources, safety behaviours, and cognitive avoidance strategies can be found in women with ED.
- Treatment for ED women with a comorbid AD should involve behavioural experiments, exposure, problem-solving training, and tolerance of emotional distress and uncertainty.

Author details

Annie Aimé[1,2*], Tanya Guitard[2] and Lise Grousseaud[2]

*Address all correspondence to: annie.aime@uqo.ca

1 Department of Psychoeducation and Psychology, Université du Québec en Outaouais, Saint-Jerome, Quebec, Canada

2 Clinique IMAVI, Gatineau, Quebec, Canada

References

[1] Hughes E, Goldschmidt A, Labuschagne Z, Loeb K, Sawyer S, Le Grange D, Eating disorders with or without comorbid depression and anxiety: similarities and differences in a clinical sample of children and adolescents. European Eating Disorders Review. 2013;21:386–394. DOI: 10.1002/erv.2234

[2] Pallister E, Waller G, Anxiety in the eating disorders: understanding the overlap. Clinical Psychology Review. 2008;28:366–386. DOI: 10.1016/j.cpr.2007.07.001

[3] Levinson C, Rodebaugh T, Social anxiety and eating disorders comorbidity: the role of negative social evaluation fears. Eating Behaviors. 2012;13:27–35. DOI: 10.1016/j.eatbeh.2011.11.006

[4] Steere J, Butler G, Cooper P, The anxiety symptoms of bulimia nervosa: a comparative study. International Journal of Eating Disorders. 1990;9:293–301. DOI: 10.1002/1098-108X(199005)9:3<293::AID-EAT2260090307>3.0.CO;2-H

[5] Webb C, Thuras P, Peterson C, Lampert J, Miller D, Crow S, Eating related anxiety in individuals with eating disorders. Eating and Weight Disorders. 2011;16:236–241.

[6] Jordan J, Joyce P, Carter F, Horn J, McIntosh V, Luty S, McKenzie J, Mulder R, Bulik C, Anxiety and psychoactive substance use disorder comorbidity in anorexia nervosa and depression. International Journal of Eating Disorders. 2003;34:211–219. DOI: 10.1002/eat.10177

[7] Goddard E, Treasure J, Anxiety and social-emotional processing in eating disorders: examination of family trios. Cognitive Therapy Research. 2013;37:890–904. DOI: 10.1007/s10608-013-9535-2

[8] Godart N, Flament M, Perdereau F, Jeammet P, Comorbidity between eating disorders and anxiety disorders: a review. International Journal of Eating Disorders. 2002;32:253–270. DOI: 10.1002/eat.10096

[9] Swinbourne J, Touyz S, The co-morbidity of eating disorders and anxiety disorders: a review. European Eating Disorders Review. 2007;15:253–274. DOI: 10.1002/erv.784

[10] Kaye W, Bulik C, Thornton L, Barbarich N, Masters K, Comorbidity of anxiety disorders with anorexia and bulimia nervosa. The American Journal of Psychiatry. 2004;161:2215–2221. DOI: 10.1176/appi.ajp.161.12.2215

[11] Godart N, Flament M, Curt F, Perdereau F, Lang F, Venisse J, Halfon O, Bizouard P, Loas G, Corcos M, Jeammet P, Fermanian J, Anxiety disorders in subjects seeking treatment for eating disorders: a DSM-IV controlled study. Psychiatry Research. 2003;117:245–258. DOI: 10.1016/S0165-178(03)00038-6

[12] Swinbourne J, Hunt C, Abbott M, Russell J, St Clare T, Touyz S, The comorbidity between eating disorders and anxiety disorders: prevalence in an eating disorder sample and anxiety disorder sample. Autralian and New Zeland Journal of Psychiatry. 2012;46:118–131. DOI: 10.1177/0004867411432071

[13] Schwalberg M, Barlow D, Algar S, Howard L, Comparison of bulimics, obese binge eaters, cosial phobics, and individuals with panic disorder on comorbidity across DSM-III-R anxiety disorders. Journal of Abnormal Psychology. 1992;101:675–681. DOI: 10.1037/0021-843X.101.4.675

[14] Wittchen H, Stein M, Kessler R, Social fears and social phobia in a community sample of adolescents and young adults: prevalence, risk factors and co-morbidity. Psychological Medicine. 1999;29:309–323.

[15] American Psychiatric Association. Diagnostic and Statistical Manual of Mental Disorders (DSM-5). 2013. Washington, DC: American Psychiatric Association.

[16] Ostrovsky N, Swencionis C, Wylie-Rosett J, Isasi, C, Social anxiety and disordered overeating: an association among overweight and obese individuals. Eating Behaviors. 2013;14:145–148. DOI: 10.1016/j.eatbeh.2013.01.009

[17] Boujut E, Koleck M, Bergès D, Bourgeois M, The prevalence of anxiety-depressive disorders in patients consulting for eating disorders: a comparison of four eating disorders subtypes. Annales Médico-Psychologiques. 2012;170:52–55. DOI: 10.1016/j.amp2011.11.007

[18] Kazelman S, Touyz S, Hunt C, Rhodes P, Does anxiety improve during weight restoration in anorexia nervosa? A systematic review. Journal of Eating Disorders. 2015;3:1–15. DOI: 10.1186/s40337-015-0046-2

[19] Steiger H, Israel M, Treatment of psychiatric comorbidities. In Grilo C M & Mitchell J E, editors. The Treatment of Eating Disorders: A clinical Handbook. New York: Guilford Press. 2010. Pp. 447–457.

[20] Raney TS, Thornton LM, Berrettini W, Crawford S, Fichter MM, Halmi KA, Johnson C, Kaplan AS, LAVia M, Mitchell J, Rotondo A, Strober M, Woodside DB, Kay WH, Bulik CM Influence of overanxious disorder of childhood on the expression of anorexia nervosa. International Journal of Eating Disorders. 2008;41:326–332. DOI: 10.1002/eat. 20508

[21] Lehoux PM, Steiger H, Jabalpurlawa S, State/trait distinctions in bulimic syndromes. International Journal of Eating Disorders, 2000;27:36–42. DOI: 10.1002/(SICI)1098-108X(200001)27:1<36::AID-EAT4>3.0.CO;2-U

[22] Schneider KL, Appelhans BM, Whited MC, Oleski J, Pagoto SL, Trait anxiety, but not trait anger, predisposes obese individuals to emotional eating. Appetite. 2010;55:701–706. DOI: 10.1016/j.appet.2010.10.006

[23] Konstantellou A, Campbell M, Eisler I, Simic M, Treasure J, Testing a cognitive model of generalized anxiety disorders in eating disorders. Journal of Anxiety Disorders. 2011;25:864–869. DOI: 10.1016/j.janxdis.2011.04.005

[24] Dugas MJ, Robichaud M, Cognitive-Behavioral Treatment for Generalized Anxiety Disorder – From Science to Practice. New York: Routledge. 2007. 247 p.

[25] Frank G, Roblek T, Shott M, Jappe L, Rollin M, Hagman J, Pryor T. Heightened fear of uncertainty in anorexia and bulimia nervosa. International Journal of Eating Disorders. 2012;45:227–232. DOI: 10.1002/eat.209929

[26] Schmidt U, Treasure J, Anorexia nervosa: valued and visible. A cognitive-interpersonal maintenance model and its implication for research and practice. British Journal of Clinical Psychology. 2006;45:343–366. DOI: 10.1348/014466505X53902

[27] Beck A, Emery G, Greenberg R, editors. Anxiety Disorders and Phobias: A Cognitive Perspective. 2nd ed. New York: Basic Books. 1985. 347 p.

[28] Beck A, Clark D, An information processing model of anxiety: automatic and strategic processes. Behaviour Research and Therapy. 1997;35:49–58.

[29] Nelson AL, Purdon C, Quigley L, Carriere J, Smilek D, Distinguishing the roles of trait and state anxiety on the nature of anxiety-related attentional biases to threat using a free viewing eye movement paradigm. Cognition and Emotion. 2015;29:504–526. DOI: 10.1080/02699931.2014.922460

[30] Villa V, Manzoni GM, Pagnini F, Castelnuovo G, Cesa GL, Molinari E. Do coping strategies discriminate eating disordered individuals better than eating disorder features? An explorative study on female inpatients with anorexia and bulimia nervosa. Journal of Clinical Psychology in Medical Settings. 2009;16:297–303. DOI: 10.1007/s10880-009-9172-9

[31] Aimé A, Sabourin S, Ratté C, The eating disturbed spectrum in relation with coping and interpersonal functioning. Eating and Weight Disorders. 2006;11:66–72. DOI: 10.1007/BF03327753

[32] Trottier K, Carter J, MacDonald E, McFarlane T, Olmsted M, Adjunctive graded body image exposure for eating disorders: A randomized controlled initial trial in clinical practice. International Journal of Eating Disorders. 2015;48:494–504. DOI: 10.1002/eat.22341

[33] Fairburn C, Cognitive Behavior Therapy and Eating Disorders. Chichester: Gilford Press. 2008. 316p. DOI: 10.1002/erv.928

[34] Polivy J, Herman P, La santé mentale et les comportements alimentaires: une relation bidirectionnelle. Revue Canadienne de santé publique. 2005;96:49–53.

[35] Groesz L, McCoy S, Carl J, Saslow L, Stewart J, Adler N, Laraia B, Epel E, What is eating you? Stress and the drive to eat. Appetite.2012;58:717–721. DOI: 10.1016/j.appet.2011.11.028

[36] Hinrichsen H, Wright F, Waller G, Meyer C, Social anxiety and coping strategies in the eating disorders. Eating Behaviors. 2003;4:117–126. DOI: 10.1016/S1471-0153(03)00016-3

[37] Bulik C, Midlife Eating Disorders. Your Journey to Recovery. New York: Walker Publishing Company. 2013.

[38] Haedt-Matt A, Keel P, Revisiting the affect regulation model of binge eating: a meta-analysis of studies using ecological momentary assessment. Psychological Bulletin. 2011;137:660–681. DOI: 10.1037/a0023660

[39] Toro J, Cervera M, Feliu M, Garriga N, Jou M, Martinez E, Toro E, Cue exposure in the treatment of resistant bulimia nervosa. International Journal of Eating Disorders. 2003;34:227–234. DOI: 10.1002/eat.10186

[40] Haynos A, Roberto C, Attia E, Examining the associations between emotion regulation difficulties, anxiety, and eating disorder severity among inpatients with anorexia nervosa. Comprehensive Psychiatry, 2015;60:93–98.

Chapter 6

Eating Disorders with Comorbid Anxiety Disorders

Cicek Hocaoglu

Additional information is available at the end of the chapter

http://dx.doi.org/10.5772/65844

Abstract

Although eating disorders and anxiety disorders (AD) are under different diagnosis categories, it is striking that they have high comorbidity and similar clinical features. The most frequently informed anxiety disorders are obsessive-compulsive disorder (OCD), social anxiety disorder (SAD) and generalized anxiety disorder (GAD). Moreover, in cases with a tendency of perfectionism, concern and harm avoidance before the diagnosis of eating disorder, the anxiety disorder is able to be failed to notice. The existence of anxiety disorder or eating disorder makes these syndromes worse. Until today, the relation in between eating disorder and AD has tried to be clarified by phenomenological, neurobiological and family studies. But even if a significant relation has been specified in phenomenological aspect in between OCD and eating disorders, the relation in between eating disorders and other AD is not clear. The existence of AD may be a risk factor in the arise of eating disorders. Therefore, diagnosis and treatment of childhood-adolescence occurring AD may prevent the development of eating disorders. The comorbidity of eating disorders and AD is negatively affecting the treatment and prognosis of the disorder. Moreover, there is limited evidence regarding the effectiveness of treatment options (medication, cognitive behavioral therapy (CBT), family therapy, dialectic behavioral therapy, interpersonal therapy) used in the treatment of cases with a diagnosis of concurrent eating disorder and anxiety disorder. In this chapter, a review of the literature on the comorbidity between eating disorders and the anxiety disorders of OCD, posttraumatic stress disorder (PTSD), SAD, GAD, simple phobia, agoraphobia and panic disorder.

Keywords: eating disorders, anxiety disorders, comorbidity

1. Introduction

Psychiatric comorbidity is defined as coexistence of more than one psychological disorder. In many studies made until today in the field of mental health, high psychiatric comorbidity rates have attracted attention [1–3]. In the case of psychiatric comorbidity, the existence of the second disorder causes more and longer hospitalization, acute state-flaming up and late response to treatment. The comorbidity of eating disorders—which have the highest risk of early death among the mental disorders—and other mental disorders has been examined in many studies [4–6]. Attention has been drawn to high comorbidity rates of especially mood disorders, personality disorders and substance abuse with eating disorders [7]. The psychiatric comorbidity is important in individuals with eating disorder. Because the symptoms of eating disorder may intensify in the existence of psychiatric comorbidity, the symptoms may become chronic and the treatment compliance of the patient may spoil. And the high mortality rates in eating disorders may be explained by this condition. For this reason, early diagnosis and treatment of other mental disorders that coexist with eating disorders will affect the course of the disorder. Although it has been reported until today by many researchers that anxiety disorders exist for once or more in the lives of about two-thirds of the individuals with eating disorder, the information regarding comorbid anxiety disorders in individuals with eating disorder is not sufficient and clear. Having significant methodological problems in studies made on this subject is making the results of the studies questionable. The selection of cases, the diagnostic criteria used and different diagnosis tools, lack of control groups with small samples and lack of preference of suitable statistical methods are among the most significant constraints of the studies. But as specified by most of the researchers, the highness of the prevalence of AD in cases with eating disorder shouldn't be forgotten. Until now, the most frequently existing anxiety disorders in cases with eating disorder are OCD, SAD and GAD, respectively. Due to the similar and coinciding symptoms of obsessive-compulsive disorder and eating disorder, it has been alleged that both mental disorders may have a common etiology. Frequent existence of both eating disorders and anxiety disorders in females and among close family members supports common genetic tendency. Although it has been informed in the studies that all the anxiety disorders are of similar rates in individuals with anorexia nervosa and bulimia nervosa diagnosis, there are conflicting results regarding which specific anxiety disorder exists the most in the sub-types of eating disorder. The studies have been mostly carried out on the individuals with anorexia nervosa (AN) and bulimia nervosa (BN) diagnosis. Eating Disorders Not Otherwise Specified (EDNOS) and binge eating disorder —which frequently exist in routine clinical implementations—have been omitted in studies made on this subject. In other words, the subject of anxiety disorders with comorbidity EDNOS and binge eating disorder has nearly never been included in the studies as different from other eating disorders. On the other hand, the prevalence of comorbid eating disorder in individuals with anxiety disorder is not clearly being known. Moreover, the information regarding the treatment approaches in the existence of comorbid anxiety disorder in individuals with eating disorder is limited. In this section, the subject of comorbidity of eating disorders and anxiety disorder has been addressed, and it has been intended for them to be discussed in light of the current literature information. From accessible studies in the literature about eating disorders

http://dx.doi.org/10.5772/65844

and comorbid AD, case selection criteria based on the diagnostic classification, the scale used in the diagnosis, the study in the control group, are included in this section: the diagnostic criteria for eating disorders and AD, diagnostic scale is not used, no control group of studies were excluded.

2. The comorbidity between eating disorders and anxiety disorders

The relation in between eating disorders and anxiety disorders has attracted the attention of the researchers for many years, and the phenomenology of anxiety and eating disorders has been examined in three perspectives until today. First, the similar clinical manifestations of eating disorders and anxiety disorders have been defined. For instance, it has been specified that there is a parallelism with OCD and cramming type of eating/vomiting periods in bulimic patients or eating rituals of anorexic patients. Second, by the studies which had covered the society and the clinical samples and which had been applied on females with eating disorder, high rates of anxiety disorders have been determined in the families of the cases. Third, in both of the CBT and pharmacological treatment approaches, it has been informed that it is effective also in the eating disorders (i.e., exposure and response prevention and fluoxetine in patients with BN) as well as the anxiety disorders [8, 9]. All these results indicate that there may be a relation in between the eating disorders and anxiety disorders. Because until today, it has been informed in many studies that the comorbidity of eating disorder and anxiety disorder exists extensively. Swinbourne et al. [10], in their study performed with 100 cases being subjected to inpatient treatment due to eating disorder and with 52 cases being treated with the diagnosis of anxiety disorder, had searched the prevalence of the comorbidity of eating disorders and anxiety disorders. In that study, the authors had determined that at least one comorbid anxiety disorder was existing in 65% of the cases being treated due to eating disorder, and that the anxiety disorder was existing before the diagnosis of eating disorder in 69% of them. The anxiety disorder diagnosis of the cases had been social anxiety disorder (42%), posttraumatic stress disorder (26%), generalized anxiety disorder (23%), obsessive-compulsive disorder (5%), panic/agoraphobia (3%) and specific phobia (2%), respectively. In the same study, it had been informed that comorbid eating disorder was existing at a rate of 13.5% in the patient group being treated due to anxiety disorder, and that eating disorder had developed after anxiety disorder in 71% of these cases [10]. The results of this study make us think that the prevalence of comorbidity of eating disorder and anxiety disorder is high. For this reason, it is required to develop clinical understanding regarding comorbidity in between eating disorders and anxiety disorders. It is required to address both mental disorders together in the clinical evaluation and treatment programs of eating disorders and anxiety disorders.

And in another study searching the relation in between anxiety frequency and eating disorders and anxiety disorders in individuals with anorexia nervosa and bulimia nervosa, the Structured Clinical Interview for DSM-IV Axis I disorders had been used. Ninety-seven cases with anorexia nervosa, 282 cases with bulimia nervosa and 293 cases with both anorexia nervosa and bulimia nervosa had been included in the study, and they had been compared with nonclinical group of women in the society. According to this, the rates of anxiety disorder in sub-types of eating disorders were similar. One or more AD has been determined along their lives in two-thirds of the individuals with eating disorder. The most frequently existing anxiety disorders are obsessive-compulsive disorder (N = 277 [41%]) and social phobia (N = 134 [20%]). Most of the participants had informed that OCD, social phobia, specific phobia and generalized anxiety disorder had started in their childhood, and that eating disorder had developed afterwards. Again in the study, attention had been drawn to the point that the ones who have eating disorder history and who are not diagnosed with anxiety disorder have tendency of perfectionism, concern, timidity and harm avoidance. The authors had specified that these syndromes may intensify in case of existence of eating disorder or anxiety disorder [11]. The results of this study have similar qualification with the results of the studies made regarding the subject. In other words, the frequency of anxiety disorders (especially OCD) in the individuals with eating disorder has been found to be higher compared with nonclinical group of women in the society. The starting of anxiety disorders before the eating disorders supports the view that anxiety disorders may be a risk factor for the development of eating disorders.

In between 1985 and 2002, Godart et al. [12] had examined all the researches searching the eating disorders with comorbidity anxiety disorders. In that study, answers had been sought for the following three questions: (1) Is there any convincing evidence regarding the anxiety disorders in women with eating disorders are existing more frequently compared with the women in the general society? (2) What are the convincing evidences regarding that there is a difference among the sub-types of eating disorders that are informed to exist along with the sub-types of anxiety disorders? (3) What is the chronology regarding the arise of both disorders? Through the studies made in different societies, the authors had specified that an increased risk had been indicated for anxiety disorders in individuals with eating disorders. In addition, studies with conflicting results had also been specified in the same study, and attention had been drawn to procedural limitations in the formation of diagnosis groups in which the control group was also included [12]. The answers of the above questions are not clear even today.

In a study with a sample group of French patients with eating disorder, the prevalence of anxiety disorders along the life and starting age of eating disorders had been searched. Sixty-three cases included in the study had been assessed by Composite International Diagnostic Interview (CIDI) and DSM-IV. It had been determined that anxiety disorder arises at least once along the life in 83% of the patients with anorexia nervosa and in 71% of the patients with bulimia nervosa. The most frequently existing one is social phobia (55% of the anorexics and 59% of the bulimics). In 75% of the patients with AN, and in 88% of the patients with BN, it had been informed that the anxiety disorder had started before the eating disorder. These results are in conformity with the studies performed in other countries. Again, the authors had specified that comorbid anxiety disorders should be considered in order to succeed in the treatment of eating disorder [13].

In the study of the same study group performed in 2003 in which 271 French women patients with anorexia nervosa and bulimia nervosa and the control group consisting of 271 healthy women had been compared, it had been determined that at least one anxiety disorder had existed in 71% of the group with eating disorder. This rate is higher than the rate of anxiety

http://dx.doi.org/10.5772/65844

disorder in the healthy control group. Again in that study, the prevalence of many of the types of anxiety disorders had been found to be higher compared to the control group with eating disorder. In 53.3% of the cases with eating disorder, the anxiety disorder exists before the start of eating disorder [14]. The results of this study supports the fact that the anxiety disorders are more frequently existing in cases with eating disorders compared with the general society, and they point out that both disorder may have common etiology and treatment approaches.

Perderea et al. [15] had searched the history of anxiety and mood disorder in the families of cases with anorexia nervosa. According to this, the authors, who had examined the studies performed on this subject in between 1980–2006, had informed that the studies had significant methodological problems and that it is not possible to reach a conclusion with the current studies.

Blinder et al. [4] had searched the DMS-IV Axis 1 comorbidity on 2436 women patients with the diagnosis of anorexia nervosa and eating disorder—not otherwise specified—who were inpatients, had determined the existence of a comorbid mental disorder in 97% of the cases. In that study, attention had been drawn to the fact that 56% of the cases had anxiety disorder. Although there was no difference in between the rates of anxiety disorder comorbidity in the sub-types of eating disorder, the comorbidity of OCD and posttraumatic stress disorder (PTSD) had been found to be statistically significantly different. It had been determined that two times more OCD was existing in cases with AN-BN (anorexia nervosa, binge-eating/purging type) and AN-R (anorexia nervosa, restricting type) diagnosis compared with the patients with BN and EDNOS. The findings of other studies—informing that OCD is being observed at an higher rate in cases with AN cases compared with BN cases—are similar [16–18]. Only in one study, higher OCD comorbidity had been informed in cases with BN compared with the cases with AN [11]. These consistent findings, regarding the association of OCD and eating disorders, are casting a light on the fact that the symptoms of OCD and eating disorders coincide. It is striking that smudge obsession and cleaning or hand-washing compulsions are more frequently being observed in cases with eating disorder. When the future studies are performed considering the OCD symptom groups, it will enable us better to understand the comorbidity of OCD and eating disorders.

The differences in the prevalence rates of comorbid anxiety disorders in cases with eating disorder are striking. Moreover, the studies had mostly been performed with female patient groups, and the rates relevant to male patients are not clear. Again the rate of existence of anxiety disorder in adolescent patients with eating disorder is not clearly being known. Thus, studies with wide samples in which the age and gender groups in different societies are being compared with control groups are required.

3. Obsessive-compulsive disorder (OCD)

Even if the OCD and eating disorders are under different categories, the studies have revealed that both disorder groups have some common cognitive, behavioral and personal features. Especially in the recent decades, it had been concentrated by the researchers on the close relation of these two disorder groups. AN is the first eating disorder scheme that is being associated with OCD due to its clinical features such as rigid diet programs, ruminations relevant to food, repeated weight measurements and continuous calories calculations [19]. For the first time, Palmar and Jones had specified by their study on four cases that the patients with AN may be assessed as OCD (the exteriorization of a compulsion neurosis) in respect of personal traits. They defended this thesis by the fact that the individuals with AN are always being interested with weight and food, and that they exhibit stereotypic and ritualistic behaviors during their diets, exercises and weight follow-ups [20]. As informed by Karayilan and Erol, DuBois had also defined AN as 'cachectic compulsion neurosis' in a similar manner [21]. Rothenberg (1986), 'a modern obsessive-compulsive syndrome' by defining the form of AN has noted may be a form of obsessive-compulsive disorder [22]. In clinical samples, in cases with AN-R, the prevalence of OCD along the life is varying in between 9.5–62% [23, 24]. And the prevalence of OCD along the life in cases with AN-BN is varying in between 10–66% [25, 26].

In a study performed as comparing with the control group, the prevalence of OCD in cases with AN had been found higher compared with the control group [27]. And for BN, the prevalence of OCD along the life had been informed to vary in between 0–42% [13, 26]. And in a study performed by comparing with the normal control group, the frequency of existence of OCD in ones having BN history either currently or in the past had been found to be higher compared with the control group [28]. But Bushnell et al. [29] had specified that there is no difference in the existence of OCD in cases with BN. In the studies comparing the OCD rates in cases with AN and BN, attention had generally been drawn to high OCD comorbidity in cases with AN. In addition, in two studies performed in Japan, higher OCD comorbidity had been informed in cases with BN [17, 30]. Matsunaga et al. [30] had specified that there are more severe mood symptoms in BN cases with OCD comorbidity compared with the BN cases without OCD comorbidity. And the qualification of the OCD symptoms in patients with eating disorder had also been searched. For instance, Fahy [31] could not find any difference in respect of obsessive-compulsive symptoms in the categories of control, suspicion, cleanliness and rumination in between the OCD groups with and without AN comorbidity, but he had indicated that obsessive-compulsive symptoms related to eating and being weighed are more prevalent in AN comorbid OCD group. And in another study, while the most frequent existing OCD symptoms were being classified as 'symmetry and order' and 'cleanliness and washing,' respectively, in AN comorbid OCD patients, they had been determined as 'cleanliness and washing' along with 'obsession and control' in patients only with OCD [32]. Matsunaga et al. [33] had determined in another study by which they had scanned the primary OCD symptoms in OCD comorbid bulimic patient group that the most prevalent symptoms were symmetry-order obsessions and controlling and arranging compulsions, and that the smudge and aggression obsessions and cleaning-washing compulsions were the secondary ones.

Bastiani et al. [34] had determined that the OCD symptoms in anorexic patients were related to 'symmetry and order,' and they had informed that the controlling compulsion of the OCD patients—consisting this comparison group of the study—was significantly higher than the AN patients along with having an extensive obsessive-compulsive symptom range.

Thiel et al. [35] had indicated that the aggressiveness obsession and controlling compulsion were being more frequently observed in patients with eating disorder, and that in the patients with the eating disorder with comorbidity OCD, symmetry obsession and arranging compulsion were more prevalent. In many studies performed relevant to eating disorder and OCD comorbidity, it had been specified that OCD starts much before the diagnosis of eating disorder [16, 36].

Fahy et al. [31] had compared the patient with OCD group with AN comorbidity with a group only with OCD in respect of starting age of disorder and had determined that the starting age of obsessive-compulsive symptoms was significantly earlier in the AN comorbid OCD group compared to the group only with OCD (average starting age of OCD 17.4 and 22.1, respectively). Again in the same study, it had been shown that the symptoms of obsessive-compulsive and eating disorder were staring nearly at the same ages in the comorbid group, and these results had been interpreted by the authors that the OCD development in late adolescence period—in which the young women are more sensitive about weight—increases the possibility of development of AN as being focused at their concerns on that point. OCD may be a risk factor for the development of eating disorder or the eating disorders, and OCD may have common neurobiological, genetic and psychological etiology. For this reason, one of the reasons being suggested in order to understand the relation of both disorders is the role of brain's serotonin activity's dysregulation in the pathophysiology of these disorders.

Considering the data of response to mediation, results of peripheric symptom study and pharmacological stimulation tests Jarry and Vaccarino [37] had concluded as follows: while the increase in the serotonin functions is increasing the primary OCD symptoms (avoidance behaviors such as washing, controlling), the lowness in the functions of serotonin is relevant to impulsivity and improper thoughts. In this text, it has been emphasized that the irregularities of serotonergic system contribute to cognitive model causing bipolar typical OCD behaviors as OCD is a thought disorder. The studies relevant to the functionality of serotonergic system in eating disorders had mostly been performed with the restrictive AN patients. Kaye [38] had found the peripheric 5-HT symptom level low in AN patients with low body mass index (BMI) and had revealed that the level of 5-HT turns to normal by correcting the weights of these patients. When the serotonin levels are considered after a long while after correcting the weights of patients with AN-R, it had been determined that they were higher compared with the AN-BN individuals with corrected weight, BN individuals and normal individuals [39].

Milos [40] had emphasized that the view of 'OCD is the result of hunger and of having low eight in AN disorder' was being supported by relating the severe thinness as the reason of distortion in the brain's serotonin activity and of increase in OCD symptoms. Based on these findings, it is being alleged that the irregularity in the serotonin functions is causing similar thought and behavior disorders in ED and OCD. Moreover, both disorders are relevant to the serotonin receptor system. Considering that the appetite is being regulated with the 5-HT1A, 5-HT1B and 5-HT2 receptors, and anxiety is being related to the 5-HT1A, 5-HT2 and 5-HT3 receptors, interaction of common receptor may be in subject in the arise of eating disorder and OCD symptoms [37]. In cases with eating disorder, OCD is negatively affecting the prognosis of eating disorder. Matsunaga et al. [30] had indicated that the psychopathology was more severe in respect of negative effect and core eating disorder symptoms in BN patients with comorbidity OCD compared to the ones without OCD. Matsunaga et al. [32] had informed that the comorbidity of OCD was causing more distortion in functionality in AN patients and increases in hospitalization rates, and had related the existence of OCD or obsessive-compulsive personality disorder (OCPD) in AN patients with severity of strain in socialization, depression and anxiety.

Thiel et al. [35] had monitored the patients with eating disorder for 30 months and had searched the effect of the existence of OCD on the results of the treatment, and they had concluded that the comorbidity of OCD doesn't significantly affect the prognosis of AN and BN. The results of a multicentered-extensive study performed by Sallet et al. [41] on the patients with OCD had shown that comorbidity of eating disorder is related to more severe obsessive-compulsive clinical symptoms, starting of compulsion at earlier ages, increase in the other axis I comorbidity, higher levels of depression and anxiety symptoms and higher suicidal attempts in these patients. When examined in respect of treatment, there are many studies proving that both the OCD and eating disorder patients respond to the selective serotonin reuptake inhibitors (SSRIs). In the pharmacology guide for anxiety, OCD and PTSD of world biological psychiatry associations' federations, fluvoxamine, sertraline and fluoxetine are being suggested primarily [42]. Kaye et al. [43] had found fluoxetine effective on restrictive AN cases in one of their studies, and in another study [44], they had indicated that fluoxetine is preventing the relapses in patients with AN.

Romano et al. [45] had determined that fluoxetine is beneficial in both the acute and chronic periods of BN disorder. Even if there is a common clinical manifestation in between the eating disorders and OCD, there are some differences. One of the most significant differences in between the OCD and eating disorders is that there is an extensive obsessive-compulsive range in cases with OCD besides the eating disorder. The compulsions decrease the anxiety in cases with OCD, and bulimic and restrictive behaviors in eating disorders function as affect regulation [46].

The extensive comorbidity rates in between eating disorder and OCD had directed the researchers to phenomenological studies in order to better understand the connection in between these two disorders. The researchers, examining the clinical features and personal traits of patients with OCD and eating disorder, had tried to explain the relation of obsessive-compulsive personality disorder by many hypotheses. Most of the patients with AN involve in decreasing the food intake, distinct activity on the body, compulsive calorie calculation along with continuous rumination relevant to food, excessive exercise and use of laxatives depending on obsessive nature of thinness in respect of clinical features [32].

The anorectics are stereotypically defined as rigid, ritualistic, perfectionist and meticulous in respect of their personality structures [35, 47, 48]. Perfectionism is the leading feature of eating disorders, and it may sometimes begin before the development of eating disorder, or it may arise as a distinct characteristic in the acute period of eating disorder, and it may even continue after treatment of eating disorder [49]. In the studies performed, the AN and BN patients tend to get higher scores in scales relevant to perfectionism compared with the healthy controls [35,

48, 50]. Kaye [51] had emphasized that the individuals with AN and BN are in conformity with perfectionist personality structure. The obsessive personality trait had been determined at higher rates in individuals with OCD and eating disorder [52].

In a retrospective study, it had been determined that patients with AN-R and AN-BP have obsessive personality structures at rates of 76 and 57%, respectively, in respect of premorbid personality traits [53]. As there are ones who allege that the obsessive-compulsive symptoms in eating disorder patients constitute a risk factor for the development of eating disorder [54, 55], there are also ones who defend that these symptoms are being exhibited as secondary phenomenon of eating disorder [56]. In the personality disorder prevalence studies performed among patients with AN, the obsessive-compulsive personality disorder (OCPD) ranks the first, and its rate is in between 17–60%. But the rate of comorbidity of OCPD and OCD is lower than expected, 6–28%. There are researchers who deem the distinctiveness of obsessional personality traits in patients with AN as the cause of development of OCD in these individuals [32]. On the other hand, the effect of prevalence of comorbid eating disorders in cases with OCD on the treatment and course of disorder is not completely being known. There are very limited studies on this subject. Tobiassen [57], in his study performed by 93 patients with a primary diagnosis of OCD, had determined higher rates of eating disorders in cases with OCD compared to the healthy group. In the same study, it had been specified that the eating disorders don't affect the treatment of cases with OCD with a higher eating disorder rate among female patients group compared with the male patients. Moreover, it has been reported that eating disorder symptoms of the cases with OCD had not decreased significantly after treatment. Until today, most of the researches had focused on the comorbid OCD in cases with eating disorder. For this reason, the future studies will search the answers of these questions.

After all, although the eating disorder and obsessive-compulsive disorder are involving as different diagnosis categories in DSM-5, their similarity in respect of high comorbidity rates and personality traits is attracting the attention of the researchers. While the obsessive and perfectionist personality traits are creating tendency for the development of OCD and eating disorder, the existence of obsessive-compulsive symptoms may be risk factor for eating disorder. The relation in between eating disorder and OCD has tried to be clarified through phenomenological, neurobiological and family studies. In phenomenological aspect, there is a significant connection in between these two disorders, but it is not possible yet to explain this connection by data regarding that it is serotonergic irregularity or hereditary tendency. The condition of OCD and eating disorder comorbidity is negatively affecting the prognosis of the primary disorder. Even if the symptoms in eating disorder relevant to diet, weight and compensative behaviors are ones similar to obsession-compulsion, the results of the current researches are not sufficient for the eating disorders to be deemed as OCD or for them to be called as variations of OCD.

4. Generalized anxiety disorder (GAD)

The relation of eating disorder and comorbid GAD had not been sufficiently searched. This subject had been addressed in a few studies. In two clinical studies, lifetime prevalence of GAD in cases with AN-R had been found 24 and 31% [13, 24]. In both studies, the rate of GAD had been determined higher than the healthy control group. But in a study, the comorbid GAD rate in cases with AN had been determined as different from the control group [58].

Walters and Kendler [59] had determined the comorbidity of GAD in cases with AN as 6.1 times more compared with the control group. In a recent clinical study performed in 2008–2012 in Sweden with an extensive sample, it had been informed that the highest psychiatric comorbidity in eating disorder cases is anxiety disorders (53%), and that GAD comes the first among anxiety disorders [60]. In the studies, the comorbidity of GAD and BN had been searched, and lifetime prevalence of GAD in cases with BN had been informed as in between 10 and 55% [61, 62]. As different from these studies, there are also studies which specify that there is no difference [24, 28, 62]. Kaye et al. [11] had informed by their studies that the comorbid GAD rate in cases with AN and BN is lower than the high rates such as 45.6 and 31.4% which had been informed by the studies of Godart et al. [14] (13 and 7%). Iwasaki et al. [17] had reported the rate of ones meeting the GAD diagnosis criteria in cases with AN and BN as 13%. In this study, it had attracted attention that GAD is generally more frequent in purging subtypes of both AN and BN even if not statistically significant. In a study, it had been alleged that GAD starts in childhood period in 75% of the female cases with BN, and the existence of GAD may be a risk factor in the development of BN [63]. These results support the fact that there exists anxiety disorder before the start of eating disorder in women with BN. Konstantellou et al. [64] had compared two groups with and without GAD diagnosis with the healthy control group. As the result of that study, attention had been drawn to the fact that the ones with eating disorder and comorbid GAD diagnosis have higher concern and avoidance scores than the other two groups. The authors had informed that there may be a common cognitive model in between eating disorder and GAD. The comorbid psychiatric disorders in adolescents with eating disorder and differences as per genders had not been sufficiently searched. Sidor et al. [65], in their study with extensive sample in which they had compared the female and male adolescents with eating disorder, had informed that the generalized anxiety rates were similar for both genders. Consequently, it is required to search in more detail the relation of GAD—being one of the most frequently existing anxiety disorders in the society—and eating disorders.

5. Posttraumatic stress disorder (PTSD)

The relation in between eating disorders and trauma has attracted the attention of the researchers. It had especially been dwelled on the subject that the childhood period traumatic stories such as childhood sexual abuse may be risk factor for the development of eating disorder [66–68]. But surprisingly the eating disorder and comorbid PTSD had been addressed in a few studies until today [69]. And in a study in which the comorbidity relevant to all the anxiety disorders had been searched in cases with eating disorder, PTSD had not even been included in the assessment [13]. In studies searching the comorbidity of PTSD in cases with eating disorder, the rate of PTSD is varying in between 11–52% [70, 71]. In a study with three clinical samples, the lifetime PTSD prevalence in cases with BN had been reported as 3% [72],

10% [62] and 30% [24]. In a study, higher rates of eating disorder had been informed for the women subjected to sexual abuse than the ones who are not subjected to it [73]. The results of this study are in conformity with the results of other studies informing that more frequent PTSD, mood disorders, substance abuse disorders, eating disorders and sexual disorders are being observed among women subjected to sexual abuse [74–76]. In a study with clinical samples, it had been informed that the diagnosis criteria of PTSD had been met in 25% of the cases with eating disorder [77]. Vierling et al. [78] had informed that there was a PTSD prevalence at a rate of 33% in the small sample patient group with eating disorder, and that there was no difference among the sub-groups with eating disorder. In the same study, it had also been emphasized that the comorbidity of PTSD has negative effects on the course of eating disorder (by reasons such as frequent problems among people, impulsivity). In adult Swedish cases having history of traumatic exposure (N = 843, mean age 27.2, 97.3% female) being followed up with the diagnosis of eating disorder, the rate of lifetime PTSD diagnosis had been determined as 24.1%. In this study, it had been informed that the diagnosis of PTSD increases the severity of eating disorder, and that the symptoms of eating disorder start within one year following the trauma [79]. Becker et al. [80], in their studies with clinical samples having eating disorder, had obtained results supporting the relation in between PTSD and eating disorders, because child sexual assault (CSA) may play a significant role in the pathology of eating disorders (specific eating disorder symptoms, specifically, bingeing, vomiting and negative body image). In a meta-analysis study performed by Smolak and Murnen [81], a relation had been found in between CSA and eating disorders. The authors had indicated that the symptoms of eating disorder increase along with CSA. In a similar manner, Jacobi et al. [82] had also specified the relation of sexual abuse and eating disorders. There are also studies informing that there is no relation in between CSA and eating disorders [83, 84]. Moreover, the rates provided in the studies for prevalence of childhood sexual abuse are very different. The reason of it is the use of different methods in the studies. In the studies searching for the comorbid PTSD rates in the sub-types of eating disorders, higher PTSD comorbidity had been informed in cases with BN [85, 86]. And in another study, three times higher PTSD comorbidity had been reported in cases with BN compared with cases with AN [11]. Only in one study, PTSD comorbidity had been informed in 8% of the cases with AN-R, and it had been specified that rate was not different from the control group [24]. Blinder et al. [4] had informed two times more PTSD diagnosis in cases with AN-BP (in women with binge/purge) compared with the cases with AN-R, BN and EDNOS. In a similar manner, the child sexual abuse had been found higher in female cases with AN-BP compared with the female cases with AN-R [87]. In ones with childhood sexual trauma history, especially bingeing and purging behaviors, may assist with affect, emotional regulating. Consequently, it is required to examine in more detail the relation of eating disorder and PTSD.

6. Simple phobia

In the studies performed until today, regarding the comorbid simple phobia in cases with eating disorder, it had been informed in between rates of 0–34% for ones with AN, and in between rates of 10–46% for ones with BN [13, 62]. Lilenfeld et al. [24], in their study in which a healthy control group was used, had concluded that there was no difference at the rate of comorbid simple phobia in cases with AN. However, there are studies informing that the rate of existence of simple phobia in cases with AN is 2–4 times more [59, 88]. Moreover, rate of existence of simple phobia by 2.37 times more had also been informed in cases with BN [88]. While lifetime simple phobia rate in cases with AN-R was 14.3% among outpatients, it had been informed as 34% among inpatients [13, 25]. And there is a study informing that this rate is 15% in cases with AN-BN [24]. In the studies performed until today, the rates relevant to the comorbidity of eating disorder and simple phobia are contradictory and not consistent. The rates of existence of simple phobia in cases with eating disorder, its effects on the primary disorder, and whether there is a difference with prevalence in the society should be searched by studies with extensive samples.

7. Agoraphobia

Different results had been obtained in the studies searching the agoraphobia in cases with eating disorder. For instance, Godart et al. [89] had informed that there are limited data in this field with varying rates in between 0–34.5% regarding the comorbidity of agoraphobia. The prevalence rate of agoraphobia in cases with AN had been found as 0% [25], it had been found as 3% in restricting subgroups [13], and as 20% in binge/purge AN [25]. In another study, attention had been drawn to lifetime high agoraphobia rates in women with AN as the result of comparison with control group (19.8% for AN-R and 27.3% for AN-BP) [14]. In a similar manner in other studies, rates of agoraphobia higher than the control group had been informed in cases with AN [27]. However, Rastam et al. [58] had informed that there was no difference in the studies. Different results from 0% [62] to 17.4% [25] had been informed for the lifetime prevalence of agoraphobia in cases with BN. In studies performed with nonclinical sample groups, the lifetime prevalence of agoraphobia had been informed in between 27–34.5% [29] for cases with BN [90]. In other studies performed as comparing with the control group, the rates of agoraphobia had been found to be high (7.5 and 17.4%) [14, 91]. In a study searching the relation of development of agoraphobia in cases with eating disorder and the family experiences, it had been informed that the mothers of the cases with agoraphobia have anxious and pessimist characteristic, and that it is affecting their relation with their children [92]. Still it is hard to completely explain the relation of eating disorders and agoraphobia.

8. Panic disorder

Different results had been informed regarding the prevalence of panic disorder in cases with eating disorder. For instance, the comorbidity of panic disorder in cases with eating disorder had been informed as 9–11% in a study, and it had been informed as 42–52% in another study [11, 93]. Panic disorder rates of 0–39% had been determined in cases with BN [62, 94]. Bushnell et al. [29], in their study in which a control group was used, had determined the lifetime panic disorder prevalence higher in cases with BN. Kendler et al. [88] had reported that three times more panic disorder exists in cases with BN compared with the control group. But Garfinkel et al. [90] had obtained different results than the results of other studies, and they had specified that the rate of panic disorder is not higher than the control group. The lifetime prevalence of panic disorder had been informed as in between 4 and 7% in cases with AN-R and as 15% in cases with AN-BN [13, 24, 25]. And in two different studies in which the control groups were used, the prevalence of panic disorder had been specified as 2–8.1% in cases with AN [27, 58]. Walters and Kendler [59], in their studies performed with a nonclinical sample, had determined that individuals with 'possible anorexia' have the risk of panic disorder by 3.4 times more. For today, it is hard to completely explain the relation of eating disorders and panic disorder, and its prevalence.

9. Social phobia (social anxiety disorder)

Despite having many data regarding eating problems and obsessive-compulsive pathology, clinical manifestations involving fear such as social phobia, agoraphobia and panic disorder had attracted the academic attention less [95]. Despite this, some studies indicate that social phobia is more frequent in patients with eating disorder [11, 13, 17, 23, 24, 27, 62, 93, 96]. And in some studies, it had been alleged that the comorbidity of social phobia in cases with eating disorder is more extensive than OCD, and that the social phobia may be risk factor in the etiology of eating disorder [97]. In another study, levels of social phobia in patients with AN and BN had been compared with the control group, and higher rates had been determined among control group women. The authors had pointed out the relation in between social phobia and higher levels of eating psychopathology in bulimic patients [98]. There are differences among the studies on prevalence rate of social phobia and eating disorders. In AN, the prevalence rate of social phobia had been informed as in between 16 and 88.2%. [11, 98]. And in BN, the prevalence rate of social phobia had been informed as in between 17 and 67.8%. [72, 98]. In other two studies, higher rates of social phobia had been determined in cases with AN compared with the control group [27, 24]. But in the study performed by Rastam et al. [58], it had been concluded that it was not different from the control group. In a study searching for the relation in between development of social phobia and family experiences in cases with eating disorder, it had been specified that the fathers of the cases with social anxiety are emotionally inhibited (lack of sharing emotions with the child) and unable to relate with their children, and it had been alleged that it causes tendency of development of social phobia in the children [95, 98]. Still today it is hard to completely explain the relation of eating disorders and social phobia with the current data.

Comparison of the prevalence of individuals with eating disorder and comorbid-specific AD is given in **Table 1**.

Comorbid-specific AD	Reference (year)	Subjects (N)	Summary of results
OCD	1. Laessle et al. (1989)	AN-R (21),AN-BP(20), BN (27)	Prevalence of OCD 9.5%
	2. Lilenfeld et al. (1998)	AN-R (27), BN (47)	Prevalence of OCD 62%
	3. Fornari et al. (1992)	AN-R (24),AN-BP(18), BN (21)	Prevalence of OCD 66%
	4. Halmi et al. (1991)	AN (62)	Prevalence of OCD 11.3%
GAD	1. Lilenfeld et al. (1998)	AN-R (27), BN (47)	Prevalence of GAD 31%
	2. Godart et al. (2000)	AN-R (29), BN (34)	Prevalence of GAD 24%
	3. Powers et al. (1988)	BN(30)	Prevalence of GAD 10%
	4. Schwalberg et al. (1992)	BN(20)	Prevalence of GAD 55%
	5. Godart et al. (2003)	AN (166), BN (105)	Prevalence of GAD 45.6%
PTSD	1. Gleaves et al.(1998)	AN (121), BN (103)	Prevalence of PTSD 52%
	2. Brewerten et al.(1995)	BN (59)	Prevalence of PTSD 3%
	3. Schwalberg et al. (1992)	BN (20)	Prevalence of PTSD 10%
	4. Lilenfeld et al. (1998)	AN-R (27), BN (47)	Prevalence of PTSD 30%
	5. Dansky et al. (1997)	BN (72)	Prevalence of PTSD 21.4%
	6. Turnbull et al.(1997)	AN (90), BN (54)	Prevalence of PTSD 11%
	7. Vierling et al.(2015)	AN (57), BN (26), EDNOS(18)	Prevalence of PTSD 33.9%
Simple phobia (SP)	1. Laessle et al. (1989)	AN-R (21),AN-BP(20), BN (27)	Prevalence of Simple Phobia 14.3%
	2. Lilenfeld et al. (1998)	AN-R (27), BN (47)	Prevalence of Simple Phobia 19%
	3. Schwalberg et al. (1992)	BN(20)	Prevalence of Simple Phobia 10%
	4. Godart et al. (2000)	AN-R (29), BN (34)	Prevalence of Simple Phobia 21%
Agoraphobia	1. Godart et al.(2000)	AN-R (29), BN (34)	Prevalence of Agoraphobia 3%
	2. Laessle et al. (1989)	AN-R (21), AN-BP(20), BN (27)	Prevalence of Agoraphobia 20%
	3. Halmi et al.(1991)	AN (62)	Prevalence of Agoraphobia 14.5%
	4. Bushnell et al.(1994)	BN(20)	Prevalence of Agoraphobia 27%
	5. Garfinkel et al.(1995)	BN(58)	Prevalence of Agoraphobia 34.5%
Panic disorder	1. Bushnell et al. (1994)	BN(20)	Prevalence of Panic Disorder 20%
	2. Lilenfeld et al. (1998)	AN-R (27), BN (47)	Prevalence of Panic Disorder 4%
	3. Godart et al. (2000)	AN-R (29), BN (34)	Prevalence of Panic Disorder 7%
	4. Laessle et al. (1989)	AN-R (21), AN-BP(20), BN (27)	Prevalence of Panic Disorder 15%
	5. Halmi et al. (1991)	AN (62)	Prevalence of Panic Disorder 8.1%
	6. Garfinkel et al.(1995)	BN(58)	Prevalence of Panic Disorder 20%
	7. Kendler et al. (1991)	BN (128)	Prevalence of Panic Disorder 9%
	8. Rastam et al. (1995)	AN (51)	Prevalence of Panic Disorder 2%
Social phobia	1. Hinrichson et al.(2003)	AN-R(21), AN-BP(34), BN(59)	Prevalence of Social Phobia 88.2 %
	2. Godart et al. (2000)	AN-R (29), BN (34)	Prevalence of Social Phobia 55%
	3. Halmi et al. (1991)	AN (62)	Prevalence of Social Phobia 33.9%
	4. Iwasaki et al.(2000)	AN-R(62), AN-BP(36), BN(57)	Prevalence of Social Phobia 18%
	5. Kaye et al. (2004)	AN (97), BN(282)	Prevalence of Social Phobia 16%
	6. Lilenfeld et al. (1998)	AN-R (27), BN (47)	Prevalence of Social Phobia 31%
	7. Brewerten et al. (1995)	BN (59)	Prevalence of Social Phobia 17%

Table 1. Summary of research papers investigating prevalence of individuals with eating disorder and comorbid-specific AD.

10. Treatment of eating disorders with comorbid anxiety disorders

The information on how the treatment of cases having the comorbidity of eating disorders and anxiety disorders is required to be is limited. Whether the anxiety disorder or the eating disorder should be the primary subject of treatment, or whether they should be treated together is not clear. Some researchers had alleged that it is required to concentrate on the cause of eating disorder for an effective treatment. However, if the patient is still in advanced hunger, minimal effects may be expected from such a treatment. Moreover, one of the most significant issues in especially vomiting patients is the absorption of medication. CBT may be effective for depression in these patients. However, there is no evidence to suggest that CBT is a superior treatment compared with pharmacological treatments. On the other hand, it is clear that the comorbid conditions frequently cause the intensification of symptoms and negatively affect the response of treatment for the primary disorder. It had been specified in many studies that the psychiatric comorbidity causes intensification of symptoms of eating disorder, causes it to become chronic and causes the development of resistance against the treatment [18, 99]. Specialized treatment protocols are required in patients with psychiatric comorbidity with eating disorder [100]. Boutelle [101] had suggested exposure and response prevention component in case of comorbid obsessive-compulsive disorder. However, the results of the studies are inconsistent. Some studies had informed that comorbid anxiety may cause weak response to treatment [102–106]. But these results had not been supported in other studies [8, 35]. In one study, it had been specified that there was PTSD comorbidity on four female cases with eating disorder, and first, the trauma symptoms had been addressed in the treatment. The authors had informed that the symptoms of eating disorder had started to improve, while the PTSD symptoms were improving. Moreover, in the same study they had alleged that vomiting was being used not only to gain sense of self-control but also as a tool of purging for each of the cases [107].

In case of the comorbidity of eating disorders and anxiety disorders, it is clear that the treatment of both should be addressed together though the treatment approaches are not clearly being known. For this reason, CBT, psychotherapy, support groups, psychopharmacological treatment algorithms that are customized and whose effectiveness had been proven by studies with placebo control are required for the treatment of eating disorders and anxiety disorders.

11. Conclusion

The anxiety disorders existing in cases with eating disorder are OCD, SAD and GAD, respectively. Again in the studies, there are findings that the anxiety disorders start in the childhood period and before the diagnosis of eating disorder. In other words, anxiety disorder may be assessed as a risk factor for the development of eating disorder. Moreover, the comorbidity AD in individuals with eating disorder history may increase the tendency of being more anxious and shy. This condition may cause the symptoms of eating disorder to intensify and disruption of compliance with treatment. Therefore, diagnosis and treatment of childhood-adolescence occurring AD may prevent the development of eating disorders. In the studies, it had been informed that all AD were at similar rates in individuals with a diagnosis of AN and BN. Only PTSD was approximately three times more frequent in individuals with BN and AN-BP as opposed to those with AN-R.

Despite all these, the subject relevant to comorbid anxiety disorders in individuals with eating disorder could not be completely clarified. For instance, EDNOS and binge eating disorder—which frequently exist in routine clinical implementations—have been omitted in studies made on this subject. In other words, the subject of anxiety disorders with comorbidity EDNOS and binge eating disorder has nearly never been included in the studies as different from other eating disorders. Another difficulty before the clinicians is how the cases having comorbid anxiety disorder with eating disorder will be treated, because the results of limited number of studies on this subject are not sufficient. In the future studies, the researchers should prefer reliable statistical strength, research design, standard measures and proper statistical methods. By this way, the comorbidity of eating disorders and anxiety disorders will be better understood by reaching to more consistent findings that are based on evidence. Perhaps in the future studies will be obtained results that similar or have common etiological causes of eating disorders and anxiety disorders.

Acknowledgements

I offer thanks to my family for suggesting that I write this book chapter.

Author details

Cicek Hocaoglu

Address all correspondence to: cicekh@gmail.com

Recep Tayyip Erdogan University, Medical School, Rize, Turkey

References

[1] Karpov B, Joffe G, Aaltonen K, Suvisaari J, Baryshnikov I, Näätänen P et al. Anxiety symptoms in a major mood and schizophrenia spectrum disorders. Eur Psychiatry. 2016;37:1–7. doi:10.1016/j.eurpsy.2016.04.007

[2] Duijkers JC, Vissers CT, Egger JI. Unraveling executive functioning in dual diagnosis. Front Psychol. 2016;7:979. doi:10.3389/fpsyg.2016.00979

[3] Ociskova M, Prasko J, Latalova K, Kamaradova D, Grambal A. Psychological factors and treatment effectiveness in resistant anxiety disorders in highly comorbid inpatients. Neuropsychiatr Dis Treat. 2016;12:1539–1551. doi:10.2147/NDT.S104301

[4] Blinder BJ, Cumella EJ, Sanathara VA. Psychiatric comorbidities of female in-patients with eating disorders. Psychosom Med. 2006;68:454–462.

[5] Solmi F, Hotopf M, Hatch SL, Treasure J, Micali N. Eating disorders in a multi-ethnic inner-city UK sample: prevalence, comorbidity and service use. Soc Psychiatry Psychiatr Epidemiol. 2016;51:369–381. doi:10.1007/s00127-015-1146-7.

[6] McElroy SL, Crow S, Blom TJ, Cuellar-Barboza AB, Prieto MLVeldic M, Winham SJ et al. Clinical features of bipolar spectrum with binge eating behaviour. J Affect Disord. 2016;201:95–98. doi:10.1016/j.jad.2016.05.003

[7] Counturier J. Psychiatric comorbidity in eating disorders. Can J CME. 2004;1:81–85.

[8] Bulik CM. Anxiety disorders and eating disorders: a review of their relationship. NZ J Psychol. 1995;24:51–62.

[9] Welch E, Jangmo A, Thornton LM, Norring C, von Hausswolff-Juhlin Y, Herman BK et al. Treatment-seeking patients with binge-eating disorder in the Swedish national registers: clinical course and psychiatric comorbidity. BMC Psychiatry. 2016;16:163–168. doi:10.1186/s12888-016-0840-7

[10] Swinbourne J, Hunt C, Abbott M, Russell J, St Clare T, Touyz S. The comorbidity between eating disorders and anxiety disorders: prevalence in an eating disorder sample and anxiety disorder sample. Aust NZ J Psychiatry. 2012;46:118–131. doi: 10.1177/0004867411432071

[11] Kaye WH, Bulik CM, Thornton L, Barbarich N, Masters K. Comorbidity of anxiety disorders with anorexia and bulimia nervosa. Am J Psychiatry. 2004;161:2215–2221.

[12] Godart NT, Perdereau F, Jeammet P, Flament MF. Comorbidity between eating disorders and anxiety disorders: results. Encephale. 2005;31:152–161.

[13] Godart NT, Flament MF, Lecrubier Y, Jeammet P. Anxiety disorders in anorexia nervosa and bulimia nervosa: co-morbidity and chronology of appearance. Eur Psychiatry. 2000;15:38–45.

[14] Godart NT, Flament MF, Curt F, Perdereau F, Lang F, Venisse JL et al. Anxiety disorders in subjects seeking treatment for eating disorders: a DSM-IV controlled study. Psychiatry Res. 2003;117:245–258.

[15] Perdereau F, Faucher S, Wallier J, Vibert S, Godart N. Family history of anxiety and mood disorders in anorexia nervosa: review of the literature. Eat Weight Disord. 2008;13:1–13.

[16] Thornton C, Russell J. Obsessive-compulsive comorbidity in the dieting disorders. Int J Eat Disord. 1997;21:83–87.

[17] Iwasaki Y, Matsunaga H, Kiriike N, Tanaka H, Matsui T. Comorbidity of Axis I disorders among eating-disordered subjects in Japan. Compr Psychiatry 2000;41:454–480.

[18] Bulik CM. Anxiety, depression, and eating disorders. In: Fairburn CG, Brownell KD, eds. Eating Disorders and Obesity: A Comprehensive Handbook. New York, NY: The Guilford Press; 2002.

[19] Fahy TA, Osacar A, Marks I. History of eating disorders in female patients with obsessive compulsive disorder. Int J Eat Disord. 1993;14:439–443.

[20] Palmer DH, Jones SM. Anorexia nervosa as a manifestation of obsessive neurosis. Arch Neurol Psychiatry 1939;41:856–860.

[21] Karayilan S, Erol A. Obsessive compulsive disorder and eating disorder. Turk Klin J Psychiatr Spec Top. 2012;5:76–84.

[22] Rothenberg A. Eating disorder as a modern obsessive-compulsive syndrome. Psychiatry. 1986;49:45–53.

[23] Laessle RG, Kittl S, Fichter MM, Wittchen HU, Pirke KM. Major affective disorder in anorexia nervosa and bulimia. A descriptive diagnostic study. Br J Psychiatry. 1987;151:785–789.

[24] Lilenfeld LR, Kaye WH, Greeno CG, Merikangas KR, Plotnicov K, Pollice C et al. A controlled family study of anorexia nervosa and bulimia nervosa: psychiatric disorders in first-degree relatives and effects of proband comorbidity. Arch Gen Psychiatry. 1998;55:603–610.

[25] Laessle R, Wittchen H, Fichter M, Pirke K. The significance of subgroup of bulimia and anorexia nervosa: lifetime frequency of psychiatric disorders. Int J Eat Disord. 1989;8:569–574.

[26] Fornari V, Kaplan M, Sandberg DE, Matthews M, Skolnick N, Katz J. Depressive and anxiety disorders in anorexia nervosa and bulimia nervosa. Int J Eat Disord. 1992;12:21–29.

[27] Halmi K, Eckert E, Marchi P, Sampugnaro V, Apple R, Cohen J. Co-morbidity of psychiatric diagnoses in anorexia nervosa. Arch Gen Psychiatry. 1991;48:712–718.

[28] Hudson JI, Pope HG Jr, Yurgelun-Todd D, Jonas JM, Frankenburg FR. A controlled study of lifetime prevalence of affective and other psychiatric disorders in bulimic outpatients. Am J Psychiatry. 1987;144:1283–1287.

[29] Bushnell JA, Wells JE, McKenzie JM, Hornblow AR, Oakley-Browne MA, Joyce PR. Bulimia comorbidity in the general population and in the clinic. Psychol Med. 1994;24:605–611.

[30] Matsunaga H, Miyaga A, Iwasaki H, Matsui T, Fujimoto K, Kiriike N. A comparison of clinical features among Japanese eating disordered women with obsessive compulsive disorder. Compr Psychiatry. 1999a;40:337–342.

[31] Fahy TA, Osacar A, Marks I. History of eating disorders in female patients with obsessive-compulsive disorder. Int J Eat Disord. 1993;14:439–443.

[32] Matsunaga H, Kiriike N, Iwasaki Y, Miyata A, Yamagami S, Kaye WH. Clinical characteristics in patients with anorexia nervosa and obsessive- compulsive disorder. Psychol Med. 1999;29:407–414.

[33] Matsunaga H, Kiriike N, Miyata A, Iwasaki Y, Matsui T, Fujimoto K et al. Prevalence and symptomatology of comorbid obsessive–compulsive disorder among bulimic patients. Psychiatry Clin Neurosci. 1999;53:661–666.

[34] Bastiani AM, Altemus M, Pigott TA, Rubenstein C, Weltzin TE, Kaye WH. Comparison of obsessions and compulsions in patients with anorexia nervosa and obsessive compulsive disorder. Biol Psychiatry. 1996;39:966–969.

[35] Thiel A, Züger M, Jacoby GE, Schüssler G. Thirty-month outcome in patients with anorexia or bulimia nervosa and concomitant obsessive-compulsive disorder. Am J Psychiatry. 1998;155:244–249.

[36] Milos G, Spindler A, Ruggiero G, Klaghofer R, Schnyder U. Comorbidity of obsessive-compulsive disorders and duration of eating disorders. Int J Eat Disord. 2002;31:284–289.

[37] Jarry JL, Vaccarino FJ. Eating disorder and obsessive-compulsive disorders: neurochemical and phenomenological commonalities. J Psychiatry Neurosci. 1996;21:36–48.

[38] Kaye WH, Ebert MH, Gwirstman HE, Weiss SR. Differences in brain serotonergic metabolism between nonbulimic and bulimic patients with anorexia nervosa. Am J Psychiatry. 1984; 141:1598–1601.

[39] Kaye WH, Ebert MH, Raleigh M, Lake R. Abnormalities in central nervous system monoamine metabolism in anorexia nervosa. Arch Gen Psychiatry. 1984;41:350–355.

[40] Milos G, Spindler A, Schnyder U, Fairburn CG. Instability of eating disorder diagnoses: prospective study. Br J Psychiatry. 2005;187:573–578.

[41] Sallet PC, de Alvarenga PG, Ferrao Y, de Mathis MA, Torres AR, Marques A et al. Eating disorders in patients with obsessive-compulsive disorder: prevalence and clinical correlates. Int J Eat Disord. 2010;43:315–325.

[42] Bandelow B, Zohar J, Hollander E, Kasper S, Moller HJ. World Federation of Societies of Biological Psychiatry (WFSBP) guidelines for the pharmacological treatment of anxiety, obsessive compulsive and posttraumatic stress disorders. World J Biol Psychiatry. 2002;3:171–199.

[43] Kaye WH, Weltzin TE, Hsu LKG, Bulik CM. An open trial of fluoxetine in patients with anorexia nervosa. J Clin Psychiatry. 1991;52:464–471.

[44] Kaye WH, Nagata T, Weltzin TE, Hsu LK, Sokol MS, McConaha C et al. Double-blind placebo-controlled administration of fluoxetine in restricting- and restricting-purging-type anorexia nervosa. Biol Psychiatry. 2001;49:644–652.

[45] Romano S, Halmi K, Sarkar N, Koke S, Lee J. A placebo-controlled study of fluoxetine in continued treatment of bulimia nervosa after successful acute fluoxetine treatment. Am J Psychiatry. 2002;159:96–102.

[46] Lockwood R, Lawson R, Waller G. Compulsive features in the eating disorders: a role for trauma? J Nerv Ment Dis. 2004;192:247–249.

[47] Holden NL. Is anorexia nervosa an obsessive-compulsive disorder?. Br J Psychiatry. 1990;157:1–5.

[48] Altman SE, Shankman SA. What is the association between obsessive compulsive disorder and eating disorders? Clin Psychol Rev. 2009;29:638–641.

[49] Halmi KA, Tozzi F, Thornton LM, Crow S, Fichter MM, Kaplan AS et al. The relation among perfectionism, obsessive-compulsive personality disorder and obsessive-compulsive disorder in individuals with eating disorders. Int J Eat Disord. 2005;38:371–374.

[50] Lilenfeld LR, Stein D, Bulik CM, Strober M, Plotnicov K, Pollice C et al. Personality traits among currently eating disordered, recovered and never ill first degree female relatives of bulimic and control women. Psychol Med. 2000;30:1399–1410.

[51] Kaye WH. Neurobiology of anorexia and bulimia nervosa. Physiol Behav. 2008;94:121–135.

[52] Jiménez-Murcia S, Fernández-Aranda F, Raich RM, Alonso P, Krug I, Jaurrieta N et al. Obsessive-compulsive and eating disorders: comparison of clinical and personality features. Psychiatry Clin Neurosci. 2007;61:385–391.

[53] Beumont PJV, George GCW, Smart DS. "Dieters" and "vomiters and purgers" in anorexia nervosa. Psychol Med. 1976;6:617–622.

[54] Anderluh MB, Tchanturia K, Rabe-Hesketh S, Treasure J. Childhood obsessive-compulsive personality traits in adult women with eating disorders: defining a broader eating disorder phenotype. Am J Psychiatry. 2003;160:242–247.

[55] Woodside DB, Bulik CM, Halmi KA, Fichter MM, Kaplan A, Berrettini WH et al. Personality, perfectionism, and attitudes toward eating in parents of individuals with eating disorders. Int J Eat Disord. 2002;31:290–299.

[56] Garfinkel PE, Garner DM. Anorexia Nervosa—A Multidimensional Perspective. New York: Brunner Mazel; 1982.

[57] Tobiassen LG. Eating Disorders in Obsessive-Compulsive Disorder: Prevalence and Effect on Treatment Outcome. Master's Thesis in Clinical Psychology. Norwegian University of Science and Technology. Autumn; 2013.

[58] Råstam M, Gillberg IC, Gillberg C. Anorexia nervosa 6 years after onset: Part II. Comorbid psychiatric problems. Compr Psychiatry. 1995;36:70–76.

[59] Walters EE, Kendler KS. Anorexia nervosa and anorexic-like syndromes in a population-based female twin sample. Am J Psychiatry. 1995;152:64–71.

[60] Ulfvebrand S, Birgegård A, Norring C, Högdahl L, von Hausswolff-Juhlin Y. Psychiatric comorbidity in women and men with eating disorders results from a large clinical database. Psychiatry Res. 2015;230:294–299. doi:10.1016/j.psychres.2015.09.008

[61] Powers PS, Coovert DL, Brightwell DR, Stevens BA. Other psychiatric disorders among bulimic patients. Compr Psychiatry. 1988;29:503–508.

[62] Schwalberg MD, Barlow DH, Alger SA, Howard LJ. Comparison of bulimics, obese binge eaters, social phobics, and individuals with panic disorder on comorbidity across DSM-III-R anxiety disorders. J Abnorm Psychol. 1992;101:675–681.

[63] Bulik CM, Wade TD, Kendler KS. Characteristics of monozygotic twins discordant for bulimia nervosa. Int J Eat Disord. 2001;29:1–10.

[64] Konstantellou A, Campbell M, Eisler I, Simic M, Treasure J. Testing a cognitive model of generalized anxiety disorder in the eating disorders. J Anxiety Disord. 2011;25(7): 864–869. doi:10.1016/j.janxdis.2011.04.005

[65] Sidor A, Baba CO, Marton-Vasarhelyi E, Chereches RM. Gender differences in the magnitude of the associations between eating disorders symptoms and depression and anxiety symptoms. Results from a community sample of adolescents. J Ment Health. 2015;24:294–298. doi:10.3109/09638237.2015.1022250

[66] Vize CM, Cooper PJ. Sexual abuse in patients with eating disorder, patients with depression, and normal controls. A comparative study. Br J Psychiatry. 1995;167:80–85.

[67] Fallon P. Wonderlich SA. Sexual abuse and other forms of trauma. In D.M. Garner & P.E. Garfinkel (Eds.), Handbook of Treatment for Eating Disorders (2nd ed., pp. 394–414). Guilford: New York., 1997.

[68] Johnson JG, Cohen P, Kasen S, Brook JS. Childhood adversities associated with risk for eating disorders or weight problems during adolescence or early adulthood. Am J Psychiatry. 2002;159:394–400.

[69] Black BC, DeViva J, Zayfert C. Eating disorder symptoms among female anxiety disorder patients in clinical practice: the importance of comorbidity assessment. J Anxiety Disord. 2004;18:255–275.

[70] Turnbull SJ, Troop NA, Treasure JL. The prevalence of posttraumatic stress disorder and its relation to childhood adversity in subjects with eating disorders. Eur Eat Disord Rev. 1997;5:270–277.

[71] Gleaves DH, Eberenz KP, May MC. Scope and significance of posttraumatic symptomatology among women hospitalized for an eating disorder. Int J Eat Disord. 1998;24:147–156.

[72] Brewerton TD, Lydiard RB, Herzog DB, Brotman AW, O'Neil PM, Ballenger JC. Comorbidity of axis I psychiatric disorders in bulimia nervosa. J Clin Psychiatry. 1995;56:77–80.

[73] Faravelli C, Giugni A, Salvatori S, Ricca V. Psychopathology after rape. Am J Psychiatry. 2004;161:1483–1485.

[74] Dahl S. Acute response to rape--a PTSD variant. Acta Psychiatr Scand Suppl. 1989;355:56–62.

[75] Putnam FW, Trickett PK. Psychobiological effects of sexual abuse. A longitudinal study. Ann NY Acad Sci. 1997;821:150–159.

[76] Thompson KM, Crosby RD, Wonderlich SA, Mitchell JE, Redlin J, Demuth G. Psychopathology and sexual trauma in childhood and adulthood. J Trauma Stress. 2003;16:35–38.

[77] Striegel-Moore RH, Garvin V, Dohm FA, Rosenheck R. Eating disorders in a national sample of hospitalized female and male veterans: detection rates and psychiatric comorbidity. Int J Eat Disord. 1999;25:405–414.

[78] Vierling V, Etori S, Valenti L, Lesage M, Pigeyre M, Dodin V et al. Prevalence and impact of post-traumatic stress disorder in a disordered eating population sample. Presse Med. 2015;44:e341–52. doi:10.1016/j.lpm.2015.04.039

[79] Isomaa R, Backholm K, Birgegård A. Posttraumatic stress disorder in eating disorder patients: The roles of psychological distress and timing of trauma. Psychiatry Res. 2015;230:506–510. doi:10.1016/j.psychres.2015.09.044

[80] Becker CB, DeViva JC, Zayfert C. Eating disorder symptoms among female anxiety disorder patients in clinical practice: the importance of anxiety comorbidity assessment. J Anxiety Disord. 2004;18:255–274.

[81] Smolak L, Murnen SK. A meta-analytic examination of the relationship between child sexual abuse and eating disorders. Int J Eat Disord. 2002;31:136–150.

[82] Jacobi C, Hayward C, de Zwaan M, Kraemer HC, Agras WS. Coming to terms with risk factors for eating disorders: application of risk terminology and suggestions for a general taxonomy. Psychol Bull. 2004;130:19–65.

[83] Pribor EF, Dinwiddie SH. Psychiatric correlates of incest in childhood. Am J Psychiatry. 1992;149:52–66.

[84] Rorty M, Yager J, Rossotto E. Childhood sexual, physical, and psychological abuse in bulimia nervosa. Am J Psychiatry. 1994;151:1122–1126.

[85] Dansky BS, Brewerton TD, Kilpatrick DG, O'Neil PM. The National Women's Study: relationship of victimization and posttraumatic stress disorder to bulimia nervosa. Int J Eat Disord. 1997;21:213–228.

[86] Mantero M, Crippa L. Eating Disorders and chronic post traumatic stress disorder: issues of psychopathology and comorbidity. Eur Eat Disord Rev. 2002;10:1–16.

[87] Waller G, Halek C, Crisp AH. Sexual abuse as a factor in anorexia nervosa: evidence from two separate case series. J Psychosom Res. 1993;37:873–879.

[88] Kendler KS, MacLean C, Neale M, Kessler R, Heath A, Eaves L. The genetic epidemiology of bulimia nervosa. Am J Psychiatry. 1991;148:1627–1637.

[89] Godart NT, Flament MF, Perdereau F, Jeammet P. Comorbidity between eating disorders and anxiety disorders: a review. Int J Eat Disord. 2002;32:253–270.

[90] Garfinkel PE, Kennedy SH, Kaplan AS. Views on classification and diagnosis of eating disorders. Can J Psychiatry. 1995; 40:445–456.

[91] Garfinkel PE, Lin E, Goering P, Spegg C, Goldbloom DS, Kennedy S et al. Bulimia nervosa in a Canadian community sample: prevalence and comparison of subgroups. Am J Psychiatry. 1995;152:1052–1058.

[92] Hinrichsen H, Sheffield A, Waller G. The role of parenting experiences in the development of social anxiety and agoraphobia in the eating disorders. Eat Behav. 2007;8:285–290.

[93] Piran N, Kennedy S, Garfinkel PE, Owens M. Affective disturbance in eating disorders. J Nerv Ment Dis. 1985;173:395–400.

[94] Hudson JI, Pope HG Jr, Jonas JM, Yurgelun-Todd D. Phenomenologic relationship of eating disorders to major affective disorder. Psychiatry Res. 1983;9:345–354.

[95] Hinrichsen H, Waller G, van Gerko K. Social anxiety and agoraphobia in the eating disorders: associations with eating attitudes and behaviours. Eat Behav. 2004;5:285–290.

[96] Powers PS, Coovert DL, Brightwell DR, Stevens BA. Other psychiatric disorders among bulimic patients. Compr Psychiatry. 1988;29:503–508.

[97] Black Becker C, DeViva J, Zayfert C. Eating disorder symptoms among female anxiety disorder patients in clinical practice: the importance of comorbidity assessment. J Anxiety Disord. 2004;18:255–275.

[98] Hinrichsen H, Wright F, Waller G, Meyer C. Social anxiety and coping strategies in the eating disorders. Eat Behav. 2003;4:117–126.

[99] Blinder BJ, Chaitlin BF, Goldstein R. (Eds). The Eating Disorders: Medical and Psychological Bases of Diagnosis and Treatment. PMA Publications: New York; 1988.

[100] Woolsey MM. Eating Disorders: A Clinical Guide to Counseling and Treatment. American Dietetic Association: Chicago, 2002.

[101] Boutelle KN. The use of exposure with response prevention in a male anorexic. J Behav Ther Exp Psychiatry. 1998;29:79–84.

[102] Goodwin RD, Fitzgibbon ML. Social anxiety as a barrier to treatment for eating disorders. Int J Eat Disord. 2002;32:103–106.

[103] Fichter MM, Quadflieg N. Twelve-year course and outcome of bulimia nervosa. Psychol Med. 2004;34:1395–406.

[104] Fichter MM, Quadflieg N, Hedlund S. Twelve-year course and outcome predictors of anorexia nervosa. Int J Eat Disord. 2006;39:87–100.

[105] Thompson-Brenner H, Westen D. A naturalistic study of psychotherapy for bulimia nervosa, part 1: comorbidity and therapeutic outcome. J Nerv Ment Dis. 2005;193:573–584.

[106] Procopio CA, Holm-Denoma JM, Gordon KH, Joiner TE Jr. Two-three-year stability and interrelations of bulimotypic indicators and depressive and anxious symptoms in middle-aged women. Int J Eat Disord. 2006;39:312–319.

[107] Torem MS, Curdue K. PTSD presenting as an eating disorder. Stress Med. 1988;4:139–142.

Section 3

Course and Prognosis

Chapter 7

The Patient's Perspective: Exploring Factors that Contribute to Recovery from Eating Disorders

Fragiskos Gonidakis and
Dafni-Alexandra Karapavlou

Additional information is available at the end of the chapter

http://dx.doi.org/10.5772/65303

Abstract

Eating Disorders (EDs) are quite distinct and difficult to treat mental disorders. Remarkably, when reviewing studies on the recovery process of ED's, the patients' experience of the therapeutic process has rarely been taken into account. To address the issue of the patients perspective on their recovery a study was conducted among ED patients. The main aims of the study were to investigate treatment factors, according to the patients view, that contributed to their recovery. Also, if there was any significant improvement within the first six months of the treatment and whether subjective improvement was in accordance with objective ED improvement and finally possible, if any, differences between different diagnostic groups.

Overall, four major conclusions were produced. First, most of the patients appreciate a structured therapy in a specialized unit for EDs with a caring therapist that can form a strong therapeutic alliance with them. Second, most of the patients regard as recovery a change that goes beyond ED symptomatology to a more "holistic" improvement. Third, the patients opinion on therapy and recovery is not influenced by the diagnosis of the ED. Finally, the opinion of the patient and the objective evaluation of recovery present more similarities than differences.

Keywords: eating disorders, anorexia nervosa, bulimia nervosa, recovery, patients' perspective, therapeutic alliance, therapy

1. Introduction

Eating disorders (EDs) are a group of mental disorders that are quite distinct and difficult to treat, as they manifest through a number of unique characteristics:

a. Although they are not considered to be a type of psychosis, there are a number of patients suffering from anorexia nervosa (AN) who lack insight on and express delusional beliefs about primarily their body image [1].

b. The diagnosis of ED often does not remain stable over the years. It is not uncommon to observe a patient suffering from AN during adolescence, bulimia nervosa (BN) or other specified feeding and eating disorders (OSFEDs) during early adulthood and binge eating disorder (BED) during middle age. This has led a number of researchers to suggest a "transdiagnostic" approach to ED classification and therapy [2, 3].

c. The first line of treatment for EDs is psychotherapy [4]. The difficulty with the application of psychotherapy, however, is that when treating patients whose symptomatology is highly reinforced, as is the case with EDs, then its effectiveness is substantially reduced. Moreover, a considerable number of patients, especially those suffering from AN, drop out of therapy for a variety of reasons [5].

d. The course of EDs is long; in many cases, patients need several years to recover. Moreover, a substantial number of patients do not recover fully or even partially and run the risk of developing a chronic disorder [6, 7].

Overall, these four points stress the necessity of improving the available therapeutic interventions. It is alarming that there are published studies on AN reporting that specialized psychotherapeutic interventions are only equally or less effective than nonspecific supportive clinical management for the disorder [8]. Remarkably, when reviewing studies on the recovery process of EDs, the patient's experience of the therapeutic process has rarely been taken into account. The patient's perspective can and must play an important role on the development of new or the improvement of existing therapeutic interventions.

2. The patient's perspective of recovery from eating disorders

Over the last 20 years, patient evaluation of treatment has been a topic of a small number of studies. The earlier studies, which were published between 1990 and 2005, showed that most of the patients who were interviewed preferred individual therapy, group therapy and self-help groups than other forms of treatment, such as inpatient programs [9, 10]. Interestingly, the more "specialized" therapies, such as behavioral and family therapy, were not regarded positively by the patients [9, 10]. The majority of the patients were more satisfied when they were treated in a specialized unit for ED's or by a therapist experienced specifically in ED therapy [10, 11]. Moreover, in clinical practice, there are patients who report that their need to be understood was often not met when they were treated by therapists who were not specialized in ED. The initial focus of treatment in weight gain and nutritional restoration seemed to be regarded positively by some patients and negatively by others [11–13]. A qualitative study showed that patients suffering from an ED preferred psychological types of treatment whereas medical interventions that focused exclusively on weight were not regarded as useful [14].

A more recent study, conducted in the Netherlands, evaluated the treatment of EDs from the patients' perspective in a large community-based sample. This study showed that treatment in specialized ED centers, self-help groups and treatments with a partner were reported to be most helpful [15]. The patients reported that the communication skills of mental health professionals, the therapist/patient working alliance, contact with peers and focus of treatment on ED symptoms as well as underlying issues were the most beneficial elements of their treatment [15].

2.1. Subjective vs. objective recovery

Most of the research on the outcome of EDs has been focused on the reduction in associated symptomatology, primarily nutrition restoration, normalization of body weight and absence of purging behaviors. While the above changes are *sina qua non* for achieving remission, it has been reported that when only these somatic criteria were considered, 79% of AN patients were considered recovered; when psychological criteria were taken into account, however, the recovery rate fell to 49% [16]. Moreover, a common observation in clinical practice is that when some patients "recover" from ED symptomatology, they become extremely anxious, distressed or even depressed. It becomes obvious that a gap might exist between the "official" recovery as measured by the researchers and the subjective evaluation of being well and free of the ED's "golden cage." Noordenbos and Seubring created a list of 52 possible criteria for recovery. This list represents the domains of eating behavior, body experience, physical and psychological well-being, and emotional and social functioning. They asked therapists and expatients to select the criteria that they viewed as important for recovery from EDs [17]. Interestingly, they found that the two groups agreed on most of the criteria for recovery. Considering the patients' experience at the end of their treatment, only four criteria had been realized by more than 80% of the patients: "I do not vomit," "I do not use laxatives," "I do not use diuretics" and "I do not use slimming pills." On the other hand, it is striking that three of the five criteria for body experience had been realized by less than 50% of the patients at the end of their treatment. Finally, three criteria were evaluated by both expatients and therapists as not important for recovery: regular menstruation, dental health and intimate relationships [17].

2.2. The therapist's characteristics

According to the patients' view, the therapist and especially a feeling of trust toward the therapist were the most important elements of what they considered high-quality therapy [18, 19]. The patients believed that a good therapist needs to have "good communication skills, knowledge of and experience with EDs, the ability to facilitate engaging in a relationship with the patient, to listen to the patient, to stand beside the patient and work together, and to focus on the person and not the disorder" [18]. Therapists having specific expertise in EDs seem to be very important elements for a positive outcome of the therapy, both for the patients and their families [19]. Furthermore, the way that the therapist interacts with the patient plays a major role in the treatment's success, according to patient opinion. A positive encounter with the therapist can make the patient feel understandable, less alone, safe, valuable and in a better mood; a negative encounter can increase self-blame, loss of feeling of identity and desire to prove that she/he is "really sick," as well as decreased willingness to disclose, which can eventually lead to dropping out of therapy [20]. The "good" therapist characteristics can be summarized in four factors: "acceptance" of the individual's personality, preferences and difficulties; "vitality" in showing active interest in the patient's ideas, thoughts and problems; "challenging" the situation created by the ED symptomatology, focusing on the patient's resources, and offering active support while not pampering him/her and finally, "expertise" in the area of ED treatment so that he/she can offer security and guidance during therapy [19].

2.3. The importance of therapeutic alliance

The patient/therapist alliance has been acknowledged as a key element of the therapeutic process and a successful outcome in numerous studies across a range of treatment modalities and research settings [21]. It is not uncommon for the ED patient and therapist to have different opinions on therapeutic goals and the definition of their alliance and its dimensions. As one might expect, converging perspectives have been associated with positive outcome and vice versa [22]. Research data on the therapeutic alliance components have shown that patients view alliance in six basic components: collaborative work relationship, productive work, active commitment, bond, nondisagreement on goals/tasks and confident progress. Meanwhile, the therapists view alliance in four basic components: collaborative work relationship, therapist confidence and dedication, client commitment and confidence and client working ability [22]. Although there are similarities between the patients' and the therapists' view of therapeutic alliance, there are also differences. Patients appear to place greater emphasis on helpfulness, joint participation in the work of therapy and negative signs of the alliance [22].

Although the patient/therapist alliance has not been specifically investigated in the area of ED's research, the studies that compare the patients' and the therapists' opinions on the elements that are important for recovery from EDs have shown considerable converging perspectives [23]. Vanderlinden et al. have reported that "improving self-esteem," "improving body experience" and "learning problem solving skills" were considered core elements of the treatment by both the patients and their therapists [23].

2.4. Quality of life

The quality of life (QoL) of ED patients has been reported to be poor. Severity of ED symptomatology, especially low body mass index (BMI), but not duration of illness has been found to be predictive of low QoL [24]. Moreover, in terms of differences across diagnostic groups, individuals with a diagnosis of AN were found to have lower psychological and physical/cognitive QoL than those with an OSFED or BN diagnosis [24]. Even after long-term treatment or recovery from EDs, the expatients reported only a slight improvement in their QoL [18]. In most cases, the QoL remained poorer than controls [25, 26]. Self-image and well-being are often reported by current ED patients as the most affected areas of their QoL [18]. The patients mention that a sense of belonging, work or education, good physical health and a general sense of well-being are the most important elements of good QoL [18].

2.5. Self-efficacy

Another construct that can be explored through the patient's perspective of their ED recovery is self-efficacy. Self-efficacy has been defined as the individual's perceived ability to perform a particular behavior [27]. When considering EDs, self-efficacy can be thought of as the individual's subjective positive evaluation of his/her ability to eat without engaging in eating disordered behavior and to maintain a realistic body image [28]. There are ED studies showing that patients' self-efficacy around eating increases with treatment and is directly related with improvement in objective measurements, such as duration of hospitalization, drive for thinness and body dissatisfaction [29].

3. The study on the patients' perspective of therapy and recovery

The study was conducted among patients suffering from an ED who were treated at the Eating Disorders Unit of National and Kapodistrian University of Athens, 1st Psychiatric Department.

3.1. Aims

The main aims of the study were to investigate the following:

1. treatment factors, according to the patients' view, which contributed to their recovery;
2. the recovery criteria that had been identified by the patients during the first 6 months of their treatment;
3. if there was any significant improvement within the first 6 months of the treatment and whether subjective improvement was in accordance with objective improvement of ED symptomatology; and
4. possible differences, if any, between diagnostic groups regarding their perception of recovery and therapy.

3.2. Methodology

3.2.1. Procedure

Each patient was approached during the initial assessment interview. The diagnosis of ED was confirmed by a psychiatrist specialized in EDs according to DSM-5 criteria. It should be noted, however, that due to the fact that the Eating Disorders Unit does not treat patients suffering from BED, the diagnosis of ED was either AN, BN or OSFED. The latter group consisted mainly of anorectic-type or bulimic-type patients who did not meet the full criteria for the diagnosis of AN or BN.

During the initial interview, the body mass index (BMI) of each patient was calculated following the measurement of her/his height and body weight. Also, the questionnaires for the measurement of ED symptomatology, quality of life and demographic data were administered. After the initial interview, every patient who was eligible for treatment was assigned to a psychologist or psychiatrist specialized in cognitive behavioral therapy (CBT) for EDs. The inclusion criteria were diagnosis of an ED; age >17 years; adequate knowledge of the Greek language; and lack of psychosis, neurological disorders and substance misuse. Each therapist had weekly group supervision meetings with one of the authors (Fragiskos Gonidakis). All participants were contacted again by the main researcher (Dafni-Alexandra Karapavlou) 6 months after their first session. During the 6 months, the questionnaires on the subjective experience of therapy and recovery were administered alongside measurements of ED symptomatology and QoL Written informed consent, according to the Declaration of Helsinki, was obtained from all participants.

3.2.2. Instruments

For the objective measurement of improvement and recovery, the following questionnaires were used:

1. Eating Disorders Examination-Questionnaire (EDE-Q). The EDE-Q is a self-report questionnaire developed by Fairburn and Wilson [30]. It consists of 36 questions on eating behavior, clustered in four subscales: restraint, eating concern, shape concern and weight concern. Each question is rated on a 6-point Likert type scale and addresses the patient's last 28 days. When appropriate, respondents are requested to provide a frequency count. In a recent study by Giovazolias et al. [31], the validity of the Greek version of EDE-Q was investigated. The authors concluded that the results supported both the internal consistency, as well as the concurrent, convergent and discriminant validity of the EDE-Q global scale and its subscales.

2. World Health Organization Quality of Life Brief questionnaire (WHOQOL-BREF). The World Health Organization Quality of Life (QoL) questionnaire is a self-report inventory of QoL with 26 original items and 4 additional items, derived from the validation of the questionnaire within Greek populations [32, 33]. The items fall into four domains: (a) physical health, (b) psychological health, (c) social relationships and (d) environment. Each item is rated on a 5-point Likert type scale and score ranges between 1 and 20; higher scores indicate better QoL. The Greek version of the WHOQOL-BREF has demonstrated good internal consistency, with Cronbach's α ranging from 0.67 to 0.81 per domain [33].

For the subjective patient experience of therapy and recovery, the following questionnaires were used:

1. Criteria on Eating Disorders Treatment Questionnaire (CEDT): To assess the quality of treatment from the patients' perspective, the CEDT was developed by the authors. The CEDT was based on the third part of the "Questionnaire for Eating Problems and Treatment" developed by de la Rie et al. [18]. Participants were asked to rate 70 items on a 5-point Likert type scale to assess the importance of each item for their treatment. The 70 items covered three major domains: treatment content, professionals involved in the treatment and the mental health facility that provides the treatment. Lastly, of the 70 items on the list, participants were asked to rank the 10 most important to them.

An exploratory principal component analysis (PCA) with varimax rotation was carried out to identify relevant factors of the 70 items regarding treatment. The results indicated that CEDT consists of a 6-factor structure: acceptance and bond with therapist, mastery and eating behaviors, treatment modalities, inpatient treatment, therapy structure and focus on underlying problems. Higher scores indicate higher importance of the factor. Cronbach's alphas were calculated to determine the reliability of the six identified factors, and the psychometric properties of the six scales were satisfactory (Cronbach's αs ranging from 0.782 to 0.848).

2. Criteria for Recovery from Eating Disorders Questionnaire. Noordenbos and Seubring [17] developed the Criteria for Recovery from Eating Disorders questionnaire. For the purpose of measuring the patients' experience of recovery, they created a list of the core characteristics and consequences of EDs based on the literature and on the criteria for recovery mentioned in effect and follow-up studies. They categorized these characteristics and consequences into groups representing somatic, behavioral, psychological, emotional and social factors. This procedure resulted in a list of 52 recovery criteria: 9 items related to eating behavior, 5 items concerning body attitude, 16 items on physical recovery, 8 items on psychological well-being, 9 items on emotional state and 5 items on social adjustment. Each item is rated on a 5-point Likert type scale, with higher scores indicating better feeling of recovery. Psychometric properties of the Greek version of the questionnaire with 6 subscales were satisfactory (Cronbach's αs ranging from 0.613 to 0.885).

Finally, additional information on sociodemographic characteristics, treatment history, weight history, hospitalization and medication history was obtained through a relevant questionnaire.

4. Participants

Of the 65 patients who were approached and were eligible to participate in the study, one refused to participate, possibly due to paranoid personality traits that made her oversuspicious about the "underlying true aim" of the study. From the 64 remaining patients, 42 completed the 6-month period of therapy (dropout rate: 34.4%). Forty of the completers were female and two were male. Regarding diagnosis, 17 were suffering from anorexia nervosa (AN), 18 from bulimia nervosa (BN) and seven from OSFED. The mean age of the participants was 26.7 (ranging from 17 to 47 years old). The mean age of ED onset was 18.5 (ranging from 7 to 31 years old). The mean duration of previous treatments was 3 years and 1 month (ranging from 1 month to 16 years). Half of the participants were university students (50%).

5. Statistical analysis

The mean scores of the answers to the CEDT and the Criteria for Recovery from Eating Disorders questionnaire were used as a way of ranking the most important factors according to the patients. The EDE-Q 6-month and WHOQOL-BREF initial and 6-month measurements followed a normal distribution while the EDE-Q initial measurement did not. For this reason, a paired sample *t*-test was used only for the comparison of the WHOQOL-BREF measurements; the Wilcoxon signed-rank test was selected to assess improvement in ED symptomatology measured by EDE-Q before treatment and after 6 months.

A one-way ANOVA was performed to assess possible differences between the three ED diagnostic groups. Finally, Pearson's bivariate correlations were performed to assess possible correlations between objective and subjective perceptions of ED symptomatology improvement.

6. Results

6.1. Patients' view on the quality of treatment

Table 1 summarizes the standardized mean scores of all CEDT factors for each of the three ED diagnostic groups. All the factors were found to contribute to the quality of treatment, having high mean scores, except for the "inpatient treatment" subscale. This was probably due to the fact that most of the participants have never been hospitalized in a mental health facility. "Acceptance and bond with therapist," "therapy structure and information" and "mastery and eating behaviors" had the highest mean scores. This result indicated that participants believed that therapeutic alliance, structured psychotherapy, and focus on how to gain control over ED symptomatology were vastly contributing to their therapy successful outcome. These three subscales were followed by "treatment modalities" and "focus on underlying problems" in terms of highest mean scores. As mentioned previously, the least identified factor was "inpatient treatment." A one-way ANOVA to compare differences between AN, BN and OSFED groups did not show any significant differences between diagnostic groups with the CEDT subscales (**Table 1**).

A great variety were found in the ranking of individual CEDT treatment factors. The most often mentioned factor was "focus on the transition back to normal life." This was mentioned by 35.9% of the participants. Also, "focus on self-esteem" was mentioned by 31.1%, "focus on underlying problems" by 21.5% and "trust in therapist" by 21.4%. The factors that were not selected at all as important by any of the participants were the following: "being able to talk about religion," "being able to tell your story," "therapist with enough time," "therapist with a sense of humor," "the location for treatment should be easily reached," "explanation about somatic complaints and consequences of the eating disorder," "receiving standardized treatment," "companion as tutor/counselor," "role-playing as part of treatment" and " talking in groups."

A Pearson's bivariate correlation analysis between CEDT and the 6-month EDE-Q subscales showed that "acceptance and bond with T = therapist" was positively correlated only with patients' BMI ($r = 0.4$, $p = 0.09$), "therapy structure" with EDE-Q's weight ($r = 0.45$, $p = 0.03$) and shape concerns ($r = 0.4$, $p = 0.01$) and "inpatient treatment" with EDE-Q's eating ($r = 0.34$, $p = 0.03$), weight ($r = 0.4$, $p = 0.01$) and shape concerns ($r = 0.45$, $p = 0.03$).

CEDT factors	Diagnosis	N	Mean	Std. deviation	Minimum	Maximum	ANOVA	
							F	p
Acceptance and bond with therapist	AN	17	50.24	4.10	43.00	55.00		
	BN	18	51.00	3.71	40.00	55.00	1.1	0.3
	EDNOS	7	52.71	2.36	49.00	55.00		
	Total	42	50.98	3.72	40.00	55.00		
Mastery and eating behaviors	AN	17	47.88	3.92	39.00	53.00		
	BN	18	44.83	6.87	28.00	52.00	2.2	0.1
	EDNOS	7	49.29	4.64	42.00	55.00		
	Total	42	46.81	5.65	28.00	55.00		
Treatment modalities	AN	17	31.85	6.72	19.00	42.00		
	BN	18	27.44	8.75	15.00	42.00	2.1	0.1
	EDNOS	7	34.00	10.55	20.00	49.00		
	Total	42	30.32	8.52	15.00	49.00		
Inpatient treatment	AN	17	19.29	4.24	12.00	25.00		
	BN	18	17.94	5.79	5.00	25.00	0.3	0.8
	EDNOS	7	18.66	6.55	5.00	25.00		
	Total	42	18.61	5.25	5.00	25.00		
Therapy structure	AN	17	49.52	6.47	39.00	58.00		
	BN	18	47.44	6.27	33.00	56.00	1.3	0.3
	EDNOS	7	52.00	7.19	39.00	60.00		
	Total	42	49.04	6.55	33.00	60.00		
Underlying problems	AN	17	31.18	3.84	24.00	35.00		
	BN	18	28.94	4.99	19.00	35.00	1.3	0.3
	EDNOS	7	31.14	3.72	26.00	35.00		
	Total	42	30.21	4.40	19.00	35.00		

Table 1. Criteria for eating disorders treatment questionnaire.

6.2. Objective and subjective recovery

A Wilcoxon signed-rank test indicated that there were significant differences in the ED symptomatology scores in both the overall and subscale scores of the EDE-Q questionnaire, showing important improvement over the 6 months of treatment (**Table 2**). A paired sample *t*-test was conducted to compare QoL before and after 6 months of treatment. Significant improvement of QoL was found only in the general health scores ($t = 3.7$, $p = 0.001$) and the psychological domain scores ($t = 4.5$, $p = 0.0001$).

EDE-Q		Descriptives	Wilcoxon signed-rank test	
Subscales		**Median**	**Z**	**p**
Eating concerns	0 month	3.4	3.16	0.002
	6th month	2.4		
Restraint	0 month	4.2	3.44	0.001
	6th month	2.4		
Shape concerns	0 month	4.8	2.76	0.006
	6th month	3.7		
Weight concerns	0 month	4.5	2.74	0.006
	6th month	2.9		
Total score	0 month	4.2	3.31	0.001
	6th month	2.9		

Table 2. Change in EDE-Q scores after 6 months of treatment.

Regarding the patients' view on the criteria of recovery, "physical recovery" had the highest mean score (mean = 48.1), followed by "emotional recovery" (mean = 31.3), "psychological recovery" (mean = 30.1) and "social recovery" (mean = 29.5). The least recognized areas of improvement were "eating behavior recovery" (mean = 28.6) and "body image recovery" (mean = 14.6). Again, a one-way ANOVA to compare differences between AN, BN and OSFED groups did not show any significant differences between diagnostic groups in their perception of recovery (**Table 3**).

Criteria for recovery subscales	F score	p value
Eating behaviors recovery	0.33	0.9
Body image recovery	1.64	0.21
Physical recovery	2.87	0.07
Psychological recovery	1.1	0.35
Emotional recovery	0.6	0.6
Social recovery	1.8	0.18

Table 3. Analysis of variance of the criteria for recovery questionnaire scores, according to the diagnosis of ED.

Pearson's bivariate correlation coefficient was computed to assess the relationship between the objective symptomatology improvement, as was measured by the EDE-Q, and the subjective improvement, as was rated by the patients (**Table 4**). Overall, there was a strong correlation between the ED symptomatology and the patients' subjective experience of psychological recovery. The feelings of improvement in self-esteem and body image, as well as reduction in self-judgment and negative feelings, were correlated with ED psychopathology. Finally, Pearson's bivariate correlation coefficient was also computed to assess the relationship between the WHOQOL-BREF QoL improvement and the subjective improvement as was rated by the patients (**Table 5**). The stronger correlations were between objective social recovery and the WHOQL-BREF social relationships and overall recovery constructs and WHOQOL-BREF's psychological domain. Social recovery, emotional recovery, psychological recovery and overall recovery showed higher correlations with the improvement in the patients' QoL.

		EDE-Q				
Eating disorder recovery criteria		**Eating concern**	**Restraint**	**Shape concern**	**Weight concern**	**Total EDE-Q**
Eating behaviors recovery	r	−0.044	−0.127	−0.042	−0.024	−0.069
Body image recovery	r	**−0.408****	−0.186	**−0.391***	**−0.387***	**−0.386***
Physical recovery	r	−0.181	−0.176	−0.132	−0.107	−0.169
Psychological recovery	r	**−0.451****	**−0.386***	**−0.436****	**−0.466****	**−0.493****
Emotional recovery	r	−0.204	**−0.309***	−0.034	−0.016	−0.160
Social recovery	r	−0.264	−0.013	−0.005	0.001	−0.072

*Correlation is significant at the 0.05 level (2-tailed).
**Correlation is significant at the 0.01 level (2-tailed).

Table 4. Correlation between EDE-Q and criteria for recovery questionnaire.

WHOQOL-BREF						
Eating disorder recovery criteria		**Overall QoL**	**Physical domain**	**Psychological domain**	**Social domain**	**Environmental domain**
Eating behaviors recovery	r	−0.018	0.082	−0.048	−0.016	0.148
Body image recovery	r	0.070	**0.352***	**0.312***	0.054	−0.098
Physical recovery	r	0.109	**0.314***	0.246	0.250	0.126
Psychological recovery	r	0.298	**0.402 ****	**0.551 ****	**0.410 ****	−0.035
Emotional recovery	r	**0.423 ****	**0.386 ***	**0.387 ***	**0.468 ****	**0.444 ****
Social recovery	r	**0.551****	**0.454****	**0.452****	**0.653****	0.291

*Correlation is significant at the 0.05 level (2-tailed).
**Correlation is significant at the 0.01 level (2-tailed).

Table 5. Correlation between WHOQOL-BREF and criteria for recovery questionnaire.

7. Discussion

The first main aim of this study was to explore factors that are regarded by ED's patients as important elements of successful treatment. ED's patients stress the importance of feeling accepted and having a good relationship with their therapist. The importance of the therapeutic alliance in relation to therapy outcome is supported also by other studies [18]. Having a good relationship with the therapist and a feeling of acceptance in therapy were also found to correlate with normal BMI. Moreover, therapy structure and focus on ED recovery were considered very important by the patients. This could refect the fact that when applying for therapy, adult ED patients have often reached a point when ED symptomatology has become highly egodystonic and disruptive for their everyday life; as such, the patients are eager to experience a reduction in the severity of their symptomatology as soon as possible [34].

The second aim was to investigate the factors that the patients regard as important for their recovery. The recovery criteria that were mostly recognized by the patients were physical, emotional and psychological. From the patients' view, it seems that the improvement in ED symptomatology is mostly attributed to their perceptions of psychological recovery. This finding is supported by previous studies, which have shown that a medical, iatrogenic approach is not found helpful by patients [35].

The third aim of the study was to explore whether patients' subjective experiences of recovery were in accordance with objective improvements in ED symptomatology, as well as improvement in their QoL. More specifically, their perception of improvement in the psychological, emotional and social domains was highly correlated with improvement in the corresponding fields in their QoL, as well as in their overall QoL. This finding might suggest that when ED therapy focuses on improving the individual's psychological, emotional and social condition, this could result in reduction in ED symptomatology and QoL improvement or vice versa.

The results indicate that while there was an overall improvement in ED symptomatology during the first 6 months of treatment, some of the QoL domains did not show significant improvement. This could be explained by the short-time period between the two measurements, especially when considering that the mean duration of illness was 8.2 years.

Another point that needs to be taken into consideration is the discrepancy that might exist between the therapist's opinion and the psychometric measures that are used during the course of ED treatment [36]. It has been demonstrated that the "opinion" of the therapeutic team about the patients' treatment course has to be considered along different psychological, psychopathological and eating-related variables. Although for about 90% of the patients, there is a convergent between the therapist's clinical assessment of the therapy's outcome and the assessment by questionnaire, 10% of patients can be missclassified [36].

Finally, it was interesting that there was not any difference between the diagnostic subgroups of ED patients in regard to factors that were important to them for their therapy and recovery. This finding is in line with the notion that in the area of EDs, we could apply a transdiagnostic treatment model, as AN, BN and atypical EDs share common psychopathological mechanisms and can respond to a "universal" therapeutic process [23, 37].

8. Conclusions

"Listen to what your patient is trying to tell you" is a phrase that is very often repeated in psychotherapy training and supervision meetings. Although to listen to your patient is common ground in psychotherapy, it is a novel area of research in the field of EDs. Overall, four major conclusions came out of the literature review and the study's results. First, most of the patients appreciate a structured therapy in a specialized unit for EDs with a caring therapist who can form a strong therapeutic alliance with them. Second, most of the patients regard recovery as a change that goes beyond ED symptomatology and into a more "holistic" improvement in their psychological, physical and social well-being. Third, the patients' opinion on therapy and recovery is not influenced by the diagnosis of the ED that they are suffering from. Finally, when compared, the opinion of the patient and the evaluation from the therapist or the appropriate clinical research measurements have more similarities than differences.

Author details

Fragiskos Gonidakis* and Dafni-Alexandra Karapavlou

*Address all correspondence to: fragoni@yahoo.com

Eating Disorders Unit, 1st Department of Psychiatry, National and Kapodistrian University of Athens, Greece

References

[1] Konstantakopoulos G, Varsou E, Dikeos D, Ioannidi N, Gonidakis F, Papadimitriou G, Oulis P: Delusionality of body image beliefs in eating disorders. Psychiatry Res. 2012;200(2–3):482–488. doi: 10.1016/j.psychres.2012.03.023.

[2] Fairburn CG, Cooper Z: Eating disorders, DSM-5 and clinical reality. Br J Psychiatry. 2011;198(1):8–10. doi: 10.1192/bjp.bp.110.083881.

[3] Wade TD, Bergin JL, Martin NG, Gillespie NA, Fairburn CG: A transdiagnostic approach to understanding eating disorders. J Nerv Ment Dis. 2006;194(7):510–517.

[4] National Institute for Clinical Excellence. Eating Disorders. London: British Psychological Society and the Royal College of Psychiatrists; 2004.

[5] Campbell M: Drop-out from treatment for the eating disorders: a problem for clinicians and researchers. Eur Eat Disord Rev. 2009;17(4):239–242. doi: 10.1002/erv.93.

[6] Smink FR, van Hoeken D, Hoek HW: Epidemiology, course, and outcome of eating disorders. Curr Opin Psychiatry. 2013;26(6):543–548. doi: 10.1097/YCO.0b013e328365a24f.

[7] Keel PK, Brown TA: Update on course and outcome in eating disorders. Int J Eat Disord. 2010;43(3):195–204. doi: 10.1002/eat.20810.

[8] Carter FA, Jordan J, McIntosh VV, Luty SE, McKenzie JM, Frampton CM, Bulik CM, Joyce PR. The long-term efficacy of three psychotherapies for anorexia nervosa: a randomized, controlled trial. Int J Eat Disord. 2011;44(7):647–654. doi: 10.1002/eat.20879.

[9] Newton T, Hartley D, Sturmey P: Treatment evaluation for eating disorders by clients with eating disorders. Behav Cogn Psychother. 1993;21:371–374.

[10] Rosenvinge JH, Klusmeier AK: Treatment for eating disorders from a patient satisfaction perspective: a Norwegian replication of a British study. Eur Eat Disord Rev. 2000;8:293–300.

[11] Swain-Campbell NR, Surgenor LJ, Snell DL: An analysis of consumer perspectives following contact with an eating disorders service. Aust N Z J Psychiatry. 2001;35:99–103.

[12] Clinton D: Expectations and experiences of treatment in eating disorders. Eat Disord J Treat Prev. 2001;9:361–371.

[13] Clinton D, Bjorck C, Sohlberg S, Norring C: Patient satisfaction with treatment in eating disorders: cause for complacency or concern? Eur Eat Disord Rev. 2004;12:240–246.

[14] Bell L: What can we learn from consumer studies and qualitative research in the treatment of eating disorders? Eat Weight Disord. 2003;8:181–187.

[15] de la Rie S, Noordenbos G, Donker M, van Furth E: Evaluating the treatment of eating disorders from the patient's perspective. Int J Eat Disord. 2006;39(8):667–676.

[16] Saccomani L, Savoini M, Cirrincione M: Long term outcome of children and adolescents with anorexia nervosa: study of comorbidity. J Psychosom Res. 1998;44:565–571.

[17] Noordenbos G, Seubring A: Criteria for recovery from eating disorders according to patients and therapists. Eat Disord. 2006;14(1):41–54.

[18] de la Rie S, Noordenbos G, Donker M, van Furth E: The quality of treatment of eating disorders: a comparison of the therapists' and the patients' perspective. Int J Eat Disord. 2008;41(4):307–317.

[19] Halvorsen I, Heyerdahl S: Treatment perception in adolescent onset anorexia nervosa: retrospective views of patients and parents. Int J Eat Disord. 2007;40(7):629–639.

[20] Gulliksen KS, Espeset EM, Nordbø RH, Skårderud F, Geller J, Holte A. Preferred therapist characteristics in treatment of anorexia nervosa: the patient's perspective. Int J Eat Disord. 2012;45(8):932–941. doi: 10.1002/eat.22033.

[21] Horvath A. The therapeutic relationship: from transference to alliance. J Clin Psychol. 2000;56(2):163–173.

[22] Bachelor A: Clients' and therapists' views of the therapeutic alliance: similarities, differences and relationship to therapy outcome. Clin Psychol Psychother. 2013;20(2): 118–135. doi: 10.1002/cpp.792. Epub 2011 Nov 14.

[23] Vanderlinden J, Buis H, Pieters G, Probst M: Which elements in the treatment of eating disorders are necessary 'ingredients' in the recovery process? – a comparison between the patient's and therapist's view. Eur Eat Disord Rev. 2007;15(5):357–365.

[24] Bamford B, Sly R: Exploring quality of life in the eating disorders. Eur Eat Disord Rev. 2010;18(2):147–153. doi: 10.1002/erv.975.

[25] De la Rie SM, Noordenbos G, Van Furth EF: Quality of life and eating disorders. Qual Life Res. 2005;14:1511–1522.

[26] Padierna A, Quintana JM, Arostegui I, Gonzalez N, Horcajo MJ: Changes in health related quality of life among patients treated for eating disorders. Qual Life Res. 2002;11:542–552.

[27] Bandura A: Self-efficacy: toward a unifying theory of behavioral change. Psychol Rev. 1977;84(2):191–215.

[28] Pinto AM, Guarda AS, Heinberg LJ, DiClemente CC: Development of the eating disorder recovery self-efficacy questionnaire. Int J Eat Disord. 2006;39:376–384.

[29] Pinto AM, Heinberg LJ, Coughlin JW, Fava JL, Guarda AS: The Eating Disorder Recovery Self-Efficacy Questionnaire (EDRSQ): change with treatment and prediction of outcome. Eat Behav. 2008;9(2):143–153. doi: 10.1016/j.eatbeh.2007.07.001.

[30] Fairburn CG, Wilson GT. Binge Eating: Nature, Assessment and Treatment. New York: Guilford Press; 1993.

[31] Giovazolias T, Tsaousis I, Vallianatou C: The factor structure and psychometric properties of the Greek version of the Eating Disorders Examination Questionnaire (EDE-Q). Eur J Psychol Assess. 2013;29(3):189–196.

[32] The WHOQOL Group: Development of the World Health Organization WHOQOL-BREF quality of life assessment. Psychol Med. 2008;28(3):551–558. doi: 10.1017/S0033291798006667.

[33] Ginieri-Coccossis M, Triantafillou E, Tomaras V, Soldatos C, Mavreas V, Christodoulou G: Psychometric properties of WHOQOL-BREF in clinical and health Greek populations: incorporating new culture-relevant items. Psychiatriki. 2012;23(2):130–142.

[34] Anderluh MB, Tchanturia K, Rabe-Hesketh S, Treasure J: Childhood obsessive-compulsive personality traits in adult women with eating disorders: defining a broader eating disorder phenotype. Am J Psychiatry. 2003;160:242–247.

[35] Tozzi F, Sullivan PF, Fear JL, McKenzie J, Bulik CM: Causes and recovery in anorexia nervosa: the patient's perspective. Int J Eat Disord. 2003;33(2):143–154. doi: 10.1002/eat.10120.

[36] Jáuregui-Lobera I, Garrido-Casals O, Santiago MJ, Bolaños-Ríos P, Ruiz-Prieto I: Does the opinion of the therapeutic team match with psychometric measures during the course of eating disorders? Nutr Hosp. 2013;28:1219–1226. doi: 10.3305/nh.2013.28.4.6581.

[37] Fairburn CG, Cooper Z, Shafran R: Cognitive behaviour therapy for eating disorders: a 'transdiagnostic' theory and treatment. Behav Res Ther. 2003;41:509–528.

Section 4

Treatment

Chapter 8

Growing Up in Pain: Anorexia Nervosa and Family Therapy in a Chinese Context

Joyce L.C. Ma

Additional information is available at the end of the chapter

http://dx.doi.org/10.5772/65247

Abstract

Despite the increasing visibility and complexity of anorexia nervosa (AN) in Chinese societies such as Hong Kong, family treatment for Chinese children and youths suffering from AN has been inadequately documented in the literature. In this chapter, the author will describe conceptualization of the disorder in the light of a systemic and developmental framework; describe the process of contextualizing the symptoms of AN; identify critical issues pertinent to treatment success; and highlight the therapist's roles in the healing journey of patients with AN, using a case illustration. More importantly, the author will critically appraise, through a cultural lens, key family therapy concepts, namely emotional enmeshment versus emotional disengagement, boundary and cross-generational collusion, which have restrained the parent/s and the patient to join hands together to drive away the disorder.

Keywords: anorexia nervosa, family therapy, Chinese, growing up, pain

1. Introduction

In ancient China, a student once asked the Zen master what Zen (禪) was. The old master said, 'Eating while eating and sleeping while sleeping'. The answer was simple but unintelligible to the student. Another Zen master Joshu (Chao-Chou), when asked the same question, answered: 'your everyday life is the Tao' [1] (p. 74). The Zen master's wisdom has shed light on the fact that living an ordinary life is a blessing, but a blessing not easily achieved by most people, and particularly not by families facing anorexia nervosa (AN).

A young woman, Ann (pseudonym), a 35-year-old single mother of two young children, a 12-year-old daughter, Sarah, and a 9-year-old son, Mark, called at a university-based family centre to request family therapy service. *The young woman* explained: 'Sarah has been suffering from AN for six months. She had steadily gained weight in the hospital and was discharged a month ago. However, after she returned home, her body weight dropped rapidly. I need professional help and advice on how to help my daughter'.

Shame is the part of traditional Chinese culture; such cultural characteristics continue to shape people's help-seeking behaviour in contemporary Chinese societies such as Hong Kong [2]. Having a family member suffering from a mental disorder such as AN is perceived as a loss of face, mianzi (面子), and shameful. The results of a recent study [2] have shown that Chinese parents with children that have mental health needs preferred enlisting help from their family members, relatives and friends, rather than seeking help from helping professionals. Seeking help from mental health professionals such as family therapists was usually the last resort. Ann must have struggled hard before she called for help. I appreciated her having the courage to seek help, enquired what effect the disorder might have on her daughter's and family functioning, reiterated the need for the whole family to participate in family therapy, and reassured that I would be able to meet them in the coming week. Ann replied that she would be able to meet the therapist with her two children, but her ex-spouse, a manager in a financial company in Mainland China, would not participate in the treatment because he was residing outside Hong Kong. Ann's marriage ended up in a divorce that was initiated by her ex-husband after Ann discovered his extra marital affair.

Having worked as a mental health social worker in a psychiatric unit of a public hospital in Hong Kong before joining the university, my passion for helping children and youths with mental health needs has grown day by day; paradoxically so has my sense of professional incompetence. My search for a better practice never ceased until I got training and received my qualification in the clinical supervision of family therapy from Wai Yung Lee, the first Chinese family therapist trained by Dr. Salvador Minuchin, Master of Structural Family Therapy (SFT) [3–5]. I later received training directly from Dr. Minuchin in New York. Thereby, my professional practice was transformed from an individually oriented practice to a systemically based practice. Inspired by the classic book written by Minuchin et al. [6] and being gratefully trusted by psychiatrists of the Department of Psychiatry of our university, I had carried out two clinical research projects 19 years ago; both of these studies aimed to assess the treatment efficacy of structural family therapy (SFT) in helping Chinese families with AN in Hong Kong [7] and Shenzhen [8], respectively.

Sarah suffers from AN, a mental disorder that is believed to be closely related to growing up issues in children and youths, specifically the problem of individuation and autonomy arising from having an excessively caring mother as proposed by Bruch [9]. While appreciating Bruch's [9] ingenious contribution to expanding the conceptual understanding of AN from a biomedical model to a psychological domain, family therapists have to be vigilant regarding the mother-blaming attitude that has been implied by Bruch's [9] psychoanalytical propositions, and be open to explore the roles the father and other family members may play in contributing to an overtly close mother-daughter relationship [10, 11], an area that has been overlooked by Bruch [9].

http://dx.doi.org/10.5772/65247

It is estimated that about 0.48% of *all* children and youths aged 12–18 in the USA are diagnosed with AN. Among those being diagnosed, 90% of them are female. AN has become increasingly visible in Chinese societies such as Hong Kong [12] and Shenzhen [13].

Children and youths with AN persistently engage themselves in dieting and excessive exercise, pre-occupied with the fear of gaining weight and dissatisfaction with their body shape despite emaciation and a deterioration in their health and psychosocial well-being [14]. The aetiology of the disorder is multiple, involving the dynamic interplay of biological (e.g. temperament and coping), psychological (e.g. sense of ineffectiveness and low self-esteem) and sociocultural factors (e.g. women's status in society, slimness as the standard of beauty in society) [15]. However, it remains unclear that the more important but scarier issue is that the child or the youth feels frightened, out of control and inadequate to face the situation other than through an obsession with dieting, binging and excessive exercising.

If untreated, the disorder seriously threatens the afflicted child or youth's health, increases psychological distress and affects her schooling, family relationships and peer relationships. The child or youth would become emotionally and socially isolated [14, 16]. The family suffers too. These families are tormented by constant fights and conflicts between the parents and the afflicted child/youth over eating and non-eating at meals, marital distress between the parents, a tense family atmosphere and family dysfunction [13].

Food is the best medicine for children and youths with AN. However, the challenge faced by clinicians is how to motivate them to take charge of their health and assume recovery. Psychotherapy is the adjunct treatment. The success rate of psychotherapy has ranged from 36 to 63% [17]. In Great Britain, among all the schools of psychotherapy, family therapy has demonstrated its treatment efficacy for helping children and youths aged 18 or under with a history of illness of less than 3 years [18]. The results of our Hong Kong study [16] have shown that Chinese families of the children and youths with AN benefited from family therapy in terms of reduced symptomatology, lower psychological distress, improved family functioning and greater couple satisfaction, in addition to the families' positive subjective experiences towards family therapy reported in the post-treatment interviews [19].

In adapting the Western-based family therapy model, namely structural family therapy [4, 5], to Chinese families with AN, it is critical to review and examine the similarities and differences between the Eastern and the Western perspectives on some of the taken-for-granted family therapy concepts, namely the emotional enmeshment, boundaries and inter-generational collusion that may have different meanings in Chinese culture. This should be done looking through a cultural lens. The overtly close emotional relationship between a mother and her children is appreciated as an expression of children's filial piety and loyalty to the family. According to Xiao Jing (孝經), the Classic of Filial Piety, children are expected to obey their parents in childhood, honour the family name during adulthood and take care of their parents in their old age [20]. Sacrificing one's self-interest and personal development for the sake of the family's well-being is cherished in Chinese society. Nevertheless, the process of cultural reflexivity is harder than it appears to be, especially for a Chinese family therapist like myself who was brought up in Chinese culture, where traditional cultural values and beliefs have been too familiar and thus invisible to me.

In this chapter, I shall describe the conceptualization of the disorder in the light of a systemic developmental framework; describe the process of therapy; identify critical issues pertinent to the treatment's success; and highlight the therapist's roles in the patient's and her family's journey to recovery, using a case illustration. More importantly, a focus will be placed on the following areas: (a) understanding the patient's major issues and concerns that have been distracting her through the symptoms of AN and have made her get stuck in her growth and development; (b) critically appraising the key family therapy concepts, namely emotional enmeshment versus emotional disengagement, and boundary and cross-generational collusion, seen through a cultural lens, which have restrained the parent/s and the patient from joining hands together to drive away the disorder; and (c) on the basis of the above assessment, helping the parents and the patient to generate options and possibilities to transcend the stifling family context, which in turn would enable the patient to combat the disorder and deal with the developmental issues.

2. Family therapy and anorexia nervosa

Unlike therapists using psychotherapy oriented towards the individual who aim to effect changes in the patient's emotion, behaviour or cognition, family therapists take a totally different track in helping. Theoretically grounded in a systemic framework [21], family therapists perceive individuals and families as an integral part of the eco-environment and are in continuous interactions with the larger social contexts (e.g. school, social services and community). The underlying assumption of family therapy is that a change in the environmental context will bring about a change in the individual [4, 5]. Such change is feasible because families in distress are believed to be richer and more resourceful than what they have seen in themselves; their family lives are more complex than what has been presented in treatment [4]. During assessment and treatment, family therapists focus on assessing the consequences of the disorder on the patient and the family, rather than focusing on its cause [22].

Similar to other human behaviour, the symptoms of AN are contextually dependent, that is, a patient's behaviour would affect her immediate social context including her family, school and peers, which in turn would influence the patient's behaviour as well. To what extent has the social context—albeit the family, school or peers—contributed to the maintenance or escalation of the symptoms? In what way has the patient's symptoms impacted the family relationships and family coping? These are key clinical questions that a family therapist would bear in mind during a family assessment while listening to the family story, and observing and discerning the family drama, which is usually full of pathology, fault-finding and blaming, mostly pointing to the patient. 'She is too obstinate and so she self-starves herself; she is losing her head to keep dieting'. All this blaming would have consumed most of the family's energy and limited their ability to look for options and possibilities for better coping.

The foremost task that a family therapist has to undertake is to help transform the family's conceptualization of AN from an individual pathology to a family concern. This requires the therapist to see the situation through an interpersonal lens to conceptualize the patient's

http://dx.doi.org/10.5772/65247

symptoms [23]. If the family holds the view that the therapist is an expert able to fix the patient's pathology and that they have no role to play in the healing, they would not participate in the treatment. Such a therapeutic task could be achieved through shifting the family's care and concern from the symptoms themselves to the symptomatic family interactions that have maintained those symptoms [24]. Minuchin, Reiter and Borda [5] referred to this as a process of externalization: '… pushing the symptoms out of the symptom bearer and helping the family members to see the family's participation in constructing and maintaining the symptoms in the symptom bearer' (p. 19), which is different from the process of externalization as understood by the Narrative School [25], that is, a process of constructing AN as the common enemy of the family members, which is related to the societal standard of beauty—slimness is beautiful.

Such a therapeutic step is illustrated by the therapist's work with Ann's family.

3. Case vignette: a neglected sibling

Sarah was weighed before treatment, which is a necessary step for the therapist to monitor her body weight, assess the patient's health risk and provide feedback on the family's treatment response.

Sarah weighted 29 kg, with a height of 138 cm (body mass index, BMI, of 15), which is lower than the average of BMI 17, the normal range of a BMI for her cohort. Her BMI indicated that her symptoms were severe [14] (p. 339). Ann was slender, looked tired and slightly depressed. Sarah was a friendly teenager who greeted the therapist with a sheepish smile. She chose to sit close to her mother on a larger sofa, and Mark, the younger son, sat a bit uneasily on another sofa opposite his mother and his sister.

After listening to the mother's description of Sarah's history of the illness, I turned to Sarah to find out more about the different aspects of her life. Engaging the patient as early as possible is paramount for assessing the family [13]. In doing so, the patient would not mistakenly think that the therapist is her parent's therapist only. Sarah responded to the therapist's questions with ease. She was studying in primary 6 in a reputable school in a neighbourhood that was far away from their present home, a new town that the family moved to after the couple divorced. She had a few friends in school. She did not like to study very much and was not particularly good at any academic subject, but did well in gymnastics. Last year she was one of the Hong Kong junior athletes who competed in an international gymnastics contest. Athletes in gymnastics and dancers are high-risk groups for AN since the sport requires them to keep their body shape and be slim [26]. The information provided gave the therapist a hint to explore the likely linkage of the disorder to her favourite sport.

The therapist:: Did your dieting relate to your wish to excel in gymnastics?

Sarah:: Not really. I am unhappy and I don't want to eat when I am in a bad mood.

Therapist:: I see. Who has made you unhappy at home?

Sarah:: My mom and my younger brother, Mark. They often fight with each other. It's very noisy at home.

Ann explained embarrassingly: My son was diagnosed as suffering from attention deficit hyperactivity disorder (ADHD) and suspected Asperger's syndrome (AS) at the age of 3. He has problems in reading and writing. Ever since he started schooling, I have had to spend tremendous amount of effort and time in homework supervision, and provide remedial training at home so that he would not lag behind in his academic performance. Mark is easily distracted during study. His misbehaviour has put me at my wit's end. Sarah is different. She is self-disciplined, fairly independent and not demanding. She has taken care of her own things so well that there is no need for me to nag her. I never knew she feels she is neglected, insufficiently cared for and not loved until the psychiatrist told me about it.

The therapist nodded and turned to ask Sarah:: Do you feel so?

Sarah replied without any hesitation:: Yes. I am unhappy because my mom would never ask if I long for anything.

Ann clarified that and said:: That's untrue. I have tried my best to meet your needs in the past.

Feeling a bit upset, Sarah replied:: Yes, only if I asked for it. You seldom spend time with me and listen to what has been happening in school.

The therapist asked:: Did your mom change after the onset of your disorder?

Sarah grinned and said:: Yes, she spends more time with me; she has meals with me and hugs me until I fall asleep.

Parents of a child with special educational needs (SEN) such as Ann tend to spend more time and effort with the child with SEN than with the typically developing sibling [27] similar to what has been experienced in this family. Caring for a child with SEN was an insurmountable task for solo mothers such as Ann to be saddled with. Besides having to rear children, she was a part-time secretary. She had undoubtedly relieved her financial insecurity, but she had to pay the price of sacrificing her sleeping time and rest.

A study conducted in Spain [30] has indicated the contribution of parental bonding to development and maintenance of eating disorders (ED). About 8.6% and 12.9% of the patients perceived their parents' parenting styles as neglectful. Patients with ED who perceived a neglectful maternal parenting during their first 16 years reported higher scores in the subscales of drive for thinness and body dissatisfaction than those who perceived the affectionless control and affectionate constraint styles. Patients who perceived a father's neglectful parenting during the first 16 years indicated higher scores in bulimia and ineffectiveness in comparison to patents who perceived other styles [30].

3.1. A day in the schedule of the family

Ann and the two children usually went to sleep quite late, at around 12:00 mid-night. They woke up at 9 o'clock in the morning. Sarah took an hour to finish her breakfast, and by half

http://dx.doi.org/10.5772/65247

past 10, Ann had to take the two children to school, which was about an hour and a half of traveling. The tight schedule left them little time for lunch. Besides, she would not yet be hungry after the late breakfast. In the evening, Sarah and Mark had dinner by themselves, with their domestic helper preparing their food, and before their mother returned home at 7 o'clock. Ann's evening itinerary was full: homework supervision with Mark; story time with Mark and Sarah, respectively; and hugging and sometimes struggling with Sarah's temper tantrum until she fell asleep.

Ann did not complain about how exhausted she was. Nevertheless, her body language and her facial expression had already revealed it. The therapist felt strongly for her. It was a mission impossible for a single mother like Ann; only the Buddhist goddess Kuan Yin with a thousand hands (千手觀音) could do it.

The therapist acknowledged her difficulties: What an impossible job you are doing! It must be a heavy burden for you to look after two children, especially Mark, who has a learning difficulty, and Sarah, with an eating disorder. Did your ex-husband share in the childcare with you before the break up of your marriage?

Ann:: Not. He is a career-oriented man. He played with them after work but I had to go 'solo' supervising Mark's school work. The situation was absolutely worse when we moved to live with my husband three years ago on the Mainland. I was a stranger in the city and we had uprooted ourselves from Hong Kong. After I discovered his affair, we fought day and night to an extent that I could hardly tolerate it any more.

Ann's eyes were filling with tears. Sarah moved to comfort her mom while Mark became more irritated, restless and distractive.

Sarah elaborated:: My mom cried every day. Mom and dad fought every day.

The therapist asked empathetically:: It must have affected both of you. How did you feel at that time?

Sarah said:: We were frightened. Mark and I hid in our room but kept listening to their heated argument in the next room. My mom was depressed, angry and hysterical. She acted as if she were crazy.

The therapist turned to Mark and asked:: How crazy was your mom at that time?

Mark shrugged and said:: Like a mad woman.

Sarah said:: More than mad. She was insane.

While telling their story, Sarah moved closer and closer to her mom, like an Australian koala bear; Mark became more restless and fidgeted. He kept playing with his fingers. The family drama that had emerged reminded the therapist of the voice of Bowlby [28], who described the behavioural response of children under the threat of losing their caregiver. Apparently, the two children were trapped by the parents' marital discord and felt very nervous about losing their parents. They were in pain when seeing their mother in pain. They have become their mother's guardian angels.

The therapist asked:: It seems that both of you are on the side of your mom. Is that true?

The two children said:: Yes.

The therapist asked:: For how long have you been protecting your mom?

Sarah replied quickly:: Since my dad's disloyalty toward her.

The therapist said to Sarah in empathy:: You must share your mom's sadness a lot.

Sarah nodded and cried. Apparently part of Sarah's sadness had come from her mother's misery.

3.2. Social support of the family

Ann's younger sister, Helen, has provided strong support to the family. Ann could leave the two children in Helen's home if she was late at work. The two children liked staying in their aunt's home because they could play with their cousins. They loved their aunt; she was well educated and respectful in church. Both families were Christians, and the support given by the church to the family was strong too. Ann would seek advice from Helen should she meet any problem. What puzzled her most was that Sarah had no problem eating at Helen's home, but eating has become problematic at her own home.

3.3. Family assessment

Sarah's symptoms, when contextualized in her family setting, symbolized the yearning of a 'neglected' sibling for attention and care from the depressed and exhausted mother in a post-divorce family of a child with SEN. Unfortunately, the mother has gone through a marital crisis of being betrayed and deserted by her ex-spouse. The symptoms could be regarded as the children's expression of their anxiety, insecurity and sadness, which have been arising partly from the mother's anguish and depression, and partly from their parents' marital discord, stormy separation and divorce. Probably due to the gender difference and differences in temperament, Sarah, the sensitive, submissive and loyal child, had expressed her emotional turmoil as AN while Mark acted out his pain and suffering through distractibility and hyperactivity.

Ann had already been aware of the fact that the symptoms of AN had provided a psychological gain to Sarah—she had won back her mother's love and care. However, she came to realize the two children's emotional turmoil was in response to the parents' marital discord, separation and divorce only after she heard of the children's stories during treatment.

Refeeding Sarah has posed a great challenge for the family. The tight daily schedule of the family had given Sarah a legitimate excuse for not eating well at lunch; the mother's part-time job has hindered her from supervising Sarah's dinner too. The domestic helper was apparently not a parent substitute as indicated by Sarah's low body weight. Nevertheless, in their narratives, it was a glimmer of hope—Sarah ate well at her aunt's home. It was a mystery why Sarah ate well there but not so at her own home, one that deserved further exploration in the second session.

http://dx.doi.org/10.5772/65247

3.4. Treatment goals

The treatment goals were three-fold: the therapist would assist Ann to (a) reschedule their daily timetable to refeed Sarah and supervise her meals; (b) respond to Sarah's longing for love and care without reinforcing her regressive child-like behaviour of refusing to eat while helping Sarah to win her mother's love and concern through age-appropriate ways; and (c) foster her psychological well-being through continuing to mobilize support from her younger sister, Helen's family, and the church as well as from her religion, and by doing so, help reduce the psychological burden of caring for the two children with different needs.

The therapist faced two dilemmas in achieving these treatment goals: (a) whether to persuade Ann to give up her part-time job, which had provided her with financial security, personal meaning and distraction from the heavy domestic duties, or to identify the better alternative that would be for Ann to balance the dual demands of work and family and (b) while appreciating the mother's effort to take more care of Sarah's emotional needs, driven by guilt, she might lack the confidence to demand that Sarah behave maturely, if needed.

4. The family's solution to refeeding and the therapist's challenge of the rigid family script

The therapist was worried about Sarah's situation, as her weight had remained unchanged at the time of the second session. Her worry was confirmed by the mother's report. Two days before the session, Ann found out that Sarah had not taken any meals for a whole day. Desperate and totally frustrated, she took Sarah to the emergency department of a nearby hospital to ask for hospitalization. The doctor agreed to admit Sarah to the hospital, but Sarah pleaded to have a last chance at self-help by living at her aunt's home rather than being hospitalized, which was acceptable to her mother as well as the doctor. The therapist perceived it to be the right time to unveil the mystery of why refeeding seemed to be more promising at the aunt's home than at the family home.

4.1. Different family schedules

The therapist asked with great curiosity: I am puzzled about this arrangement. Sarah, there must be differences between staying at home and living with your aunt's family. Can you tell us the differences?

Sarah said: It is quite different. In their family (Helen's), they sleep earlier and eat earlier. All the children have to sleep at 10:00 p.m., whether you like it or not. I can wake up earlier and have my breakfast earlier; in doing so, I feel hungry at lunch and can take in more food then.

Ann protested mildly: Why can't you do that at home?

Sarah defended jokingly: You're my mom and Helen isn't. I dare not disobey her.

It was amazing that the mother and the daughter had already identified their way to refeeding, when only the week before, the therapist had kept worrying about how to help reschedule the family routine to ensure adequate parental supervision at mealtimes.

4.2. Different parenting styles

Jauregui Lobera et al., [30] have found that the stereotyped parenting styles among families of patients with ED were characterised by low care and high control during the first 16 years and the same parenting styles could be applicable to current styles of the mothers. To what extent is this true to Sarah's family?

Further inquiry about the difference in the parenting styles among Sarah's father, mother and her aunt Helen had revealed that in the eyes of Sarah, her father had played with them in the past. Her mother had taken care of their daily life, but her aunt was firmer than her parents in relating to her. She appreciated her father's providing autonomy and space, and her mother's being remarkably capable of attending to the details of their life and her aunt's firmness in limit-setting.

Ann welcomed Sarah's short stay with her younger sister since it did provide a temporary refuge for her, relieved her from the caring burden, and enabled her to have more time to take care of Mark. She did not feel she was being undermined by such an arrangement. Since childhood, she had known fully well that Helen was more capable than her. In reflection, Ann perceived herself to be as capable as Helen in limit setting with her children when she was not lethargic and moody. She had already quitted her part-time job to have more time for the family and herself.

4.3. Challenging the rigid family script

Sarah's weight had increased 1 kg by the third session, indicating her stay with her aunt had taken effect. This had allowed room for the therapist to shift the focus of the work from fostering parental supervision during mealtimes to the rigid family script—albeit each of the family members had to sacrifice their personal needs in order to help Mark, the child with SEN. Such an issue was naturally brought up when Sarah told the therapist that she preferred staying at her aunt's home rather than returning home sometimes.

Ann, the mother, explained to the therapist: She (Sarah) felt very bored at home.

The therapist turned to ask Sarah: How come? I remember that you like playing the piano.

Sarah said: It's because I couldn't do it. I didn't want to disturb and distract Mark from doing his homework.

The therapist asked in great puzzlement: I am confused and I don't understand. What do you mean?

Sarah explained: Mark did his homework in the sitting room, where our piano is. If I practiced my music, Mark would not concentrate on his school work.

http://dx.doi.org/10.5772/65247

The therapist continued asking: I see. Does your mom ask you to sacrifice your hobby to help Mark?

Ann cut in and said: No. I've never made such a demand. She is too eager to please me and be a good girl. That's the problem. (Ann sighed!)

At this point the therapist perceived it to be the right moment to invite Ann, the mother, to talk directly to Sarah, her daughter on this issue.

Sarah asked her mom: Is it really true that there's no need for me to ask for permission if I want to watch television?

Ann replied reassuringly: Yes, as long as you ask Mark to do his homework in his room.

Sarah looked at her mother with an unbelievable gaze.

Ann reassured her daughter with care and concern: Yes, I don't want you to feel that you have no say at home.

The mother's repeated reassurance was extremely crucial for Sarah, who has been shaped by the family context to suppress her own needs to accommodate the special learning needs of her younger brother. Was Mark really a child with a big problem?

On the contrary, Mark was quite a smart child. He liked to make observations and conduct different experiments. For instance, during bathing, he tested the effect of heat on water. He studied each part of his toys and reassembled them to understand their operational mechanisms. He concentrated deeply on scientific experiments and observations. He became distractive and inattentive only when learning Chinese and English. After hearing the strengths of Mark from Ann and Sarah, the therapist said: 'Thanks for telling me so much about him. Otherwise I would misunderstand him as a problem child'.

The reframing of Mark from a problem child in the family to a child with his own unique strengths and talents had allowed the therapist to be more forceful in challenging the rigid family script that Sarah, the elder sister, should sacrifice her personal needs for her younger brother, Mark, a child with SEN. The therapist ended the session by asking Mark and Sarah if they could work out their own way of relating to each other in a mutually fulfilling manner, rather than turning to their mother for advice and approval. Both of them responded to the therapist's suggestion with their witty smiles.

5. Key treatment strategies

The clinical case reported above has illustrated the fundamental treatment principle and strategies of SFT, that is, to help shift the family's conceptualization of their difficulty from the symptoms and pathology, in our instance, Sarah's AN, to the stifling familial context that has maintained or escalated the symptoms [24]. That shift, if it had been achieved, would have enabled the family to actively participate in treatment to change the undesirable family context and discover the multiple meanings of the disorder at the individual and familial levels.

Our case has provided anecdotal evidence in a Chinese context to support the results of Jauregui Lobera et al.,'s study [30] that the ED symptoms are associated with neglectful parenting. In Sarah's family, her symptoms can be understood as the expression of an unfulfilled need of a neglected sibling for parental care and concern in a post-divorce family of a child with SEN; The disorder has symbolized Sarah's emotional response towards her mother's anguish and depression at a deeper level as well.

The excessively close relationship between Ann and her two children, Sarah and Mark, can be attributed partly to the strong parental bonding [30], changing family shape, that is, a post-divorce family and their experience of being abandoned by the father, and partly to the gendered division of labour between man and woman in the family before the divorce. Nevertheless, the family structure discerned can also be interpreted culturally as arising from the children's filial piety towards their lonely and sorrowful mother and their loyalty to the family. Having recognized the cultural meaning, the therapist had more empathy towards them. Her awareness of the power of our cultural forces in shaping people's beliefs, emotional expressions and coping is heightened; it also points the way to assist the family to transcend cultural constraints to have more options and possibilities for living a better life.

Minuchin et al.'s [5] multi-layered self has guided the therapist to discover that Mark, an inattentive and distractive child, is a child with great curiosity and concentration regarding scientific observation and inquiry. In understanding each person's personality and strengths within the family, the therapist has successfully joined Mark, a child with SEN, and challenged the inflexible family script—that each of the family members has to sacrifice their personal needs, hobby and leisure activities to help him.

A review of the family's daily schedule has assisted the family to find their own idiosyncratic way of refeeding Sarah. Sarah gained body weight steadily from the third session onwards. At the end of the treatment (total no. of sessions offered = 9), Sarah's body weight had increased from 29 to 38 kg (BMI = 20).

With the shift in the family definition of their presented problem, the next step in treatment for families with two parents is to, on the one hand, collaborate with the parents through empowerment and the instilment of hope for refeeding the patient with AN, and on the other hand, to encourage the patient to elicit help and assistance from her parents to drive away the disorder [13]. Paternal engagement is of great clinical utility in helping Chinese families since the father is often the head of the family. The therapist would find means to actively engage the previously less involved or absent father in the treatment and childcare such as meal supervision, mediating the mother-daughter conflicts, and providing emotional support to his spouse and the patient [11].

The parents' resistance to collaborating together in helping may indicate the need to explore their marital relationship and the history of their upbringing. A few Chinese parents had experienced extreme poverty, massive famine and starvation during the Cultural Revolution in China in the 1960s and 1970s, and they tended to respond to their daughter's self-starvation with rage and hostility [11]. An empathetic understanding of their upbringing and its linkage to their here-and-now emotional response would help clear up the misunderstanding between

http://dx.doi.org/10.5772/65247

the parents and the patient and reduce their hostility. Couple therapy may be required for a few parents with marital problems [13].

However, in helping post-divorce families such as Ann's family, in which the father's involvement is minimal due to his living far away, the therapist would need to search for an alternative treatment strategy to replace the strategy of parental collaboration. The family's temporary measure to place Sarah in the care of her aunt's home has underscored the importance of kinship as a family resource for Chinese families. According to traditional Chinese culture, the concept of family *jia* (家) refers to the kinship and the extended family, rather than just the immediate household [29]. Hence, the therapist would need to identify the healer/s of the family not only within the household itself but also among close relatives of the family. A similar treatment principle would be applicable for families with different family shapes (e.g. blended families) in Chinese societies.

Handling unresolved conflicts (e.g. mother-daughter conflicts) and relapses by preventing the emergence of the symptomatic cycle is an integral part of the treatment process, while supporting the patient's individual development and transformation is paramount [13]. All these can be achieved through continued collaboration with the family and the patient. In view of the life-threatening nature of the disorder, family therapists without any medical training should not hesitate to seek medical back up from a doctor experienced in managing patients with AN. Collaborating with a family-oriented social worker in the community, who would actively take up the role of a case-manager to mobilize community resources for the family (e.g. multi-problem families), would definitely facilitate the patient's and the family's journey of healing.

Being a part of the therapeutic system, the therapist has to be watchful of how his or her own response has influenced the family, which in turn would also affect the therapist's responses. An artful use of self and a continued discovery of the multiple layered of self [4] would help to overcome therapeutic impasses and challenges that have arisen from treatment. The more readily the therapist could move away from his/ her comfort zone to deal with family conflicts and intense emotions in the family with courage and mindfulness, the greater the likelihood he or she would be able to achieve the goal of helping.

6. Conclusion

Family therapists assist the family and the patient to use their resources and strengths to transcend the stifling familial context and drive away the disorder. However, similar to the learning experience of a Zen student [1], the family's healing is a process of self-discovery. A Zen master cannot give enlightenment to his student and so it is with the therapist. A therapist, at the best, is only a participant observer [5] in treatment and a companion on their journey of recovery.

Author details

Joyce L.C. Ma

Address all correspondence to: joycelai@swk.cuhk.edu.hk

AAMFT, Department of Social Work, The Chinese University of Hong Kong, Hong Kong, China

References

[1] Suzuki DT. An introduction to Zen Buddhism. Great Britain: Clays Ltd., St Ives PLC; 1949. 54 p.

[2] Ma JLC, Lai K, Lo WK. Perceived social support in Chinese parents of children with attention deficit hyperactivity disorder in a Chinese context: Implications for social work practice. Social Work in Mental Health. 2016; 1533–2993. DOI: 10.1080/15332985.2016.1159643

[3] Minuchin S, Nichols MP. Family healing: Tales of hope and renewal from family therapy. New York: The Free Press; 1993. 287 p.

[4] Minuchin S, Nichols MP, Lee WY. Assessing families and couples: From symptoms to system. Boston, MA: Pearson Education, Inc.; 2007. 224 p.

[5] Minuchin S, Reiter MD, Borda C. The craft of family therapy: Challenging certainties. New York and London: Routledge; 2014. 248 p.

[6] Minuchin S, Rosman B, Baker L. Psychosomatic families: Anorexia nervosa in context. New York: Harvard University Press; 1978. 351 p.

[7] Ma JLC, Lai K. The applicability of family therapy for Chinese children and adolescents suffering from anorexia nervosa in a Chinese context: A preliminary study. Social Work in Mental Health. 2009; 7(4): 402–423.

[8] Ma JLC. Perceived process of change in family therapy for eating disorders in Shenzhen, China: A qualitative study. Journal of Family Psychotherapy. 2012; 23(3): 184–201. DOI: 10.1080/08975353.2012.705638

[9] Bruch H. Eating disorders. New York: Guilford Press; 1973.

[10] Nichols MP. Inside family therapy: A case study in family healing. MA, USA: Allyn and Bacon; 1999. 242 p.

[11] Ma JLC. The roles of father in the recovery of Chinese young persons with eating disorders in two Chinese cities, Hong Kong and Shenzhen. Journal of Family Therapy. 2015; 37(1): 61–78.

[12] Lee S, Lee AM. Disordered eating in three communities of China: A comparative study of female high school students in Hong Kong, Shenzhen, and rural Hunan. International Journal of Eating Disorder. 1999; 27: 317–327.

[13] Ma JLC. Anorexia nervosa and family therapy in a Chinese context. Hong Kong: The Chinese University Press; 2011. 284 p.

[14] American Psychiatric Association. Diagnostic and Statistics Manual V. Washington, USA: APA; 2013.

[15] Ogden J. The psychology of eating. Cambridge, MA: Blackwell; 2003.

[16] Ma JLC, Lai K. Applicability of family therapy for Chinese children and adolescents suffering from anorexia nervosa in a Chinese context: A preliminary study. Social Work in Mental Health. 2009; 7(4): 402–423. DOI: 10.1080/15332980802237750

[17] Lock J, Le Grange D, Agras WS, Dare C. Treatment manual for anorexia nervosa: A family-based approach. New York: Guilford Press; 2004. 270 p.

[18] Russell GFM, Dare C, Eisler I, Le Grange. Controlled trials of family treatment in anorexia nervosa. In: Russell GFM, Dare C, Eisler I, Le Grange PDF, editors. Psychobiology and treatment of anorexia nervosa and bulimia. New York: Psychiatric Press; 1992. p. 149–170.

[19] Ma JLC, Lai K. Perceived treatment effectiveness of family therapy for Chinese patients suffering from anorexia nervosa: A qualitative inquiry. Journal of Family Social Work. 2006; 10(2): 59–74.

[20] Jing X. Classic of filial piety. In: Legge J. (Trans.). The Chinese classics. Hong Kong: Hong Kong University Press; 1960. Vol. 1–5.

[21] Bronfenbrenner U. The ecology of human development. Cambridge, MA: Harvard University Press; 1979. 352 p.

[22] Eisler I. The empirical and theoretical base of family therapy and multiple family day therapy for adolescent anorexia nervosa. Journal of Family Therapy. 2005; 27: 104–131.

[23] Tomm K, George SS, Wulff D, Strong T. Patterns in interpersonal interactions: Inviting relational understandings for therapeutic change. Routledge. 2014. 284 p.

[24] Micucci JA. The adolescent in family therapy. New York: Guilford Press; 1998.

[25] Maisel R, Epston D, Borden A. Biting the hand that starves you. New York: W. W. Norton and Company; 2004. 336 p.

[26] Piran, N. On the move from tertiary to secondary and primary prevention: Working with an elite dance school. In: Piran N, Levine MP, Steiner-Adair C, editors. Preventing eating disorders. New York: Brunner/Mazel; 1999. pp. 256–269.

[27] Sicile-Kira C. The effects of autism in families and partner relationships. Family Therapy Magazine. 2008; May/June: 18–22.

[28] Bowlby J. Attachment and loss, Volume III. Great Britain: Penguin Education; 1980.

[29] Wen CI, Chang YH, Chang LY, Chu C. Family structure and its related variables: A case of Taipei. In: Yi CC, Chu C, editors. Social phenomena in Taiwan: An analysis. Taipei: Institute of Social Science and Philosophy, Academia Sinica Press; 1989. pp. 1–24.

[30] Jauregui Lobera I, Bolanos Rios P, Garrido Casals O. Parenting styles and eating disorders. Journal of Psychiatric and Mental Health Nursing. 2011; 18: 728–735.

Chapter 9

Eating Disorders: A Treatment Apart. The Unique Use of the Therapist's Self in the Treatment of Eating Disorders

Abigail H. Natenshon

Additional information is available at the end of the chapter

http://dx.doi.org/10.5772/65697

Abstract

Treatment skills that serve general mental health practice, though applicable to eating disorder care, by themselves will not suffice to meet the uniquely pressing demands and requirements of treating these life-threatening disorders. Eating disorders adversely influence every aspect of human functioning, demanding a comprehensive and integrative approach to care. Because eating disorders disrupt the patient's relationship with self and others, the quality of the therapist's versatile and integrative use of self within the therapeutic relationship can become the single most significant intervention in achieving successful healing outcomes. The intensity of professional challenges within the treatment process reflects the urgency behind the patient's need to heal. Treatment efficacy is achieved through the therapist's commitment to a timely, intentional, and practicable fulfillment of clearly established goals, uniquely tailored to each patient and eating disorder. The self-integrated psychotherapist, as case manager, is required to manage a complex landscape of pathology and strengths, regression and healing, diverse professional and familial resources, transference and countertransference phenomena and, with skillful proficiency, traditional as well as nontraditional (neurophysiological) treatment interventions and approaches to care. This chapter highlights key elements in the therapist's V.I.A.B.L.E. (Versatile, Integrative, Action-oriented, outcome-Based, Loving, and Educative) use of self in facilitating the healing of the eating disordered patient and malnourished brain.

Keywords: eating disorders and neurobiology, anorexia nervosa, bulimia nervosa, binge eating disorder, eating disorder treatment, eating disorder recovery, the eating disorder therapist's unique use of self, managing eating disorder resistance to healing, mindfulness in psychotherapy, the VIABLE eating disorder practitioner, family's role in eating disorder treatment, integrative psychotherapy, somatosensory education, neurophysiological treatment interventions, outpatient team in eating disorder treatment, milieu treatment for eating disorders, emotionally integrated therapist, psychotherapeutic relationship in eating disorder treatment, set point weight theory, mind-brain-body connection in eating disorder treatment, Feldenkrais Method of Somatic Education©, trauma-informed yoga, body image, self image

1. Introduction

Although considered mental health disorders, eating disorders (ED) carry dire physiological risks and complications resulting from severe and prolonged dietary restriction [1]. Ranking among the 10 leading causes of disability among young women [2], they have the highest mortality rate of any psychiatric disorder [3–5]. Symptom presentation is diverse and unique to each patient, demanding an equally diverse and integrative treatment process and path to recovery. Though the agenda of any treatment process will be responsive to the demands of the therapeutic moment, it is the eating disorder practitioner's focused intentionality, goal clarity, and sustained vision of complete and comprehensive recovery that best serve the process. *Every* moment of care is a pivotal moment in care, demanding precision in judgment and incisive decision-making to avoid, or redirect, a treatment process that may have gone off course or become ineffective. The work of conducting ED treatment can be as challenging for the therapist as for the patient. Both patient and professional face the challenges of tolerating and accommodating the ambiguities and frustrations of an inevitably unpredictable, yet critical, healing process. By modeling steadfast commitment to treatment engagement and goals through a mindful therapeutic attachment, therapists empower and embolden their ED patients to follow their lead.

2. Eating disorders are diseases

With disease origins in genetics and in brain structure and function, the risk of death by suicide in patients with Anorexia nervosa (AN) is 57–58 times the expected rate in similar age and gender populations [6]. Crude mortality from suicide or medical complications from starvation or compensatory behaviors associated with the illness is 9% [7, 8]. The impact of ED symptomatology on the individual is wide-ranging and potentially irreversible. Through the loss of muscle mass, the malnourished heart decreases in size, affecting heart rate and blood pressure. The main causes of sudden death in ED are those related to cardiovascular complications [9]. Twenty-five percent of individuals with AN experience a chronic or continuously relapsing course [7, 8].

Cerebral atrophy due to enduring AN was initially thought to lead to an irreversible reduction in gray matter volume [10]. It was later proven that long-term weight restoration might eventually lead to a restoration of gray matter and structural normalcy, though not to fully normalized functionality [11]. Anorexic patients with amenorrhea or irregular menses, even after structural brain changes had been resolved, displayed significant cognitive deficits across

http://dx.doi.org/10.5772/65697

a range of tasks [12]. Co-occurring conditions central to the ED diagnostic process carry significant implications for ED treatment and prognosis. Depression, anxiety, mood disorders, attention-deficit/hyperactivity disorder (ADHD), posttraumatic stress disorder (PTSD), diabetes, food allergies, gastrological disorders, addictions, and personality disorders create the warp and weft of the integrative fabric of these disorders.

Low weight and higher cortisol levels are correlated with greater structural brain abnormalities [13]. Malnutrition is of particular concern during the critical stages of early brain development in childhood, adolescence, and young adulthood. "Epidemiology and diagnosis, medical complications, nutritional concerns, psychological issues, treatment, and treatment outcome for adolescents [and children] with ED differ from those for adults, with particular emphasis on pivotal medical and developmental issues unique to the peripubertal period" [14]. Profound and diverse emotional effects of ED on mind and body can be deeply traumatic to patients who in many cases are too young and emotionally undeveloped to have acquired the skills required to cope with the challenges of disease, as well as recovery, processes. The development of new cases of ED has been steadily increasing since 1950 [15, 16]. Children under the age of 12 admitted to the hospital for ED rose 119% in less than a decade [17].

Since the fourteenth century, with the first diagnosis of AN, there has been "historical drift" in the rapid acceleration in new presentations of eating-related pathology as seen in symptom variability and gender representation [17]. Diagnoses have become increasingly differentiated and refined in their definition. Forms of AN have become distinguishable as "restrictive, or purging type." Bulimia nervosa (BN) is diagnosable as "purging, or restrictive type," the diagnostic differentiation denoting distinctive personality characteristics. Eating disorders not otherwise specified (EDNOS) and binge eating disorder (BED) are examples of the evolution of eating disorder pathology. Binge eating disorder is the most likely ED diagnosis to be missed, as the intermittent patterns of binging and starvation result in a normal and constant weight. The onus is on the enlightened clinician to probe actively, and with sensitivity and reassurance during diagnostic assessments to uncover these and other hidden ED, as well as related problems that might include activity disorders/excessive exercise with the intention to lose weight, orthorexia, diabulimia, body image disturbances, night eating syndrome (NES), rumination, chew and spit (CHSP), body dysmorphic disorder, etc.

Of particular significance within the ED field, historical progression is evident in the introduction of the diagnosis "avoidant/restrictive food intake disorder" (ARFID), replacing feeding disorder of infancy and early childhood in the American Psychiatric Associations' Diagnostic and Statistical Manual of Mental Disorders, Fifth Edition [18]. The manual describes ARFID as "an eating or feeding disturbance (e.g., apparent lack of interest in eating, food-avoidance based on the sensory character of food, and/or concern about aversive consequences of eating) as manifested by persistent failure to meet appropriate nutritional and/or energy needs." Pediatricians all too frequently miss this diagnosis in infants, children, and adolescents whose patterns of weight and height appear to be normal on growth charts. It is left to ED experts to recognize and understand these atypical "picky eating" disorders, so as to guide increasing numbers of patients and parents to early diagnosis and integrative treatment options. The ever-changing course of ED presentation demands the practitioner's commitment to professional continuing education, intellectual curiosity, and the willingness to recognize and accommodate the evolution of developments within the ED field through clinical responsiveness within mainstream practice.

3. ED treatment is a treatment apart

Ironically, it is the rare graduate school of mental health practice that offers curriculum specialty training in the treatment of ED. A student studying for her Master's degree at a highly reputed school of social work inquired as to why the absence of ED-related courses. She was told that specialty training was "unnecessary and redundant" based on the proliferation of generic courses that address the emotional issues underlying and driving these diseases. These educators and administrators were of the mind that the methodology for treating ED consists of "techniques and approaches indistinguishable from those offered by *any* highly skilled mental health clinician." This widespread misconception is not uncommon in teaching curriculums that fail to recognize ED as neurophysiological, and potentially lethal, diseases in their own right.

In actual fact, clinical strategies, techniques, and methodologies for ED treatment management and recovery are, in many respects, *not* unlike those that are applicable to more generalist types of mental health care. However, the lethality of these disorders, the integrative nature and demands of their treatment, and the need for the therapist's unique use of self in confronting the challenges they present, clearly set these diseases apart in their manner of treatment. "Though in some respects elusive, the tools of this treatment trade are actually supremely accessible; in many respects they are disarmingly simple and hardly strangers to us. We know them all; we know how to implement them. We have only to learn *why, how* and *when* to offer *which* of our previously acquired techniques and skills. The outcomes we seek lie in the use of *self* in response to the unique demands of the ED patient and treatment moment [19]".

If not actively healing, ED pathology becomes increasingly entrenched, reshaping the structure and function of the brain. By fragmenting the patient's core self and taking over its role as "director of operations," the ED creates radical changes within the patient's personality and physiology. Compounding treatment challenges, parents or life partners of ED patients invariably find themselves confused and helpless in the face of their loved one's emotional withdrawal. The typical ED patient's ambivalence about, and resistance to recovering puts therapists and patients at cross-purposes from their very first treatment encounter, and beyond. The ED therapist comes to the treatment process seeking a commitment to a recovery process that will restore life quality and reintegrate the patient's fragmented core self. The patient typically enters the treatment process denying disease, or clinging to the ED for his or her very survival. Emotionally flexible therapists need to use themselves deftly, exercising nuanced creativity and skills in facilitating and sustaining a meaningful therapeutic connection capable of evoking the patient's motivation to heal.

3.1. The ED therapist requires a flexible use of self within the ED treatment process

For those who believe that the best therapist to treat an eating disorder is one who has suffered from an ED, I would counter that assumption with the notion that one need not be a horse in order to become a horse doctor. Approximately one-third of all ED practitioners have struggled with, and recovered from, a clinical ED. "The lifetime prevalence of an ED among professionals was 33.2% for females, and 2.23% for males. Note that 38.8% of treatment facilities reported hiring clinicians with a history of an ED" [20]. Practitioners who have suffered an ED are likely to have developed an exquisite sensitivity to the experience of ED patients. However, just as easily they could find themselves experiencing what is known as countertransference, an emotional reaction of the therapist to the subject's contribution. Triggered by the resonance of dormant issues, countertransference reactions could impede the quality of therapeutic responsiveness.

The empathic, emotionally integrated and developmentally evolved ED therapist who is a seasoned and sensitive veteran of life and its challenges within *any* context, should be qualified to manage and competently treat these disorders. The practitioner's *own* self-integration and emotional flexibility is a springboard for "response-ability," preparing him to intercept and accommodate the unexpected curve balls of the ED recovery process. In particular, it is the practitioner's skillful use of self within a trusting and mindful therapeutic connection that enhances the patient's internal strengths, evoking her faith in her own capacity to heal, and in the treatment process as a vehicle for change. In accruing self-trust within this connection, the patient ultimately comes to rely on her own newly acquired, sustainable coping capacities that far outweigh the benefits of her past reliance on her ED, now becoming irrelevant and obsolete.

Like the patients they treat, therapists too, strive to grow and develop as human beings throughout the course of personal and professional life experiences. The effective eating disorder practitioner will have accessed and encountered himself, putting his own emotional and cognitive "house in order" in preparation to access and connect with the patient who seeks to accomplish the very same goal. Through self-reflection and self-acceptance, the emotionally flexible therapist becomes capable of retrieving and integrating the emotional aspects of his own psyche that may have been lost, denied, avoided, or repressed in the creation of his or her own self-integrity. Through an active and palpable presence within the therapeutic moment, the therapist's self-integration inspires healthy role modeling. The ED patient's successes will be dependent not only upon *what* the therapist thinks and knows, but on modeling after *the way* he thinks, acts, and responds.

Though diverse and broad-spectrum ED treatment techniques and strategies enhance learning and change, healing occurs essentially through the *process of the recovery journey* itself. Emotional, cognitive, and behavioral learning required for recovery is enhanced within the framework of a powerfully human and loving therapeutic connection. The therapist's use of self within the context of the therapeutic relationship can be seen as the global positioning system (GPS) that charts the route to full recovery, replete with "rerouting" directions for the inevitability of wrong turns and setbacks as part of the journey. Ultimately, patients acquire the practice and resiliency they need to navigate life's roads confidently on their own. The ED healing process becomes a metaphor for life itself… for human tasks that evolve toward maturational development through the stimulus of learning within the context of nourishing human relationships. It is not uncommon for recovered individuals to express gratitude for having had the opportunity to define, refine, and refresh the "gestalt" of their very existence through the process of ED healing.

3.2. Treating ED is not for the weak at heart

As the treatment process is steeped in patient resistance and denial, and often complicated by mood, personality, and attachment disorders, the ED patient population is capable of arousing intense emotions within practitioners. The ED corrodes the patient's internal strengths, impairing judgment and the capacity to benefit from treatment. The ED individual fears giving up a disorder that (falsely) promises a guarantee of competency and self-control in the face of life's exigencies and unpredictability. Even on the verge of full recovery, patients describe a sense of "longing" for their ED. ED therapists need to prioritize attention to the patient's potential to return, by default, to old behavioral symptoms, such as recurring weight loss or stagnation, binging and purging, excessive exercise, etc particularly at times of stress, even after a healthy eating lifestyle appears to be securely in place.

It is not atypical to find that parents of teen or child ED patients will feel more needy of the therapist's attention, coaching, guidance, and support then does the identified patient. Therapists who treat ED individuals do well to have achieved a substantial degree of comfort and competency in treating complex family systems, as it is incumbent upon the practitioner who treats the individual patient to treat the family system as well. ED treatment occurs in clinical offices for 1 or 2 hours per week. The recovery process happens at home, 24/7, in the company of the entire family system, every member impacted by the ED's presence. If uninformed, well-intentioned family members may inadvertently enable problems in attempting to eradicate them. Involved parents and enlightened siblings are a boon to the struggling child, treatment team, and recovery process. Therapists need to empower parents by offering permission and courage to stand up to the child who, through the voice of the ED, may attempt to dictate the parameters of care, at home and in the treatment office; ie. "I will not discuss eating, because it will make me feel more anxious and I will cry." "I don't have a problem and I don't need treatment. I can handle this myself."

3.3. Countertransference phenomena can contribute to treatment resistance

Within the context of the countertransference phenomenon (where the person in treatment redirects feelings for others onto the therapist), self-awareness, honest intention, and clear boundaries become the therapist's parachute. The capacity to remain vulnerable and receptive to others, the benchmark of our humanity, allows therapists to stay real, encourage trust in the treatment relationship, and facilitate learning. Through self-awareness and attention to the treatment process, therapists need to resist the temptation to collude with the resistant patient who consciously or unconsciously deflects the focus of attention in treatment away from the tough challenges of food talk, symptom abatement, and recovery demands. Therapists need to contain their desire to "fix" the overly dependent patient's problems by being overly ready to prescribe answers and solutions, a message implying that easy short cuts can resolve

http://dx.doi.org/10.5772/65697

complex problems simply. "There is a time for expert opinion, but not in the place of first building the patient's own motivation as an active, not passive, participant" [21].

The countertransference phenomenon need not be an impediment to treatment, but can function as a vehicle for the patient's learning. When faced with emotional challenges within the treatment context, as practitioners, we need to do precisely what we counsel our patients to do; that being, to take control where we can, and where control evades us, to cope as best we can in an effort to achieve treatment goals. Miscommunications and misunderstandings are common fare within any in-depth human relationship. During times of patient discontent, the practitioner does well to readily encourage feedback of all types, particularly when it is negative, modeling transparency and a sincere willingness to accept responsibility and seek problem solutions through discussion and accommodation. Complaints typically contain invaluable learning for the patient, as well as the practitioner. Intention and goals need to be shared, and the patient's honesty applauded. The therapist's response through self-disclosure needs to be purposeful, motivated by the intention to enhance the patient's self-awareness, learning, and change. When effective, it can deepen the patient's access to affect and the promotion of self-regulation. "Following self-disclosure, the therapist should immediately shift the focus back to the patient and her response" [22]. The following is an excerpt from a letter I wrote to a codependent parent of an 11-year-old anorexic patient, who corroborated with this child's choice to leave treatment precipitously.

> "...In considering N's leaving treatment at this juncture, what becomes apparent to me is that her malnourished brain is not equipped to make rational decisions of this sort on her own. I believe she is frightened to the point of panic, and understandably so, at the thought of meeting the required demands of recovery from a disease she feels she cannot live without. In leaving this treatment relationship, however, it appears that she is 'shooting the messenger.'
>
> In a situation like this, it is the parents' trust in, and support for, the therapist and therapy process that carries the day. One of the factors that leads to, and exacerbates N's ED is her feeling of being out of control, overly powerful, and therefore unsafe within her own skin. By giving in to her unrealistic ploy to avoid treatment, a parent becomes an unintentional enabler of the ED. Flip side, the parent who can remain steadfast in understanding and supporting the treatment process becomes an invaluable advocate for both child and recovery. The eating disorder has to be confronted, and in the process, so must N. In observing her response to outpatient care, I believe a higher level of care would be an appropriate alternative for her under these circumstances."

4. Achieving "VIABLE-ity" in eating disorder practice

Along with clarity of intention, relentless urgency of purpose, and an integrative, goal-driven vision of successful recovery outcomes, the ED specialist exhibits distinguishing qualities represented in the acronym V.I.A.B.L.E. [19], which stands for Versatile, Integrative, Action-oriented, outcome-Based, Loving, and Educative. It goes without saying that though all of the characteristics described here are essential qualities of ED practitioners, many have broad applicability to skillful generalists, as well. General psychotherapy skills alone, however, are insufficient to manage the lethality of the ED, the unique complexity of the treatment and recovery processes, and in many instances, the depth of the victims' resistance to healing.

5. Seeking V.I.A.B.L.E. treatment through the therapist's Versatility

5.1. Utilize diverse treatment approaches, modalities, and strategies within ED treatment

Approaches to treatment are determined by (1) the nature of the disease and its unique symptom presentation, (2) the age of the patient, (3) the patient's physical and developmental status, and (4) the overall emotional health and availability of the patient's family system. The technically skilled and seasoned ED psychotherapist needs to be capable of integrating traditional "best practice" methodologies with alternative types of interventions, to accommodate the diverse nature of ED pathology which impacts behavior, emotions, cognition, sensation, mood, physiology, nutrition, and the neuroplastic brain. The versatile practitioner's use of dialectical behavior therapy (DBT) and cognitive behavioral therapy (CBT) treatment techniques and strategies is designed to systematically ameliorate distortions within the patient's cognition, self-perception, and judgment. The assignment of behavioral tasks to counteract habitual, ritualistic, and entrenched thoughts and actions inspires new learning, the motivation to heal, and accountability within the change process, while creating new neuronal pathways in the recovering brain. The recent advent of mindfulness-based cognitive behavioral therapy (MCBT), designed to help people who suffer from repeated bouts of depression and chronic unhappiness, combines the ideas of cognitive therapy with meditative practices and attitudes. Dialectical behavior therapy (DBT), too, incorporates the quality of mindfulness as a central component of treatment.

The Maudsley Method of Family-Based Therapy (FBT), not to be confused with conjoint family systems therapy, has been considered a "best" evidence-based practice for treating eating disorders in young children and families. The method follows a manualized protocol dictating the roles that parents need to assume in their child's refeeding process. Early phases of FBT minimize the significance of the therapeutic connection between the practitioner and child where the child is not yet developmentally capable of separation from parents, or is too emotionally undeveloped to absorb and benefit from the values and insights imparted through treatment. In the latter phases of FBT, as the child becomes developmentally more self-reliant and present, the relational context of the therapist/child connection becomes increasingly relevant.

Acceptance and commitment therapy (ACT) is a branch of cognitive therapy that acknowledges the centrality of the therapy relationship. Successful outcomes are achieved through acceptance and mindfulness strategies, coupled with commitment and behavioral change strategies, which result in psychological flexibility. "ACT focuses on full acceptance of present experience and mindfully letting go of obstacles as clients identify and pursue their life goals"

http://dx.doi.org/10.5772/65697

[22]. Such mindfulness strategies in psychotherapy cultivate moment-to-moment awareness as a curative mechanism that serves most forms of psychotherapy across the board [22]. By attending to their own experience in the present moment, therapists become more open to, and accepting of, whatever awareness emerges in that experience and in the experience of the other, to include body sensations, affects, and thoughts. Current studies suggest that in successful treatment alliances, therapists are perceived as being warm, understanding, and accepting, approaching their patients with an open, collaborative attitude. In developing these qualities, mindfulness qualities in psychotherapy practice deepen the therapeutic relationship [23].

The transdiagnostic approach to eating disorders, Unified Protocol (UP) is an emotion-focused cognitive-behavioral treatment developed to be applicable across the full range of anxiety and related disorders. Consisting of four core modules, it increases emotional awareness, facilitates flexibility in appraisals, identifies and prevents behavioral and emotional avoidance, and provides situational and interoceptive exposure to emotional cues [24]. "Clinicians are often faced with the difficult task of treating individuals with complex clinical presentations that require them to use multiple protocols or to tackle several problems at once, with little empirical data to guide them. Transdiagnostic treatments may help eliminate the need for multiple diagnosis-specific treatment manuals and simplify treatment planning, overall" [25–27].

Motivational interviewing is also highly relevant to ED treatment in light of ongoing ambivalence about, and fear of, recovery that essentially immobilizes patients, particularly within the precontemplative stage of treatment. Through motivational strategies and tools, family involvement, therapist-patient relationship quality, the use of medication, and behavioral contracts, therapists assess and shepherd readiness for change by suggesting realistic goals that the patient feels are within her reach. Therapists do well to use the patient's own incentives and logic, impaired as they may be, as a place to start: "So, am I understanding correctly that you believe the more weight you lose, the more popular you become at school? Are you saying that in the throes of your disease now, you are feeling increasingly happier and more secure?"

5.2. Enhance the partnership between patient and brain through neurophysiological treatment approaches

Among the more novel adjunctive treatments for ED are those that occur through enhancing the vibrant partnership between patient and brain. Like a beaver building a dam to change the distribution of water in the aftermath of natural forces, the patient who is inspired by the therapist to "put aside an obsessive focus on the past in order to reconsider, rethink, and re-create the course and flow of the present, has a hand in mindfully creating a far-reaching and lasting influence on brain structure and function to affect the future" [22].

ED are disorders of self-sensing and self-perception. Anorexic patients experience an altered capacity to process and integrate bodily signals. Their sensation of body parts is distorted, experienced as dissociated from their holistic and perceptive dimensions [28]. In stimulating regions of the brain that lie beyond the scope of talk therapy, neurophysiological treatment interventions that integrate brain, body, and mind have been shown to increase sensory awareness and self-awareness, both elements essential to ED recovery. Twenty-first century research and imaging technology has demonstrated the neuroplastic brain's capacity to regenerate, reconfigure, and heal itself through adjunctive, noninvasive, neurophysiologically based somatosensory treatment interventions (those dealing with the embodied nervous system) by informing, integrating and healing the brain through creating connectivity between and body and brain. Various forms of somatosensory education hold the potential to facilitate recovery from ED and body image disturbances. Despite this, such practices have not yet become part of mainstream clinical ED practice.

5.2.1. The Feldenkrais Method

Dr. Moshe Feldenkrais recognized the value of systematic exploration and reorganization of sensory motor aspects of self-image during the early part of the twentieth century. Through pleasurable, sequential forms of movement with attention, *the Feldenkrais Method of Somatic Education©* stimulates sensory integration by reconnecting individuals consciously with their unconscious sensorimotor repertoire. Facilitation of the method is accomplished through the verbally guided directives of a Feldenkrais practitioner in Awareness through Movement© group lessons; or through gentle, nonverbal, hands-on Functional Integration© lessons, which connect and integrate the sensing body and brain. In a controlled study within a multimodal treatment program, ED inpatients participating in adjunctive Feldenkrais treatment were shown to increase their acceptance of, and contentment with, problematic zones of their body. Other results indicated "the development of a felt sense of self, self-confidence, and a general process of maturation of the whole personality" [29]. Easily accessible demonstrations of short and simple Feldenkrais movements have become available via the Internet for use in professional offices and patients' homes. ED therapists do well to encourage patients to reinforce mindful neurophysiological healing at home, as "sustained practice solidifies learning" [30]. Integrating body and brain leads to the integration of the total self, awakening the patient's potential for realizing new options in *all* life spheres. By verbally processing somatosensory experiences with the patient either during the movement experience, or in its aftermath, therapists help patients fully understand how the functions of somatic education parallel and complement the functions of the psychotherapy process by increasing awareness of a sense of mind/body wholeness and a unified perception of self.

5.2.2. Trauma-Informed Yoga

Trauma-informed yoga regulates the nervous system, bringing it from a dysregulated state to a unified, centered state. Unprocessed traumatic memories stored in the brain become recycled when triggered, creating imbalanced patterns of nervous system activation. Yoga naturally regulates the overwhelmed nervous system by bringing unconscious content from trauma-related neurological and muscular patterns into consciousness. Teaching the use of breath, which evokes self-regulation, and facilitating close attention to present-moment awareness of self, yoga shifts sympathetic nervous system arousal to a balanced parasympathetic sense of calm and relaxation. Yoga has been shown to promote affect tolerance of physical and sensory experiences associated with fear and helplessness [31]. The trauma-informed yoga practitioner needs to conduct a full assessment of the patient's nervous system imbalances in order to provide postural movements that accommodate the individual's unique needs. For ED patients suffering from co-occurring substance abuse or addictions, yoga-breathing practices may be useful in counteracting all types of urges brought on by environmental triggers that could result in relapse [31].

5.2.3. *Eye Movement Desensitization Reprocessing*

A growing body of research points to *eye movement desensitization and reprocessing* (EMDR) as a highly successful, (mindful) method for treating a variety of conditions, including trauma [32]. Traumatic experience becomes locked in the brain and body. As an integrative psychotherapy approach involving interpersonal, experiential, and body-centered techniques, EMDR processes traumatic memory stored in the brain. Given the direct correlation between the trauma of sexual abuse and the onset of ED, this methodology can be considered a helpful adjunctive resource in the treatment of ED.

5.2.4. *Neurofeedback training*

Parts of the traumatized brain remain out of synch with other parts of the brain, leaving the trauma victim unable to take in neutral information without fear, and unable to learn freely from life experience. *Neurofeedback training* (NFT) represents an effective alternative for modifying neurophysiological activity in the brain that contributes to specified impaired cognitive processing and emotional and behavioral dysregulation. Noninvasive instruments measure physiological activity, then "feed back" information to the user, a process that enables individuals to reverse the effects of trauma and depression by integrating brain function, and allowing the patient to change the course of neurophysiological activity to improve health and performance.

5.2.5. *Transcranial magnetic stimulation*

Another form of noninvasive technological brain intervention that has been used successfully with ED patients includes *transcranial magnetic stimulation* (TMS), which sends low dose magnetic pulses to parts of the brain associated with unrelenting depression. The technique has been shown to ease depression and improve mood when medication has been insufficient to relieve depressive symptoms for patients with a severe and enduring ED (SEED).

5.3. Manage resistance by tapping into personal and external resources

The process of recovery typically feels worse to the patient than does the pathology of disease. It is up to the psychotherapist to penetrate and break through treatment resistance to facilitate patient engagement, from the very first meeting, and throughout the recovery process. Treatment resistance can be seen in the patient's failure to: (1) recognize and accept the ED diagnosis, (2) engage in the treatment process, (3) attend sessions consistently, (4) attempt to comply with food plans, and (5) include parents and family in treatment where appropriate. When resistance and/or accompanying denial interferes with the treatment process, the mindful and empathic therapeutic connection and the creative use of diverse resources can become motivational. Tools existing within the clinician's "professional toolbox" include the following:

5.3.1. Tool #1: Recognize and celebrate the patient's internal strengths

As early as the first diagnostic session, the therapist's capacities to inspire, build, and nurture trust in the therapy relationship and treatment process lays the groundwork for treatment engagement, patient self-acceptance, and healing. Instilling trust in the patient's existing strengths and potential for growth, particularly at treatment outset, is the glue that upholds and sustains an otherwise fragile, tentative, and ambivalent precontemplative treatment connection and process. Planting the seeds of self-trust ultimately provides patients the stamina to sustain recovery efforts through challenging treatment junctures. Reframing a situation can recapture, refresh, and restore the healing process through trust development. As an example, by empathically reframing the ED to be the patient's well-intentioned bid for self-survival, the therapist dismantles her fears that she is crazy and culpable. In addition, it inspires hope in the implication that she will soon become capable of discovering more reliable, less self-destructive means of coping with discomfort and adversity.

Positive change can be identified in the demonstration of the patient's: (1) growing commitment to treatment, (2) connection with the therapist, (3) capacity to identify feelings, (4) increased capacity to recognize and verbally communicate needs, (5) growing independence and self-determination, (6) healthy eating lifestyle, (7) improved coping capacities, and (8) improved quality of daily function. By recognizing and acknowledging the elusive or disguised nature of recovery progress, personal growth, and resiliency, therapists evoke optimism and incentive to heal. Constructive life lessons frequently reside in mistakes, if not failures.

> J returned from college with a sad confession. She had begun to slide back into her purging patterns. "I'm a failure" was her message, clear and simple. Her doctor and nutritionist had both read her the riot act. Her lesson from me was not about how to eat better or become more disciplined, but about how to view the situation from a more positive and realistic framework, helping her to differentiate normative recovery patterns from significant relapse. "So," I observed, "Let's take a look at what *has* changed!" I helped her see that she had become more ready to be honest with herself and with others, more acutely aware of precipitants to her regressions. Her digressions had become more contained; now isolated incidents, they were no longer the start of extended patterns of dysfunction. General problem-solving in other life spheres improved, as had her relationships with others. Increasingly aware of her needs and feelings, she was becoming increasingly assertive in communicating those needs, both within, and outside of, treatment sessions. She was, in fact, progressing well in her ED recovery.

http://dx.doi.org/10.5772/65697

5.3.2. Tool #2: Rally your forces: tap into the network of family resources

Though baffled, fearful, and generally uninformed, by default, parents and families become witnesses to their child's struggles in kitchens, bathrooms, grocery stores, and restaurants. Parents need to learn to understand the disease, its effects on their child, and the unpredictability (and necessity) of the recovery process. They need knowledge, guidance, and skills to respond effectively, and with sensitivity, to their child's efforts to recover, and to mediate the effects of the ED on the greater family system, particularly at meal times. Life partners of ED individuals, as well, need to learn to interpret the significance of changes they see, or may not see, throughout the course of treatment, be they in the form of progress or regression, or both. Family members need to keep pace with the ongoing development of the recovering individual's strengths, which will influence the ever-changing nature of their support for their loved one throughout the treatment process. When the psychotherapist takes on the dual roles of individual and family therapist, treatment efficacy becomes streamlined, simultaneously guiding the family along the same continuum of growth and change that the identified patient travels, and at the same pace. Treating family members conjointly with the identified patient avoids the potential for the practitioner to breach confidentiality by enabling family members to speak for themselves, openly, willingly, and face to face.

5.3.3. Tool #3: Consider a referral to a psychopharmacologist for a medication evaluation

Psychopharmacological medication is meant to help people feel, and function, better. If and when medications fail to result in either or both of these outcomes, it is clearly time for the psychotherapist to recommend a medication reevaluation, or possibly, a second opinion. When a treatment process is stagnating or regressive, a medication reassessment holds the potential to break through neurochemical barriers in the brain that contribute to entrenched resistance to healing. The psychopharmacological specialist in the treatment of ED seeks to balance brain chemistries, optimize brain function, and facilitate the patient's potential to benefit from the treatment experience. Malnutrition, co-occurring mood disorders, depression, anxiety/obsessive compulsive disorder (OCD), and ADHD (in some cases brought on by the disease itself) highlight the importance of the input of a skillful psychopharmacologist as part of the ED outpatient professional team. Medications are not meant to provide a cure, but to facilitate healing through the psychotherapy process. It is important to recognize that until the starving brain has been refed, the benefits of using medication will be less than optimal.

ED patients commonly resist consideration of the medication option, fearing the unknown, the possible side effect of weight gain, or taking the "easy way out" in the face of an ED that demands willful deprivation and self-discipline. Some patients are afraid to "contaminate" their body. Others, who consider medication to be the "last resort," fear that they will ultimately discover themselves to be beyond help. It is critical for the knowledgeable psychotherapist to reduce the patient's (and family's) resistance to the medication option by preparing them for the medication evaluation, describing benefits and possible side effects of relevant medications, establishing realistic expectations, quieting fears, etc.

Because of the breadth of factors that contribute to and co-occur with ED, psychopharmacologists need to diagnose mental health status fully, and in depth, before providing medication.

Though fluoxetine (prozac) has been shown to be beneficial in treating AN and BN, medications affecting serotonin neurotransmitters can be contraindicated, creating suicidal tendencies in cases where there may be a yet undiscovered underlying mood disorder. Stimulants prescribed for ADHD can suppress appetites in patients with AN. Hormone replacement therapy, commonly prescribed for anorexic patients, does not enhance bone density, but masks the loss of natural menses. "The commonly prescribed use of estrogens for anorexic patients to bring on a period in seeking bone density enhancement may create a false picture indicating that the skeleton is being protected against osteoporosis. Thus, the motivation to regain weight, and adhere to treatment of the ED, may be reduced. Hormone and oral contraceptive therapy should not be prescribed for young women with amenorrhea and concurrent ED. The most important intervention is to restore menstrual periods through increased nutrition" [33].

6. V.I.A.B.L.E. treatment incorporates an Integrative style of thought and action

6.1. Sustain a "big-picture" perspective through envisioning, and seeking, a complete ED recovery

ED therapists need to be myopic, even while functioning as visionaries. The seasoned ED practitioner integrates knowledge with instinct, intention with flexibility, and diversity within structure, holding onto the "big picture" of disease and recovery even while attending to the small details of behavioral change. With ED, small changes become the stuff of vast transformations. In validating the patient's feelings, thoughts, and ideas, the therapist makes sense of them for the patient within the larger picture of the disorder, of the narrative of her life, and of her relationships with food, self, and loved ones.

As integrationists, ED therapists piece together submerged and disparate facets of the patient's personality to foster the re-creation of the patient's true and authentic integrated self. In uncovering, discovering, differentiating, then reintegrating all parts of the patient's exiled self, disclosed and undisclosed, systematically and intentionally, the 1000 piece puzzle of the patient's holistic self slowly reassembles itself into an integrative fabric through the recovery process. As integrationists, practitioners play diverse roles in the life of the ED patient, as teacher, mentor, cheerleader, confidant, case manager, and "parent" in supporting and containing the patient to her point of readiness for flight into recovery as an autonomous, independently functioning, self-possessed, self-regulated, human being.

6.2. Be prepared to "understudy" multiple roles within the treatment team

In taking on the responsibility of case manager, it is up to the outpatient ED psychotherapist to put together an outpatient team of expert treatment professionals capable of tending to the broad-based needs of the ED patient throughout the course of care. Defying compartmentalization, ED symptoms need to be recognized and professionally managed by every member of the team. Wearing diverse professional "hats," each team member acts as a representative of the wider healing process, capable of mediating all spheres of pathology. Particularly in

http://dx.doi.org/10.5772/65697

smaller, less diverse, rural communities, where trained and experienced professionals may not be readily accessible, the need for an integration of knowledge, skill sets, and a multifaceted use of self becomes particularly critical. Members of the professional team, including medical doctor, psychopharmacologist, individual/family therapist, and nutritionist, need to understand and "understudy" each other's parts, learning essentially to "speak each other's lines" as needed, fluently, throughout the treatment process.

As an example, where an at-risk anorexic child patient resists treatment engagement with the outpatient psychotherapist, the familiar and authoritative pediatrician may step in to become active in monitoring weight and vital signs regularly, actively demanding accountability and improvement. In the absence of timely change, the pediatrician's recommendation for a higher level of care potentially carries the day. In response to a patient who is starving herself, my nutritionist team partner would typically ask the patient to consider the fact that she is abusing herself, inquiring "what that might be about." Following such an exchange, she would attend to the issue of introducing behavioral change into the patient's eating lifestyle. Even in the latter stages of recovery, there is rarely a session that goes by without my inquiring about how one's eating-related progress is going.

6.3. Encourage families and life partners to become advocates for recovery

Apart from parents of child patients, life partners and siblings become witnesses, and potentially effective supporters of ED recovery as well, when properly prepared for the task. Siblings of adolescents with AN have been shown to demonstrate poorer psychosocial adjustment than their peers, both before and after the identified patient's FBT recovery efforts. Clinicians and parents need to become aware of sibling difficulties and to offer additional support if required [34].

When a family member contacts me by phone or email to discuss concerns about his or her loved one's recovery, my response is always inclusive, welcoming them to attend conjoint family sessions for open and mutual discussions. The patient who refuses to participate in an occasional conjoint meeting with family or partner raises a therapeutic issue that demands attention and resolution.

Any concerns about privacy disclosures or confidentiality breaches when the family joins the individual patient in conjoint family treatment become unfounded, a non-issue, as family members are brought together to air their *own* immediate concerns and issues, willingly, and by choice, to one another. Except in extreme instances of dysfunction within family systems, parents or spouses need to become part of the fabric of treatment, in various ways, to varying degrees, and at various points within the healing process.

In those instances where a married ED patient enters treatment, the marital dyad becomes the primary family system. Involving the spouse in treatment potentially enriches and facilitates the identified patient's recovery.

> C. was a compulsive exerciser, waking at 3:00 AM to make time for eight hours of exercise daily. She would fulfill her computer-based employment responsibilities while exercising on machines. Interfering with the lives of family members in the

context of daily living and travel, her compulsions began to undermine her marriage. Ultimately, C's husband felt compelled to supercede the eating disorder by taking control of his wife's behaviors, threatening to leave the marriage if she did not comply with his directives to give up exercise completely. Having done so, as she restored her weight, her extreme body image discomfort finally prompted her to seek ED treatment. This patient refused to consider taking medication to diminish her anxiety, compulsions and occasional panic attacks.

It became apparent that C's husband needed to attend a conjoint couple's therapy session to become educated about her need for a gradual increase in her own *self*-regulation as part of her recovery. The session facilitated a plan for a treatment arrangement at home allowing her to attempt to return very gradually to a normal degree of exercise in the hope of overcoming her compulsive urges towards extremes in behaviors and thinking *in all areas of life*. Conjoint sessions provided the backdrop for a more complete recovery and a healthier, stronger marriage.

6.4. Integrate diverse treatment milieus and levels of care when necessary

Levels of care for ED treatment range from the most restrictive (hospitals and long-term residential facilitates) to less restrictive alternatives (group partial hospital programs (PHPs), intensive outpatient programs (IOPs), and individual outpatient therapy with an outpatient team of ED experts providing therapeutic, medical, psychopharmacological and nutritional services to individuals and families. The latter is the least restrictive outpatient level of care, allowing the patient to remain in her home environment with the support of loved ones, fulfilling her life roles at school or work, side by side with friends. A higher level of care becomes a consideration primarily when the patient faces immediate physiological or emotional risk, requires forcible refeeding, or when the outpatient team alternative proves unworkable due to the patient's treatment resistance or progress stagnation. Higher levels of group care enforce refeeding, provide cognitive and behavioral immersion, offer emotional exposure to peer support, and enhance internal strengths and coping resources, ultimately setting the stage for the patient to make subsequent long term progress through recovery efforts within less restrictive outpatient care.

Choosing the appropriate care level, at the right time, can optimize the course of treatment for each individual patient, impacting one's engagement in treatment, one's time spent in treatment, the nature of the weight gain process, and the extent to which emotional goals are attained. In some instances, the referral to a higher level of care, at the right moment, could potentially insure that the window of readiness for treatment engagement and healing is captured rather than lost forever. In transitioning into or out of a program successfully patients and parents need preparation to understand what to expect and to establish realistic goals for themselves within the upcoming experience.

A pediatrician who universally prescribes higher levels of care as a child's initial entry into ED treatment in order to "save parents time and money," believes it is more efficacious to bypass the option of diagnostic assessment through an

http://dx.doi.org/10.5772/65697

outpatient treatment team of ED professionals. Such a universal prescription misleadingly implies that restrictive environments are more beneficial than those permitting recovery within the context of daily living; that all patients, and all recoveries, are alike; and that restrictive treatment programs "cure" ED patients.

7. Seeking V.I.A.B.L.E. treatment through an Action-oriented treatment style

7.1. Any ED diagnosis can be considered a call to action

An ED waits for no one. Unless it is healing, the condition is progressing. The diagnosis of an ED is frequently elusive. Through a deep understanding of these diseases, seasoned therapists develop a capacity to anticipate or intuit their presence, a skill rooted in diagnostic acuity. Within the context of human connection, the astute therapist reads 'between the lines' of the therapeutic moment, guiding an inquiry and early detection of physiological, developmental and emotional gaps in the patient's psyche and body image.

> E was a 29-year-old woman who began treatment with me for depression and relationship problems. In response to her description of her college days where she spoke of herself as being perfectionistic, highly compulsive, and depressed, I chose to wonder aloud if she had ever struggled with an ED or other eating related issues. "My God!" she responded. "How did you know? I have never told a soul!" By understanding the emotional configuration of her personality, I was able to intuit and surmise the possible existence of a past or ongoing ED. In learning that my hunch had been correct, I better understood the breadth and depth of her treatment needs.

Learning to identify suspicious clusters of symptoms potentially shines a light on existing, future, or past ED that might otherwise have remained undisclosed. In making the educated guess, therapists learn to "connect the dots" of conversation and affect. At times, making an eating disorder diagnosis can be much like observing a disparate grouping of stars and seeing a constellation. By anticipating the unspoken (based on information that *has* been offered), by discerning which topics require further investigation, and by actively probing the possibility of earlier patterns of behavioral impulsivity and compulsions such as self-mutilation/cutting, childhood shoplifting, promiscuity, substance abuse, and excessive exercise, therapists become capable of revealing hidden, or yet undisclosed, underlying ED and co-occurring conditions.

7.2. ED require an active, purposeful, and on-going diagnostic process

ED offer little leeway for cursory assessment of both the disease and recovery status, throughout the course of treatment. An ongoing diagnostic assessment of recovery, which may be considered the flipside of an ongoing diagnostic assessment of pathology, enriches the treatment process, motivating new directions for growth and change. Assessment of recovery status might reveal a possible resurgence of resistance and regression, which could signify a worsening pathology. Recovery derailments can be gradual or sudden, temporary or enduring, minor or significant, at times warranting consideration of a higher level of care or tapping additional personal and professional resources (family, team, psychopharmacological medication) for support, as needed. Effective ED treatment demands *ongoing* positive change in the form of recovery progress, both immediate and long term, behavioral and emotional, throughout the duration of care.

7.3. In managing a moving target, ED practitioners dare not take their hands off the wheel

The ED therapist moves and motivates people with the intention of moving and motivating the healing process. Authoritative action, not to be confused with authoritarian demands, produces desired outcomes. Micromanagement and the imposition of directives, judgments, projections, or boundary intrusions replicate the role of the overly controlling ED, denying the patient self-determination, a most pivotal component of recovery. In response to the momentum behind a forward-moving disease, therapists need to carefully monitor, then shepherd, the pacing of recovery change. Except in the case of young children who are developmentally unprepared to take on the tasks of self-determination throughout recovery, or of highly resistant patients whose malnourished brains have impaired their capacity to make responsible decisions, the use of "*soft power*" can produce positive outcomes. The nonjudgmental therapist's radical acceptance of the patient can redirect the forces of resistance..

> An 18-year-old anorexic patient declared, "I can fix myself. I don't need therapy." I replied, "I'm all for that plan. You are, and will always be, the primary person responsible for your own recovery. I am basically here as a coach, cheerleader and collaborator. So why don't you try to follow your own meal plan this week, and let's talk about how things go when we meet again. Be sure to journal your efforts, so together we can gauge your progress and determine your next steps.

7.3.1. Taking action demands courage in ED patients as well as practitioners

Action-based behavioral tasks and strategies, such as the patient's journaling, or in-office meals eaten in the company of the therapist, create accountability, and can become strong motivators for change. As important diagnostic tools, such strategies can shed light on an elusive process of ED recovery change.

> A recovering anorexic patient, who had made brilliant progress in integrating regular and nutritious meals into her life, spoke of having skipped lunch three times one week because of mounting stressors at work. After legitimizing her urges, and identifying the feelings that evoked them, I discussed the normalcy of an occasional and intermittent regression during eating disorder recovery, not to be considered a relapse. I requested that she attempt to resume eating lunches daily and journal her efforts and struggles, successes and failures, to be assessed together in our quest for understanding and problem-resolution during our next meeting. In another instance of an anorexic patient's strong resistance to considering the inclusion of lunch into her eating lifestyle, I planned to conduct the next

http://dx.doi.org/10.5772/65697

few sessions over lunch together, side by side, in-office or at a restaurant, supporting her efforts, providing exposure, processing fears.

Actively engaged practitioners model energy, initiative, and resolve. A study showed that when therapists make referrals to higher levels of care and encourage patient follow through, of those patients who were offered a phone number, 37% made contact; when the counselor took initiative to place the referral call for the client, 82% completed the referral [21]. The therapist who chooses to remain passive, nondirective, or more like a friend by avoiding tough therapeutic issues in an effort to protect the patient's comfortability and trust, enables the ED. "Toughness" is a sign of a practitioner's clear intention to support positive change.

In reminiscing about her ED treatment, a recovered patient once commented, "You knew things that were in my head and heart even before I did, and you recognized what I was capable of doing even before I did. Best of all, I couldn't get away with anything because you knew the drill, and were not afraid to challenge me."

Healing therapeutic connections ride on the therapist's capacity to sustain the fragile balance between discomfort and learning, and between learning and change.

8. Seeking V.I.A.B.L.E. outcome-Based treatment

8.1. If at first you do not succeed, try something different

If one technique does not work, it is incumbent upon the practitioner to find another that will. As a therapist, I am a Machiavellian proponent of doing what works, whatever that may entail. Nontraditional, "outside-the-box" treatment alternatives have been shown through evidence-based controlled studies to carry the potential to achieve positive outcomes for ED. If an intervention works for a single individual, offering that option to other ED individuals becomes a legitimate and viable option.

At age 13, M and her mother attended outpatient therapy sessions together for several months and saw a pediatrician and nutritionist weekly. Despite this, her AN remained intractable. Whatever weight she was able to gain, she readily lost. Still, she resisted medication and a higher level of care. Insisting that she could 'recover on her own,' her resistance to recovery intensified and she began to miss therapy sessions. In my effort to rescue a now fragile treatment process, I offered M the unique opportunity to discontinue therapy temporarily, going it on her own, utilizing the knowledge that she had already gleaned through treatment to date. This plan stipulated the singular requirement that she see her doctor weekly for monitoring of weight and vital signs. I also extended an invitation to her mother to attend coaching sessions with me regularly, without M, which she readily accepted. Feeling 'heard,' and grateful to be allowed to try her own hand at recovery, after 3 weeks, M requested permission to join her mother in her return to treatment.

> In her absence from treatment, M made peace with the idea of seeking a higher level of care. She ultimately agreed to attend an intensive after-school outpatient program, under the stipulation that if she did not gain sufficient weight there, she would enter a higher-level full-day partial hospital program. Having been offered an opportunity for self-determination, M felt an enhanced sense of trust and connection with me. Prior to starting higher-level care, she reached out to me on several occasions for my support and reassurance about what was now her own decision.

8.2. The proactive therapist sustains a clearly boundaried, but palpable, presence in the heat of the treatment trenches

> T was a 12 year old who had begun her descent into AN; at the start of her session, she sat in the car, bawling. Her mother rang my doorbell to ask what to do, as her daughter refused to get out of the car for her third therapy session. I instructed her to return to the car and speak with her daughter, setting clear but loving limits, and making authoritative demands… T would either come into the session to continue her outpatient work, or she would need to enter an ED program. Crying hysterically, T refused to get out of the car. At that point, I donned my boots and jacket and began this session on the street, in front of my office, in the snow. I told her how relieved and optimistic I felt to see that she was finally beginning to get in touch with her feelings, which made her so much more accessible to getting the help she so richly deserved. Reframing and educating, meeting and joining with her where she was, I applauded her integrity and courage in expressing herself. Standing up to her mother would hopefully become a prelude to standing up to her ED. Feeling genuinely understood, T began to experience hope and a sense of relief as she followed me into my office that day, where we proceeded to have a break-through session. [19]

8.3. Rules, like therapists, require flexibility

In an imperfect world of ED treatment and recovery, hard and fast rules may occasionally need to be bent in offering the most practicable solutions for patients. In nuanced decision-making, ED therapists become models of thought and action.

> An intake therapist at a renowned outpatient treatment center refused to assess a patient for admission because she needed two more pounds to reach her 'safe' body mass index goal. This patient was asked to attend an in-patient program to restore her weight first, in the interest of "optimizing the therapy process." Though motivated to achieve recovery through a higher level of care to support her re-feeding efforts, the patient became caught up in a catch-22. She would either have to enter a financially prohibitive in-patient milieu, or gain the required pounds in a less restrictive environment. Both alternatives were daunting to her. Though declared medically stable by a medical doctor who was monitoring her weekly, her recovery efforts floundered.

By disregarding the "psycho" and "social" aspects of the bio/psycho/social disease, this intake counselor placed too much emphasis on the criteria of weight alone in determining the patient's preparedness for treatment. This diagnostic assessment needed to take into consideration the patient's readiness and motivation for recovery, her financial constraints, and her medical monitoring, in addition to her weight. A short-term weekly contract for a stipulated amount of weight gain, in-program, might have been a more appropriate and workable alternative.

8.4. Don't stop until you are there. Advocate proactively within health policy systems

As neurobiological disorders with their origin in genetics, EDs were declared legitimate "biologically based mental illnesses" by the Academy for ED in 2006, deserving of medical insurance coverage. Congress succeeded in eliminating discrimination in health care coverage against people who have mental health disorders in the passage of the Emergency Economic Stabilization Act of 2008, which took effect in 2010. Despite these advancements, insurance coverage for ED treatment remains spotty, with some companies denying coverage totally and others denying longevity of coverage. Some insurance companies appear to be more amenable to providing coverage for diagnostic codes that indicate less serious, more ephemeral, types of diagnoses. In some instances, companies have considered the normal weight ED patient not appropriate for coverage.

In dealing with insurance companies, advocacy from personal and professional mentors needs to be active and focused. Communications need to be traced to the top of the bureaucratic pyramid in seeking assurance that the company assumes appropriate responsibility for its decision against coverage for the ED patient, particularly if a patient's health is at risk. The insurance company needs to be made aware of their liability if they refuse to cover a patient who dies for lack of care. Most insurance carriers allow families to appeal the refusal of coverage, and some now hire in-house employees to assist consumers in such appeals. Most higher-level ED programs and facilities offer the assistance of a specialized coordinator/advocate, hired to intercede and develop trusting relationships with insurance companies for the benefit of patients. Some residential programs offer scholarships for patients who would otherwise be unable to afford to take advantage of a costly, but life-saving, treatment milieu.

9. Seeking V.I.A.B.L.E. treatment through the Loving/caring therapeutic relationship

9.1. The treatment relationship as an intervention

According to Daniel Siegel, "Relationships are woven into the fabric of our inner world. We come to know our own minds through our interactions with others" [35]. Emotional, cognitive, and behavioral learning is enhanced within the framework of a powerfully human and loving therapeutic connection. "Love is not something that we generate; it is found in the activity of intimately attending" [22]. Because ED are disorders of relationship and attachment, the quality of relational connection or attunement between the ED therapist and patient is pivotal. The healing connection between therapist and eating disordered patient becomes the prototype and practice ground for all healthy relationships, as the conduit for the return of the ED patient's exiled core-self. Though the patient's resistance to letting go of the disorder may be a primary source of the ED clinician's initial treatment challenges, the quality of the therapy relationship is frequently the "deal breaker" when ED treatment fails. Conversely, it can be the quality of the treatment connection that transforms the therapist's goals and intentions into fertile seeds of successful outcomes within a safe and trusting treatment environment. Studies have found that "...the model of therapy simply does not make much difference in therapy outcome. Empathy accounts for as much and probably more outcome variance than does specific intervention" [22]. Empathy not only helps the patient to feel better and feel "felt," it may create a new state of activation with coherence in the moment that improves the capacity for self-regulation [35].

The foundation of the healing therapeutic connection exists within brain physiology. Neuroimaging studies of structural brain changes associated with the process of relationship within psychotherapy demonstrate that relational experiences in psychotherapeutic treatment result in detectable changes in the brain. "The aim of the talking cure...from the neurobiological point of view is to extend the functional sphere of influence of the prefrontal lobes" [30]. "The intention of therapy is to work through the effects of isolation and disconnection, as they play out in life and in therapy, toward the goal of reconnection and restoration of mutual connection. For the patient, this results in a greater capacity to act, increased clarity, enhanced self-worth, and the desire for more connection, while remaining present and accessible in his or her shared humanity" [22]. According to Christopher Germer, "Given that there is little empirical evidence that (treatment) effectiveness improves with experience, continuing education, licensing, professional degree, clinical supervision, or any other marker of professionalism, and given the importance of the therapeutic relationship, the larger challenge is to find a way to help cultivate the qualities of excellent therapists" [22].

9.2. Engage in strategies that reinforce the strength of therapeutic connections

Mindfulness in psychotherapeutic practice creates strong connections between people. The mindfulness process requires the therapist's and patient's attention and "presence" within the treatment moment, where the inception of psychotherapeutic change takes place. Daniel Siegel describes presence as "being aware, in a receptive state of what is happening as it is happening. This receptivity correlates with a brain state in which there is intentionality, awareness, conscientiousness, and nonjudgmentalism in interacting with others, promoting rewarding relationships" [36]. Mindfulness in psychotherapy practice allows patients a greater capacity to choose whether to act on one's urges, a concept that is particularly relevant to the treatment of BN, characterized by impulsivity and self-dysregulation. Mindfulness in psychotherapy stimulates the patient's ever-changing neuroplastic brain to learn. As the brain learns, people change and heal; as people change and heal, the brain alters in structure and function, ultimately stimulating further changes.

http://dx.doi.org/10.5772/65697

Recognizing and addressing the patient's newly emerging, fledgling strengths throughout the course of treatment reinforces the patient's self-acceptance and empowerment, facilitating trust in the therapeutic connection, but not without reservations. Low self-esteem and the fear of becoming fat and out of control render some ED individuals wary about trusting the therapist's positive affirmations. In the face of a complimentary observation, the self-hating patient may distrust the accuracy of the therapist's perceptions. ED patients may also fear (1) recovery from a much coveted disorder, (2) the therapist's terminating treatment before she feels ready, and (3) being expected to demonstrate strength and competency that she does not possess. Through a deeply sensitive understanding of the ED mind, and carefully worded subtleties of self-expression, the knowledgeable practitioner can avoid making well-intentioned comments that might inadvertently raise anxiety or stimulate regression in the ED patient.

> "You are looking great," can all too easily be interpreted as "You have gained weight and look fat." "You don't have too much weight to gain," a comment offered as encouragement to an anorexic teen with a dysregulated eating lifestyle, would clinch the patient's belief that she is already fat and that continuing to follow her meal plan would only make her fatter. A pediatrician mentioned the "benefits of eating fatty acids" in encouraging the inclusion of fish in an anorexic adolescent's diet; that patient resolved never to eat fish again.

It is never too late to repair a moment of distortion by investigating and processing it, clarifying and resolving misinterpretations, either as they occur, or after they have happened. The therapist's full transparency behind a misconstrued but well-intentioned comment can deter a patient's anxiety and potential for recovery derailment. Patients feel reassured and become capable of developing increasing trust in the therapist who substantiates positive comments by citing the origin of a complimentary observation and the thought process behind it.

> "Here's what has led me to remark about what I see as your substantive progress and the growing strengths you have achieved." Is there any part of what I am saying that you might accept as being an accurate description of yourself?

> "You know, when I offer positive feedback to you, I am aware that it must be difficult for you to hear because of how poorly you think of yourself. Can you tell me what it feels like for you to hear the positive things I am saying about you?"

It is not unusual for patients who may idealize their therapist to forego sharing what they consider to be shameful self-revelations, for fear of giving rise to judgment or disapproval. Therapists might anticipate and diffuse such a dynamic by wondering aloud "if such a thing might ever happen within our own treatment relationship." Welcoming a potential problem by putting it 'on the table' can stave off its occurrence, creating an atmosphere of total acceptance.

Another strategic tool that therapists might use to nurture and reinforce a genuinely caring connection with patient and family is to offer ready accessibility between sessions when needed, throughout care, always within the confines of exquisitely honed professional boundaries. I invite and welcome contact with patients who are in crisis, and with parents who have inquires or observations that deserve immediate attention. The process of learning and change exists in life, both within, and beyond, the therapeutic hour.

10. Seeking V.I.A.B.L.E. treatment through Education of self and others

10.1. Myth busting

The impact of ED pathology on the malnourished brain typically fosters cognitive distortions and illogical beliefs, which give rise to self-destructive thoughts and actions. ED therapists need to anticipate and address cognitive distortions, myths, and misconceptions about ED, educating patients and parents about the realities of these disorders, and their impact on the brain, mind, and body. Educating oneself first is prerequisite to educating others. Because misconceptions about ED are widespread, it is essential for professionals to know, and patients to learn, what is true and what is not. EDs are not exclusively female disorders, nor are they disorders of childhood. "Ten million men will suffer from an ED in their lifetime, and 13% of women over 50 have ED symptoms. Note that 70% of them will not seek treatment due to stigma, as well as lack of education, diagnosis, and access to care [37]." Two misconceptions that prevent ED individuals from seeking recovery assistance are the beliefs that ED are addictions, and therefore they are incurable. In fact, the genetic clusters in familial deoxyribonucleic acid (DNA) that predispose an individual to ED onset may contain substance and 'process' addictions, which are addictions to activities. However, ED are *not* addictions (primary, relapsing diseases of the brain). In addition, EDs are curable in approximately 80% of patients who receive effective care and who are willing to seek complete recovery [37].

10.2. Take responsibility for recognizing what you may not know

A professional's lack of education about ED and their treatment can be misleading and potentially dangerous for the ED patient in recovery.

> An anorexic patient spent three years with a highly regarded psychiatrist who refused to acknowledge her ED as a pivotal aspect of her personhood or treatment. His theory was that "her symptoms were too complex to be an ED." He perceived the ED symptoms as being tangential and secondary to other "more core" co-occurring problems, assuming that once these were treated and resolved, the ED would disappear. She ultimately left this therapist to seek specialized ED treatment. His parting warning was, "Don't let anyone "treat you like an ED patient. Your problem is much deeper than that." This physician was right in his allusion to the fact that her problems ran deep and wide, though wrong in thinking that an ED diagnosis and treatment would exclude the recognition and treatment of a myriad of commonly co-occurring conditions. In the face of a complex and integrative system of comorbidity, attention to one's eating lifestyle and weight-regulation issues not only saves lives, but also can provide a behavioral foothold in unmasking, and simultaneously treating, co-occurring problems.

http://dx.doi.org/10.5772/65697

10.3. Understand the role of weight in eating disorder treatment and recovery

The role of weight in the diagnosis and treatment of ED is perhaps the most misleading of all the commonly held misunderstandings about ED and their recovery. Patients need to understand that severe and prolonged dietary restriction and weight loss can lead to serious physical and neurological complications. At the same time, they need to understand that weight restoration alone in an underweight ED individual is not a predictable criterion for recovery. Most patients and parents, and all too many professionals, believe that the *only* requirement for medical rehabilitation for an ED is removing the immediate danger of death due to malnutrition. This is not the case. In fact, electrolyte imbalances due to purging behaviors in a normal weight ED patient can lead to sudden death.

Weight "restoration," is not to be confused with weight "gain." They both represent one single strand of the larger fabric of ED healing. Weight gain and normalizing blood tests and vital signs are significant in indicating *improved* eating and brain function, marking the patient's *potential* to achieve a full, integrative ED recovery, cognitively, emotionally, physically, and neurophysiologically. For the anorexic patient, full and *sustainable* weight restoration to the body's "set point," along with restoration of the menses and hormonal normalization, will ultimately normalize brain function and development. Attaining one's set point weight, marking full weight restoration and a normalized function of brain and body, leads to the reversal of amenorrhea. Each person has a set point weight to which he or she naturally gravitates. Bodily fluctuation from that point may diverge a few pounds in either direction, but the fit body at its set point weight will rarely gain or lose weight beyond its natural range.

> I conceptualize the set point weight as being like an ocean's tide. When the moon is new, gravitational forces may not exert a pull on a body of water as strongly as when the moon is full. The rising tide, be it slightly higher or lower, always approaches, (but does not exceed,) a certain point on the shore... with the exception of tropical storms or other natural forces. The set point weight is equally consistent, expected to fluctuate ever so slightly, but always hovering close to the water line." [19]

It is ultimately the patient's healthy and fearless relationship with food, restoration of weight to set point, normal hormonal health, and reintegration of the fragmented core self that become the cornerstone of a full ED recovery.

Regular weigh-ins can be an important accountability tool for the underweight patient. Patients who fear that any amount of weight gain will lead to the loss of self-control through binging and obesity, do best when weighed "blind," so their weight remains undisclosed to them, even while available to clinicians and parents when appropriate. It is counterproductive for clinicians to identify an "ideal weight" or to offer anorexic patients the "carrot" of reaching a specific "target weight" as their goal. The body mass index (BMI) has been proven an unreliable reflection of a healthy nutritional state [38]. No one, not a nutritionist, patient, or physician, can set an arbitrary target weight and expect its achievement to lead to recovery. The *body alone*, through the process of ingesting healthy, balanced, regular meals, is the only accurate determiner of its ideal weight for its own unique structure and function.

If a nutritionist or physician says, "It is important for you to gain another five pounds (to reach the low end of normal on the growth charts,) the patient hears," "Five pounds is all I need to gain in order to get everybody off my back;" "Five pounds gained will still allow me to stay skinny without being considered sick. If I gain 6 pounds, I will have become fat." Patients' misconceptions about food and weight need to be corrected. Such false notions include: food is fattening; the more one eats, the more weight one gains; when it comes to food, less is more; healthy eating is fat-free and sugar-free eating. Patients and families need to learn that food restriction damages the functions of the healthy metabolism, which burns calories and fat.

10.4. Understand that "almost recovered" is not synonymous with ED recovery

Within the context of eating disorder recovery, "almost recovered" does not apply. The term "relapse" should not to be confused with the patient's *choice* not to recover to one's set point weight during treatment. Full recovery, marked by the reintegration of the core self and the emotional flexibility that comes with it, obsoletes the usefulness of an ED as a coping tool. Where there has been a full ED recovery, ensuing life crises may at times evoke a brief return to disordered behaviors, but such regressions will invariably be temporary, if not momentary. Most will be reversible through the ex-patient's coping skills or through a few "refresher" treatment sessions. This, in light of the reality that no small change in the direction of healing is lost on the receptive brain. Having learned to walk does not preclude one's capacity to crawl, though the evolutionary benefits of becoming upright and using feet for locomotion clearly creates the brain's incentive to *continue* to use the most efficacious and practicable alternative. "So smart is the brain, when we permit it, even after doing something a million times the wrong way, doing it right even one time feels so good that the brain-body system recognizes it immediately as right" [39].

10.5. ED practitioners need to educate patients and families about the importance of the brain, mind, and body connection

In treating the ED patient, practitioners also treat the patient's brain. The ED professional community needs to develop a greater breadth and depth of understanding of the organ that they treat. In addition, they need to educate their patients to do the same, in recognizing the brain's role in evoking ED pathology and in fostering ED recovery. The brain is an *embodied* system, extending beyond its skull case [32]. Sensory receptors throughout the body communicate with the cranial brain via the spinal cord through "bottom up" stimulation. By educating patients and families about the ever-increasing accessibility of neurophysiological interventions available for mainstream ED practice, the vast potential to create a brain/body partnership in healing can provide direction, optimism, and a sense of "can-do" within the process of recovery.

Human experience affects brain change, and brain change, in turn, affects human experience. In light of the diversity of symptom presentation and bio-psychosocial consequences of ED, the integration of a variety of differentiated treatment approaches and clinical interventions best accommodate the integrative needs and demands of the ED patient within the treatment

http://dx.doi.org/10.5772/65697

moment. The more varied and integrative the experience, the greater is the possibility of changes facilitating the healing reintegration of the fragmented self. ED treatment techniques such as the Feldenkrais Method, trauma-informed yoga, Nia, dance therapy, and Tai Chi, in offering movement with attention, access the more primitive subcortical regions of the brain where talk therapies do not reach, thereby globally upgrading and integrating brain function.

10.6. Partially recovered ex-patients may subsequently return to ED treatment to complete the tasks of full recovery

Practitioners cannot be assured that skill mastery and an expert use of self, alone, will guarantee successful recovery outcomes within the first round of treatment efforts. Some partially recovered patients may choose to terminate treatment prematurely, feeling emotionally unprepared or unwilling to face and resolve the underlying emotional issues driving the disorder. Other patients, who have made significant progress in the recovery of healthy eating behaviors, may choose not to fully restore their weight to set point range. In both instances, they will leave treatment with their ED in tow. In order to sustain recovery gains, recovery must be within all spheres of pathology.

Life experience can be a potent teacher to those who have left treatment to practice and hone their new coping skills on their own. Recovered patients come to realize the extent of the residual ED's limitations on happiness within their present lives. Where the eating disorder treatment relationship has been of quality and the work meaningful, partially recovered ex-patients may return to psychotherapy for relatively short stints when needed, after months or even years have passed, seeking to resolve emotional tasks left unfinished. Resuming treatment a second time around holds great potential for the patient to develop a healthier relationship with self and others, fully closing the circle of a complete recovery. The return to "refresher" treatment has particular potency within the first two years following termination of initial treatment efforts.

10.6.1. Case study 1

> N, a highly effective businesswoman, after struggling with her anorexia for 20 years, was able to recover a healthy enough eating lifestyle to adequately nourish her brain and body through her first round of care, which included treatment programs and extensive outpatient treatment. She found safety, however, in her decision to cling to remnants of her disease, so she never stopped restricting certain foods, and continued to obsess over distortions in body image. Ultimately, she became embroiled in an emotionally abusive love relationship with a bully who kept her as enslaved emotionally as did the tyranny of her eating disorder. N returned to treatment to hone and build upon the skills she had previously acquired, to develop the courage and wherewithal to stand up to, and free herself from, the victimization of this love relationship. In recognizing how her relationship with this man paralleled the nature of her connection to her ED, she developed an increased sense of self-determination, and ultimately, empowerment to leave him. Breaking out of her habitual patterns of co-dependency and powerlessness

facilitated her self-esteem, upgrading her life quality and moving her closer to a full ED recovery.

10.6.2. Case study 2

An adult anorexic female who had developed seizures as a result of malnutrition, precipitously left ED treatment after developing a healthy eating lifestyle that restored much of her lost weight, and ultimately put an end to her seizures. It appeared that she was not ready to respond to my encouragement to complete her recovery by working through critical issues of low self-esteem and co-dependent passivity within her important life relationships. Having left treatment without fully recovering, she developed other self-destructive habits (mild addiction processes) to replace her ED behaviors. Three years went by before she sought treatment again to work through relationship problems with her defiant teenage son and with her husband, who wished for a deeper emotional connection and expressions of intimacy.

Having matured and mastered the changes she had begun to achieve in her initial round of care, she returned to care having become developmentally ready to augment and practice, through life experience, the emotional strides she had made in her earlier ED treatment. She came to understand that her precipitous departure from her initial treatment was based on her feelings of worthlessness and the sense that she did not deserve to improve the quality of her existence more than she had done. Her renewed treatment reinforced her self-esteem, self-determination, and self-integration. Her marriage became stronger as she became stronger, her son began to heal through her newly empowered parenting, and she achieved a state of self-forgiveness and self-acceptance that led to an unfamiliar, but genuine, sense of well-being. The self that had been lost to her for so long had made a palpable comeback, leaving her feeling happier and fully grounded. No longer feeling socially awkward, timid, and insecure with others, her renewed spontaneity, emotional courage, and empowered flexibility led her to the sense that she had become "a new person."

10.7. Take care of yourself as a practitioner

Where a patient's enduring symptoms of pathology stem from the characterological nature of personality structure, expectations for recovery and growth may show less promise in some cases. Characterological disturbances in ED patients are generally less amenable to change, despite the therapist's expertise and commitment to the patient and treatment process. Such diagnoses are hard to discern, especially in youngsters, and may remain unknown, hidden, or otherwise undefined during much of the treatment process. Though characterological personality dysfunctions carry significant consequences for treatment, prognosis, and interpersonal dynamics within the therapeutic attachment, their presence does not necessarily preclude ED recovery, nor the achievement of substantive maturational gains and emotional

http://dx.doi.org/10.5772/65697

development throughout the process of treatment. In facing the challenges of treating these complex disorders and personalities, therapists need to learn to take as good care of themselves as they do of their patients, keeping expectation for themselves, as well as their patients, realistic. In such cases, professional consultation can be affirming and validating, enlightening one's work, refreshing one's awareness that each patient carries his or her own genetic and biologically determined predilections toward healthy or unhealthy functioning that must be taken into consideration, respected, and managed.

In treating the adolescent brain, unpredictable and acting out behaviors become the norm. Practitioners need to recognize and accommodate the not yet fully formed adolescent brain under the influence of emerging hormones, which will be less capable of positive responsiveness to treatment as seen in the patient's less than responsible judgment, choices, and behaviors. Treating ED adolescents begs the question of how to distinguish the chaotic and underdeveloped functioning of a normal adolescent brain, from the malnourished ED brain that awaits refeeding, or from the brain of a young patient with serious mental health conditions that might ultimately warrant a diagnosis of characterological personality dysfunction(s). The distinction, which typically will remain unclear during adolescence, essentially lies in the *extent* of disruptive and disingenuous functioning in the context of the patient's daily life. Conditions that may connote a more serious prognosis for adolescents include: an irrevocable quality of manipulating others; an extreme lack of empathy for loved ones; a refusal to appreciate the consequences of one's actions; and a cognitive structure that is based upon persistent lying. Asking all adolescent patients to stretch beyond the reach of their brain development best serves their treatment. Therapists need to approach the adolescent patient with clear expectations and requirements, firmly backed by empathy [17].

11. Conclusion

Current data suggests that eating disorder recovery lies in a complex interplay between weight status, normalization of stress hormones, and global hormonal well-being for optimal brain function and ongoing brain maturation [17]. Four core principles of effective eating disorder treatment include: (1) changing the neurobiological context, to include nutritional rehabilitation, weight normalization and stability, without the interruption of compensatory behaviors as symptom substitutions; (2) treating psychiatric comorbidities to remission; (3) addressing external environmental changes; and (4) connecting to maintenance factors for recovery [17].

Unique requirements of the emotionally evolved, flexible, and integrated eating disordered psychotherapist find their roots in one's commitment to a steadfast clarity of intention and purpose throughout an action-based, goal-driven treatment dynamic. Setting the facile eating disorder therapist apart from the generalist psychotherapist is his capacity to master, and then transcend, left-brain technical skills through right-brain empathic intuition in neurophysiological connection with the patient's right brain. The practitioner's self-acceptance precedes his capacity for full acceptance of the ED patient. It takes a special kind of professional to find gratification in a journey that is typically as arduous as it is extensive. It is the "phoenix" of the patient's reemerging unified self that arises "out of the ashes" of a debilitating disease, however, that makes the treatment of eating disorders as gratifying, and at times, as joyful, as it is challenging.

Acknowledgements

I extend my deepest appreciation to my husband Lou, and my talented daughter, Elizabeth, who edited this chapter skillfully and with love.

Abbreviations

AN	anorexia nervosa
ADHD	attention deficit/hyperactivity disorder
PTSD	posttraumatic stress disorder
BN	bulimia nervosa
EDNOS	eating disorder not otherwise specified
NES	night eating syndrome
CHSP	chew and spit
BDD	body dysmorphic disorder
ARFID	avoidant/restrictive food intake disorder
BED	binge eating disorder
ED	eating disordered
GPS	global positioning system
DBT	dialectical behavior therapy
CBT	cognitive behavioral therapy
MCBT	mindfulness-based cognitive behavioral therapy
FBT	family-based therapy
ACT	acceptance and commitment therapy
UP	unified protocol (transdiagnostic approach to ED treatment)
TMS	transcranial magnetic stimulation
SEED	severe and enduring eating disorder
OCD	obsessive compulsive disorder
DNA	deoxyribonucleic acid
EMDR	eye movement desensitization and reprocessing
NFT	neurofeedback training

PHP partial-hospital program

IOP intensive outpatient program

GCFP Guild Certified Feldenkrais Practitioner

BMI body mass index

Author details

Abigail H. Natenshon

Address all correspondence to: abigailnatenshon@gmail.com

TreatingEatingDisorders.com, Highland Park, Illinois, USA

References

[1] Garner DM. Psychoeducational Principles in the Treatment of Eating Disorders. In DM Garner & PE Garfinkel (Eds.), Handbook for Treatment of Eating Disorders. New York: Guilford Press; 1997. pp. 145–177.

[2] Mathers CD, Vos ET, Stevenson CE, Begg SJ. The Australian Burden of Disease Study: measuring the loss of health from diseases, injuries and risk factors. Med J Aust. 2000;172:592–596. [PubMed]

[3] Harris EC, Barraclough B. Excess mortality of mental disorder. Br J Psychiatry. 1998;173:11–53. [PubMed]

[4] Millar HR, Wardell F, Vyvyan JP, Naji SA, Prescott GJ, Eagles JM. Anorexia nervosa mortality in Northeast Scotland, 1965–1999. Am J Psychiatry. 2005;162:753–757. [PubMed]

[5] Sullivan PF. Mortality in anorexia nervosa. Am J Psychiatry. 1995;152:1073–1074. [PubMed]

[6] Zerwas S, Lund BC, Von Holle A, Thornton LM, Berrettini WH, Brandt H, Crawford S, Fichter MM, Halmi KA, Johnson C, Kaplan AS, La Vie M, Mitchell J, Rotonda A, Strober M, Woodsine DB, Kaye WH, Bulik CMJ. Factors associated with recovery from anorexia nervosa. J Psychiatr Res. 2013;47(7):972–979. doi: 10.1016/j.jpsychires.2013.02.011

[7] Berkman ND, Lohr KN, Bulik CM. Outcomes of eating disorders: a systematic review of the literature. Int J Eat Disord. 2007;40:293–309. [PubMed]

[8] Steinhausen HC. The outcome of anorexia nervosa in the 20th century. Am J Psychiatry. 2002;159:1284–1293. [PubMed]

[9] Jauregui-Garrido B, Jauregui-Lobera I. Sudden death in eating disorders. Vasc Health Risk Manag. 2012;8:91–98. Published online 2012 Feb 15. doi: 10.2147/VHRM.S28652

[10] Parigi AD, Schur E. Brain Imaging Behavioral Medicine and Clinical Neuroscience. In: RA Cohen & LH Sweet LH (Eds.), Eating Disorders. New York: Springer; 2011. pp. 184–186.

[11] Roberto CA, Mayer LE, Brickman AM, Barnes A, Muraskin J, Yeung LK, Steffener J, Sy M, Hirsch J, Stern Y, Walsh BT. Brain tissue volume changes following weight gain in adults with anorexia nervosa. Int J Eat Disord. 44(5):406–411. doi: 10.1002/eat.20840. Epub 2010 May 19.

[12] Taber KH, Murphy DD, Blurton-Jones MM, Hurley RA. An update on estrogen: higher cognitive function, receptor mapping, neurotrophic effects. J Neuropsychiatry Clin Neurosci. 2001;13(3):313–317.

[13] Chui HT, Christensen BK, Zipursky RB, Richards BA, Hanratty MK, Kabani NJ, Mikulis DJ, Katzman DK. Cognitive function and brain structure in females with a history of adolescent-onset anorexia nervosa. Pediatrics. 2008;122(2):e426-37. doi: 10.1542/peds. 2008-0170

[14] Fisher M, Golden NH, Katzman DK, Kreipe RE, Rees J, Schebendach MA, Sigman G, Ammerman S, Hoberman HM. Eating disorders in adolescents: a background paper. J Adolesc Health. 1995;16:420–437.

[15] Hudson J, Hiripi E, Pope HG, Kessler RC. The prevalence and correlates of eating disorders in the National Comorbidity Survey Replication. Biol Psychiatry. 2007;61(3): 348–358. doi: 10.1016/j.biopsych.2006.03.040

[16] Striegel-Moore RH, Franko D. Epidemiology of binge eating disorder. Int J Eat Disord. 2003;34 Suppl:S19–S29.

[17] Bermudez O. ARFID: some new twists and some old themes. In: 2016 Eating Recovery Center Learning from the Leaders: Current Issues and Innovative Interventions in Eating Disorder Treatment; April 2016.

[18] American Psychiatric Association. Diagnostic and Statistical Manual of Mental Disorders. 5th ed. Arlington, VA: American Psychiatric Publishing; 2013.

[19] Natenshon AH. Doing What Works: An Integrative System for the Treatment of Eating Disorders from Diagnosis to Recovery. Washington, D.C. NASW Press; 2009.

[20] Barbarich NC. Lifetime prevalence of eating disorders among professionals in the field. J Treat Prevent. 2002;10:305–312.

[21] Miller WR, Rollnick S. Motivation Interviewing: Preparing people to change addictive Behavior. New York, N. Y. Guilford Press; 1991. 68 p.

[22] Germer C, Siegel RD, Fulton PR (Eds). Mindfulness and Psychotherapy. New York, N.Y. Guilford Press; 2005. p.285.

[23] Pollack SM, Siegel RD, Pedulla D. Three Ways to Bring Mindfulness into Therapy. Greater Good Science Center; September 8, 2014.

[24] Farchione TJ, Fairholme CP, Ellard KK, Boisseau CL, Thompson-Hollands J, Carl JR, Gallagher MW, Barlow DH. Unified Protocol for transdiagnostic treatment of emotional disorders: a randomized controlled trial. Behav Ther. 2012;43(3): 666–678. doi: 10.1016/j.beth.2012.01.001

[25] Fairburn CG. Cognitive Behavioral Therapy and Eating Disorders. New York, N.Y. Guilford Press; 2008.

[26] Fairburn CG, Cooper Z, Shafran R. Cognitive behaviour therapy for eating disorders: a "transdiagnostic" theory and treatment. Behav Res Ther. 2003;41(5):509–528.

[27] Fairburn CG, Cooper Z, Doll HA, O'Connor ME, Bohn K, Hawker, DM, Wales JA, Palmer RL. Transdiagnostic cognitive-behavioral therapy for patients with eating disorders: a two-site trial with 60-week follow-up. Am J Psychiatry. 2009;166(3):311–319. doi: 10.1176/appi.ajp.2008.08040608. Epub 2008 Dec 15.

[28] Gaudio S, Brooks SJ, Riva G. Nonvisual multisensory impairment of body perception in anorexia nervosa: a systematic review of neuropsychological studies. PLoS One. 2014;9(10). DOI: 10.1371/journal.pone.0110087

[29] Laumer U, Bauer M, Fichter M, Milz H. Therapeutic effects of the Feldenkrais Method (awareness through movement) in eating disorders. Feldenkrais Res J. 2004;1:170–180.

[30] Doidge N. The Brain's Way of Healing. Remarkable Discoveries and Recoveries from the Frontiers of Neuroplasticity. New York: Viking; 2015. 233 p.

[31] Van der Kolk BA, Stone L, West J, Rhodes A, Emerson D, Suvak M, Spinazzola J. Yoga as an adjunctive treatment for posttraumatic stress disorder: a randomized controlled trial. J Clin Psychiatry. 2014;75(6):e559-65. doi: 10.4088/JCP.13m08561

[32] Korn D, Leeds AM. Preliminary evidence of efficacy of EMDR resource development and installation in the stabilization phase of treatment of complex posttraumatic stress disorder. J Clin Psychol. 2002;58(12):1465–1487. doi:10.1002/jclp.10099

[33] Bergstrom I, Crisby M, Engstrom AM, Holcke M, Fored M, Jakobsson KP, Of Sandberg AM. Women with anorexia nervosa should not be treated with estrogen or birth control pills in a bone-sparing effect. Acta Obstet Gynecol Scand. 2013;92(8):877–880. doi: 10.1111/aogs.12178. Epub 2013 Jun 15.

[34] van Langenberg T, Sawyer SH, LeGrange D, Hughes HK. Psychosocial well-being of siblings of adolescents with anorexia nervosa. Eur Eat Disord Rev. 2016 Aug 8. doi: 10.1002/erv.2469. [Epub ahead of print]

[35] Siegel DJ. An interpersonal neurobiology approach to psychotherapy. Psychiatr Ann. 2006;36(4):63.

[36] Siegel DJ. The Science and Art of Presence: How being open and receptive to life cultivates well-being. Mindsight Digit J. 2016; 2.

[37] https://www.nationaleatingdisorders.org/get-facts-eating-disorders

[38] Tomiyama AJ, Hunger JM, Nguyen-Cuu J, Well C. Misclassification of cardiometabolic health when using body mass index categories in NHANE 2005-2012. Int J Obesity. 2016;40:883–886. doi;10.1038/ijo.2016.17

[39] Feldenkrais MP. Body and Mature Behavior. London: Routledge and Kegan Paul; 1949; New York: International Universities Press, 1950 softcover edition, out of print.

Chapter 10

EMDR in Anorexia Nervosa: From a Theoretical Framework to the Treatment Guidelines

Maria Zaccagnino, Cristina Civilotti,
Martina Cussino, Chiara Callerame and
Isabel Fernandez

Additional information is available at the end of the chapter

http://dx.doi.org/10.5772/65695

Abstract

Studies on the risks and on the positive factors implied in the onset of anorexia nervosa (AN) have reported the role of an insecure or disorganized state of mind (SoM) with respect to attachment. We compare the effects of eyes movement desensitization and reprocessing (EMDR) approach with cognitive behavioral therapy (CBT) in the treatment of AN in terms of SoMs, reflective function (RF), and narrative coherence (Coh). Our results are part of a broader observational clinical comparative study of the two approaches, and it is based on the Adult Attachment Interview (AAI) outcomes. Differences in terms of belongingness to a secure group and an unsecure group before and after the treatments in EMDR and CBT group have been reported through McNemar's test. The generalized linear model (GLM) repeated-measures multivariate ANOVA (RM-MANOVA) has been selected. Our results suggest that EMDR allows an active reprocessing of traumatic memories related to family dynamics and to eating behaviors, which could enable a positive resolution of eating disorder (ED) symptoms. The emotional reprocessing of unresolved attachment issues can allow a better modulation of the control-related rigidity that is a commonality between AN patients.

Keywords: EMDR, anorexia, psychotherapy, eating disorders, reflective function, narrative coherence

1. Introduction

Anorexia nervosa (AN) has been described in 1978 by Bruch [1] as a "Golden Cage," the condition of being trapped in a perfection mask, threatened by a persistent sense of losing control. A deep anguish is expressed through a constant check on body image, on food, and on weight, to obtain a sense of independency and a definition of the self. Emotional and psychological suffering, along with the consequent interruptions of a coherent narrative that occur during the development process, generates a set of specific features, such as a misperception of body size, an impaired sense of satiety, and problems with personal relations and with the regulation of emotions and misconception of the sexual role [2]. The idea of dealing with overwhelming emotions can be frightening, and a strong control seems the only way to manage or avoid them.

In modern Western society, the frequency and severity of eating disorders (EDs) are becoming a severe and worrisome phenomenon, which, nowadays, is showing even worse long-term outcomes [3, 4]. The study of the developmental aspects in the etiopathogenetic evolution of EDs, it is essential to prevent, cure, and manage this debilitating form of suffering. EDs can be considered as a composite and eclectic psychiatric condition, affected by a social and cultural world, increasingly focused on the physical aspects and on the "cult of thinness" [2, 5]. In the last years, the constant access to the social platform and media is changing the social context. Internet multiplies exposure to contents that can, on the one hand, disturb the relationship with the body self-image and, on the other hand, worsen significantly the psychological functioning in people who already have a fragile personality structure. In particular, social media have recently been included among the factors that contribute to ED [6]. A vision that considers only the psychosocial aspect, however, seems to be reductive [2, 7]. Considering AN as a direct response to the mass media mandates can be misleading because, for example, ED (and specifically AN) appear to be cross-cultural [8].

To date, there are numerous interpretative models regarding the onset of AN, defining several orders of potentially interacting risks and maintenance factors. In terms of environmental factors at the macrosystem level, there is a higher incidence of AN in cultures or environments where art, fashion, and mass media spread the idea that thinness is a symbol of beauty, charm, health, and success [2, 9]. Focusing to microsystem, according to the studies of Stice conducted on a sample of adolescent girls [10], the development of an ED is influenced by some parenting attitudes as, for example, a familiar criticism on weight and search of mothers of thinness. Parenting bonding style is often characterized by low care and high control, with a percentage comprise between 8.6 and 12.9 of AN patients that describe the relation with caregivers as neglectful [11]. In this context, we underline two main key concepts, before introducing the concept of attachment. Firstly, it seems necessary to improve current theories that infer a direct causality between parental behaviors, in particular on the mother side, with the development of AN. Simplistic and linear theories potentially generate, in addition to an enormous sense of guilt, confusion on possible origins, and consequences of AN in the quality of life and in family relationships. Secondly, it is important to recognize the role of the family environment, without critical judgments and without reducing the source heterogeneity observed in AN patients.

http://dx.doi.org/10.5772/65695

Pioneer in this context was the work of Minuchin, psychiatrist and family therapist, who in 1978 focused on the families of AN patients referring them as "psychosomatic" and describing them as stuck, imprisoned, characterized by excessive worrying and protection, rigidity, and with the habit to not solve, but rather avoid, conflicts [12]. Minuchin et al.'s work has provided over the years the foundations for research and for the treatment of EDs, influencing the scientific and therapeutic communities to consider families not only as a problem source but also as a possible source of resources and solutions.

In between micro- and macrosystem, the role of peer groups seems to have a potential role in the onset of ED. Conversations between teenagers regarding diets and weight can move from the simple exchange of information and advice, passing for the promotion of membership in the group, to regulatory standards. Moreover, the subjects of ridicule or exclusion show higher levels of body dissatisfaction, low self-esteem, and depressive symptoms [13].

While acknowledging the difficulty to distinguish between genetic and environmental factors in the family context, it seems that a part of influence on the genesis of the disorder is due to genetic factors and that 38–55% of monozygotic twins are more at risk of incurring in AN than in dizygotic [14, 15].

The interpretative models, as well as the therapeutic models of intervention, do not seem to be able to disregard a complex and multicausal vision, which takes into account the multiplicity of aspects involved in the onset of the disorder and root in the individual's history an important component of causality in the onset of an ED. Schmidt and Treasure [16] proposed a maintenance model of AN combining intra- and interpersonal aspects while many studies stress the importance of emotional factors in the onset and in the perpetration of the disorder. Studies concerning risks and positive factors implied in the onset of ED, for example, identify the importance of some individual and family risk factors such as deficit to the development of self-esteem, identity, and independence; the presence of pathologies in the cognitive sphere; and excessive concern on body weight. Moreover, in the families of ED patients, it is likely the presence of affective disorders, substance abuses, extreme criticisms, examples of eating disorders, and impaired attachment relationships between parents and children [17–19].

1.1. Attachment theory and anorexia nervosa

Compared to 20 years ago, when it was still reported the need to increase the scientific evidence of the link between attachment and the development of EDs [20], the literature that currently supports an influence of insecure attachment in the onset of EDs is very rich. Attachment insecurity represents a vulnerability factor related to anorexia, such as body mass index (BMI), dissatisfaction with body image, pressure to diet, and food restrictions [21–24].

Many studies emphasized how prolonged stress (abuse, physical or psychological maltreatment, neglect) experienced during early stages of life could cause the interruption of the development of self-regulatory processes and may lead to the onset of psychological deficits closely related to EDs [25–27]. In a study with anorexic children were seen a low dyadic reciprocity, high levels of maternal intrusiveness, frequent conflicts, the presence of negative emotions, and a lack of pleasure in the interactive patterns between mothers and children [28].

Schore [29, 30] reports that the relational traumas can be characterized by a conscious or unconscious shared fear-based interaction between the child and the caregiver. The author reports the effects of early trauma to the child self-organization focusing on the child-adult relation instead of specific events. Complex PTSD (C-PTSD) has been defined by Herman [31] as a clinical frame of the patients which had experienced a series of microtraumas (small T traumas, as defined by Shapiro [32], that reiterate in a considerable time span. The microtraumas can derive from several factors, such as emotional neglect, experiences of rejection, humiliation, and physical violence. This particular type of early and complex trauma is characterized by the paradoxical and simultaneous activation of both attack and defense systems. Consequently, the integrative function of consciousness can collapse increasing the child's fragility and the risk of the developing dissociative phenomena. The traumatic emotions dissociated from consciousness can also lead to different states of fragmented ego [33].

A definition of "traumatic development" [34] is related to the presence of a constant threat or danger within the attachment relation with the caregivers, from which it is not possible to escape. The effect of the microtraumas accumulates, resulting in a compromised individual development [35]. DSM-V [36] defines, instead, a "traumatic event" (Big T traumas) as a single or a few events of a short-time span in which the subject life, or the life of a beloved one, has been in danger (car accidents, natural disasters, sexual or physical abuse, terrorist activities, war, etc.). C-PTSD recognizes the painful consequences of strong emotions related to disturbing powerless experiences, which characterize each traumatic experience [34]. "Small T traumas" are much more common in nowadays society; still, they are more difficult to report clinically. To construct an efficient clinical framework, the emotional consequences of early stage relational traumas have to be well defined. The destabilizing consequences of continuous small T traumas can result into relevant and long-standing disorders.

In the disorganized attachment pattern, the caregiver's behavior may be characterized by frequent and frightening abusive attitudes causing the child to experience states of "fright without solution" that can lead to experience a growing and pervasive anguish and terror. The child is thus in the paradoxical situation of being terrorized by the secure base [34, 37].

These findings are in line with a recent study conducted by Keiser Permanente, the Adverse Childhood Experiences (ACEs) Study, which underlines how the exposure to Adverse Childhood Experiences (ACEs) including abuse, neglect, and household dysfunction is associated with multiple long-term physical and mental health problems [38, 39]. When adverse experiences remain unresolved and unprocessed over time and not metabolized by the brain, a "mnemonic network" is formed, mainly composed of all the perceptions, body sensations, emotions, and expectations linked to memories of traumatic events. In AN patients, a dysregulation of HPA axis activity seems to be present. Recent studies suggest that ACES may contribute to the emerging and maintaining process of this dysregulation [40, 41].

Some subjects with histories of traumatic events manifest little or no emotions linked to their relational traumas, and they tend to generalize such mechanism while interpreting the surrounding world. The negative and overwhelming emotions related to traumatic stresses are extremely difficult to manage; for this reason, people might initiate ED behaviors (such as self-starvation, overeating, and vomiting) as a coping strategy [25]. Once triggered, both dissociative reactions and alterations in eating behaviors tend to persist with considerable impact on physical, emotional, and relational development, leading to possible long-lasting pathological outcomes. In this perspective, the compulsive use of bingeing or the refusal of food can become an attempt to escape or regulate negative intolerable feelings or intrusive thoughts related to the traumatic memory. In many studies, Rhodes and Kroger [42] found higher levels of maternal overprotectiveness in childhood and higher levels of separation anxiety in the EDs sample of young women compared with a healthy control group. Other studies on samples of women with ED have shown that the most serious symptoms of childhood separation anxiety and styles of insecure attachment are preserved compared to samples of healthy women [19]. The family environment in which ED subjects grew appears to be characterized by a low level of cohesion and a low propensity for individual growth: It is therefore likely that these families have difficulties to sustain their children in the normal separation-individuation process [43]. Moreover, the presence of turbulence in the emotional processing in the caregivers, such as unresolved losses, can be transmitted to offspring becoming a risk factor in the development of AN [18].

Therapeutic approaches adopted in current clinical settings for EDs, often do not deal with past traumatic experiences, focusing more on the present and on behavioral symptoms. The risk is to neglect developmental factors that could trigger the maintenance of the vicious circle of AN. It is thus evident the requirement, in a therapeutic approach, to consider factors of the life story of the patient, especially focusing on the attachment. The impairment might have triggered the dissociative behavior leading to specific controlling strategies. Focusing on the attachment allows a psychotherapist to emphasize and understand the role of the control on the patient sense of self protection.

1.1.1. The emerging of the control part

Typically, AN patients are violent self-criticists, intolerant to the slightest transgression of the rules, and with no compassion for themselves. In a kind of "emotional totalitarianism" [44], a continuous monitoring of weight and food assumes a dichotomous structure, such as been skinny/fat, good/bad, and powerful/powerless. There is no possibility to explore the world without encountering a severe internal or external judgment. Obsessive-compulsive traits [45] consist in a very high self-expectations and a self-imposed perfectionism. These characteristics are considered by international scientific literature as decisive for the preservation of the disease and for the resistance to its treatment [45–47]. Lawrence [48] has been one of the firsts to investigate the AN as a problem related to the control part. The fear to gain weight or to lose the management on the desire of food is the symptom that hides a deep terror. The emotional suffering can be considered as a component of the non-metabolized memories that consist in maladaptive sensations, beliefs, and images. Any present reminder can activate the non-metabolized memories, leading to dysfunctional emotional regulation and behavioral responses [26, 49]. AN patients consider the control of themselves an absolute must, while the lose of control is understood to be a complete and irreversible failure on a personal and moral level. The constant attention to the body and to the quantity of eaten food is completely debilitating, even if it provides an apparent control on the reality.

Self-imposed constrictions that do not derive from a social surrounding are a determinant factor for the preservation of the psychopathology and for the resistance to its treatment [46]. The control inhibits the skill to explore the interpersonal relations. The inner conflict in anorexic people lies between the desire to be perfect and the fear of the consequential expectations, between the fear to not be sufficient and the terror that no one will ever accept them in case of failure. These patients live in a constant ambivalence: On one side, they have the fear to achieve their ideals and on the other the fear to not reach them. The paradox of the control consists exactly in this: When one feels in despair for being out of control, the need to use this form of control compensation emerges. The control is therefore a central factor in the studies focused on the correlation between the ED and the difficulties to manage emotions. It is clearly involved in the mechanism of avoidance of negative effects, in the possibility of being generally self-aware, in the recognitions and acceptance of the related emotions, in the tendency towards impulsive behaviors, in the ritualization, in the abuse of stereotypes, and in the failure to recognize feasible strategies to manage and contain such behaviors.

In neurobiological research, it has been underlined how the alimentation in AN is connected with specific cerebral modifications that involve the neuronal network to manage the control. It has been observed that, in the AN patient's brain, it is present in a lower activation of specific areas of the limbic system, which is also involved in the elaboration of emotions. Higher brain activation, instead, has been detected in the areas related to the control, with an inhibition of appetite and on the general skill to define values. A 2013 study [50] compared the differences of the brain volume of AN patients and a reference group composed of healthy individuals. A consistent brain size reduction in the grey matter and in the white matter, with an increasing level of cerebrospinal fluid, has been reported in AN patients. The temporal and occipital lobes manifest a higher sensitivity, and a grey matter reduction in the group of patients currently affected by the psychopathology. Other studies reported further reductions in the brain volume, especially in the temporal and parietal cortex and the midbrain area. The modification in the brain network for the cognitive control seems to be partially responsible for the lack of mental flexibility in AN patients. In the study of Lao-Kaim et al.[51], it has been reported that people affected by AN have diffuse alterations of the executive functions. The reduced cognitive flexibility seems to be linked to an abnormal function of the front parietal, which manages the direction of the control, inwards or outwards. Frontal-striatal modifications have been reported to limit also the procedural knowledge. The two aspects suggest that the perseverations and the lack of flexibility characteristic of people affected by AN can block multiple process of higher order, from the learning ability to the control. These factors influence the patients at a lower cognitive level contributing to preserve the disorder.

The latest evidence obtained in neurobiology and the progressive establishment of the research on the attachment relations showed that possible ED sources are of traumatic nature and that early traumas can increase the vulnerability of children from dissociative disorders. The consequent generation of dissociative states can then result in difficult emotion management, leading to the generation of dysfunctional control strategies. Hereby, AN patients can reach the point to prefer to risk their life than give up their control [52].

http://dx.doi.org/10.5772/65695

1.2. Therapeutic approaches

As reported in several studies, precise indications on the efficacy of AN treatment are limited [53–55].

In young patients, it seems that family-based treatments are the most effective [54–57]. A well-known approach in the scientific literature is the Maudsley family-based treatment (FBT). It combines cognitive behavioral therapy (CBT) with systemic-relational intervention, and it is an intensive outpatient treatment aimed to normalize the weight of adolescents affected by AN. The FBT is generally a short clinical program aimed to improve family functioning and to prepare families of adolescents with EDs to support the recovery of the weight in everyday life through educational activities and skills training [58].

In adult population, no specific psychotherapy approach can be considered as an elective method in treating AN, even if there is evidence regarding the efficacy of interpersonal psychotherapy (IPT) and cognitive behavioral therapy (CBT) [54, 59–61]. In particular, CBT is today one of the most investigated approaches, and in light of the recent results, it appears to present the highest efficiency in terms of number of dropout [60, 62] and clinical outcomes [63]. The approach has been therefore selected, in the present work, as a reference to compare the effects obtained by AN patients. Recent researches have shown that CBT enhanced (CBT-E), a specific form of CBT proposed by Fairburn [64], can improve ED symptomatology in adults and youth, focusing mainly on the behavioral level of the disease [65–67].

Despite that CBT and FBT are the most commonly used approaches; we would mention some potential limitations. Scientific studies are, in fact, numerically scarce, and their methodology has to be improved [66]. High dropout rates [67] are reported, and ED patients seem resistant to the creation of a positive therapeutic relationship [68]. Moreover, CBT and FBT do not prioritize the ontogenetic aspect of the disease and the influence of the past experiences in the onset and in the maintenance of the ED. Given the previously introduced relationship between insecure attachment and EDs, we infer that a therapeutic approachable to consider a large time span and the consequential evolution of the disorder is auspicable and necessary to treat the disorders both in prevention and in the treatment phase. Hereby, ED symptoms shall be also evaluated as potential manifestations of traumatic events and of insecure attachments [21, 22, 68–70].

1.2.1. Eyes movement desensitization and reprocessing (EMDR)

As stated from the EMDR International Association (EMDRIA; www.emdria.org), the EMDR is a widely recognized evidence-based psychotherapy implementation. It has firstly been applied to relieve post-traumatic stress disorder (PTSD) symptomatology, and it has evolved to an integrated approach in psychotherapy. Positive results are reported in the scientific scenario also in the treatment of several psychiatric conditions, mental health difficulties, and psychosomatic problems. The paradigm, on which EMDR is grounded, adaptive information processing (AIP), is transverse to the different therapeutic approaches, and it can be integrated with different clinical traditions [71]. The AIP model is based on the assumption that every person, under normal conditions, possesses an innate neurobiological ability that allows processing and transforming incoming information in adaptive material, which functionally integrates the experience and past information. Traumatic materials can prejudice the subjective integrative capacity of assimilating these experiences in an adaptive way. The eight-phase, three-branched (the past, present and future) process of EMDR re-enables the normal information processing and integration [72].

The main purpose of EMDR is to help a patient to access the unresolved memory and to metabolize it, to turn from a "frozen memory" to the one integrated, neutral, and healthier [73]. In other words, the patient is asked to concentrate on the emotionally disturbing material and, at the same time, to focus on an external stimulus which usually consists in eye movements or other kind of bilateral stimulation, such as tapping or bilateral auditory tones. During this process, the patient is advised to concentrate on thoughts, feelings, or images which emerge. With the proceeding of the treatment, the patient is able to create associations with more adaptive material, until the traumatic memories are integrated in a coherent way [74]. Briefly, the EMDR appears to be able to transform the emotional experience into cognitive experience [75].

In this chapter, we report a specific protocol inserted in a framework linked to the traumatic spectrum. Focus is posed on the analysis and on the elaboration of early relational traumas and on the consequent negative judgments on the self (e.g., *"I do not deserve," "I worth nothing," "I am not enough"*). One of the basic concept of the implementation of EMDR approach with AN patients is to investigate where and how the symptomatology and the patient's part of control have originated, focusing on its protective function. A gradual approach permits the patient to progressively feel those difficult emotions that have been considered unmanageable by the patient.

2. The pilot study

In light of these considerations, a pilot study was conducted with the aim to compare the usefulness of EMDR related to standard CBT in the treatment of AN in terms of adult representations with respect to attachment.

The hypothesis in this study is that, as the EMDR protocol helps to access and process traumatic memories with an adaptive resolution, the patient will become able to recognize them in the past, promoting an effective reprocessing of the disturbing memories, obtaining an improvement of the AN symptomatology related to the control part.

2.1. Methods

The results presented in this chapter are part of a broader observational clinical comparative study of two active interventions—EMDR therapy and CBT [76]—and are here strictly focused on the important issue of attachment implications. On the whole, the study was carried out over a period of twelve months. AN patients were eligible to receive up to 48 individual therapy sessions of 50 min with an experienced psychotherapist over a maximum 1-year period. The average number of therapy sessions received by each participant during the trial was 36 sessions without any patient dropouts from the treatment.

The AN patients were selected from a pool of people who demanded for treatment in a period of 12 months in a clinical center specialized in AN disorder treatment (Centro di terapia EMDR specializzato in anoressia e disturbidell' alimentazione, Milano, Italy).

This study was conducted in a private practice setting, in accordance with the Declaration of Helsinki, under the recommendations and upon the approval of the Research Guidelines of the Centro di Ricerca e Studi in Psicotraumatologia (CRSP) of Bovisio Masciago, MB, Italy, and of the art. Ten of the "National Board of Italian Psychologists Code of Ethics for the Psychologist" regulate research activities for Italian psychologists in private practices (http://www.psy.it/normativa/italy/code_of_ethics_eng.html). The administration of AAI at T0 and at T1 was part of the routine procedure for monitoring the psychotherapeutic process. Before taking part in the research project, all AN patients received complete information concerning the rationale of the study design and provided a written informed consent for their participation in the study. All participants knew their right to withdraw their consensus or their data from the study at any time. Eligibility of patients who express the interest to participate in the study was determined via the EMDR clinical guidelines [73].

Four psychotherapists were involved in the process: two for the EMDR and two for the CBT. They are clinical psychologists qualified as cognitive behavioral psychotherapists who had at least 5 years of clinical experience. EMDR therapists were certified by the accrediting association in Italy (Italian Association of EMDR) to practice the EMDR.

2.2. Interventions

The EMDR treatment followed anorexia nervosa protocol [77] focused on relational traumas and on clinical work with the control part: 2 sessions of resource development prior to EMDR reprocessing and 30–46 sessions of EMDR treatment over the span of one year's time. The main hypothesis is that traumas (both big T and small T traumas) contribute to the development of dysfunctional regulation strategies. Since the control and perfectionism are essential parts of the onset and for the maintenance of dysfunctional cycles in AN, the protocol focuses in creating links between the different parts and help the patients to legitimize them. Moreover, in AN patients, it is possible to detect a fragmentation of the self. Hereby, within the AN-EMDR protocol, it has been included a treatment of different ego states [78].

The CBT treatment was constituted of 32–48 sessions and was provided following manual-based CBT guidelines [62]. The treatment involved three phases: The first is focused on the strategies to address behavioral dysfunction relating eating and weight that enhance the risk of relapse; the second consists in the implementation of cognitive restructuring techniques; and the third is the co-construction of a scheme-based approach in order to address a comprehensive range of relevant issues that widen beyond eating and weight (e.g., relational issues, developmental problems, mood disorder, low self-esteem).

2.3. Participants

Participants were 20 Italian adolescent and young adult patients (average age: 18.80 years, SD = 2.04 for EMDR and 19.70 years, SD = 2.86 for CBT). The selection criteria were female subjects aged 15–25 years, with a DSM-V diagnosis of AN. Exclusion criteria were inability to speak or read Italian, understand the interview questions, the presence of metabolic pathology interfering with eating or digestion (e.g., diabetes) and psychotic disorder.

2.4. Tools

The entire set of questionnaires included the Adverse Childhood Experiences Questionnaire (ACE-Q; [38]—only at T0), the Adult Attachment Interview (AAI), [79], the Eating Disorders Inventory-3 (EDI-3) [80], the Symptom Checklist-Revised (SCL-90-R; [81]), and the Difficulties in Emotion Regulation Scale (DERS; [82]). In this section, the focus is on the ACE-Q, on the AAI, and on the related Reflective Function (RF) and Coherence (Coh) Scale. Further results not relevant in the present investigation are reported elsewhere [76].

The 10 ACE questions assess childhood mistreatments in terms of childhood emotional, physical, and sexual abuse or neglect, and household dysfunction, such as parent violence, substance abuse, parental separation, and incarceration.

The AAI is a semi-structured interview, which assesses adults' state of mind (SoM) in respect of childhood attachment relationships. Throughout 18–21 questions, patients were invited to recover attachment-related autobiographical memories from early childhood (until 12 years) and to evaluate these memories with their current perspective. The interviews were transcribed verbatim and coded by the principal investigator (M.Z.), who was blind respect to the psychotherapeutic approach followed by the AN patients. In this study, we used the Main and Goldwyn's [83] coding system. M.Z. was trained in the Main and Goldwyn AAI coding system [84] by D. Jacobvitz and N. Dazzi and certified as highly reliable by Main and Hesse. The coding system of the AAI [79] classifies the attachment SoMs in three main groups: free or autonomous (F), dismissing (Ds), and entangled or preoccupied (E). Moreover, a further classification which considers eventual incoherent narrative, presence of lapses in the monitoring of the discourse, monitoring of reasoning while recalling one or more traumatic experiences (such as abuses or losses) has been implemented to uncover a partial or absent level of processing of these memories. The interviews are rated on the nine-point Unresolved Scale. A score above 5 is interpreted with a primary unresolved classification (followed by a secondary classification of F, Ds, or E category); a score below 5 is interpreted as a secondary unresolved classification.

The Reflective Functioning Scale [85], assessed by M.Z., was employed in the AAI transcripts. It estimates the degree of complexity of the subject's model of mind and how the patient is competent to reflect about her/himself and others' SoMs. The RF scale is reported as a unique overall score in a range from 1 to 9.

2.5. Statistical analysis

The results were analyzed by the use of the Statistical Package for the Social Sciences (SPSS). Differences in terms of belongingness to a secure group or to an unsecure group between T0 and T1 in EMDR and CBT sections were compared by use of the McNemar's test. The p value was calculated with the continuity correction. One generalized linear model (GLM) repeated-measures multivariate ANOVA (RM-MANOVA) was used to investigate both the main effects and interactions for BMI and RF in the AAI at T0 and at T1, between and within EMDR and CBT groups. For the "within-subjects" part, the treatment results have been reported as a function of treatment time (defined as the psychotherapy sessions from T0 to T1), while for the "between-subjects" part, a comparison between EMDR and CBT psychotherapies is reported. When a correlation has been found, investigation on the possible sources has been executed. Two independent t-tests for the significant scores across intervention type at T0 and at T1, using within-group descriptors.

2.6. Results

2.6.1. Description of the sample at T0

Student's t-test analysis on the samples at T0 revealed the absence of significant differences between EMDR and CBT patients in terms of age, BMI, Coh, and RF score at baseline (all $p > 0.05$). Seventy-five percentage of our sample had three or more ACE (80% in the EMDR group and 70% in the CBT group). In both groups, the ACEs reported in our sample consisted the following: being insulted, put down or humiliated by parents during childhood, growing up in a context where a member had some forms of psychopathologies. At T0, all patients but one (in the CBT group) had an insecure SoM: In the EMDR group, five patients were DS, four were E, and one was U/DS. In the CBT group, one patient was F, four were Ds, three were E, and two were U/Ds. No patients had a secondary U classification.

2.6.2. Differences between T0 and T1 in EMDR and CBT groups

Both treatments (EMDR and CBT) resulted in an increase of BMI and the RM-MANOVA yielded a significant pre/post-main-effect ($V = 0.966$, $F (1, 18) = 515.003$, $p < 0.001$). A significant interaction was found between T0 and T1 and the treatment condition ($V = 0.830$, $F (1, 18) = 88.022$, $p < 0.001$). It emerges that in the EMDR group, the scores at T1 were significantly better than at T0.

Concerning the SoM with respect to attachment, in the EMDR group at T1, 7 on 10 patients became "earned secured," whereas in the CBT group, only one patient move from an unsecure to a secure SoM and the two patients classified as primary. Unresolved continued to have an U classification after 1 year of treatment. The exact McNemar's test reported a statistically significant difference in the proportion of secure SoM pre- and post-intervention in the EMDR group ($p = 0.027$), whereas the difference in terms of becoming secured attached in the CBT group is not meaningful.

Both EMDR and CBT patients have reported higher scores on Coh and RF scales with a significant pre/post-main-effect (respectively, Coh: $V = 0.859$, $F(1,18) = 109.696$, $p < 0.001$, and RF: $V = 0.637$, $F(1,18) = 31.610$, $p < 0.001$) and a remarkable interaction between the pre/post-measures and the treatment conditions (respectively, Coh: $V = 0.438$, $F(1,18) = 14.049$, $p = 0.001$

and RF: V = 0.723, F(1,18) = 47.087, $p < 0.001$). For both scales, the only statistically relevant improvement has been found in the EMDR group (Coh: mean difference between T0 and T1 in the EMDR group:-2.4, SEM = 0.163; 95% CI [-2.769,-2.031], $p < 0.001$; mean difference between T0 and T1 in the CBT group: not statistically significant; RF: mean difference between T0 and T1 in the EMDR group:-2, SEM = 0.298; 95% CI [-2.674,-1.326], $p < 0.001$ and mean difference between T0 and T1 in the CBT group: not statistically significant) (**Table 1**).

	T0				T1				
	EMDR		Control		EMDR		Control		
	M	DS	M	DS	M	DS	M	DS	Sig.
Body mass index (BMI)	14.95	1.35	15.04	1.33	18.98	1.22	17.28	1.34	*§
AAI-Coh	3.4	0.52	3.5	0.52	5.8	0.63	4	0.67	*§
AAI-RF	4.5	0.85	4.4	1.17	6.5	0.97	4.8	1.03	*§

*Significant pre/post-effect, independent of the type of treatment (CBT or EMDR).
§Significant group (CBT vs. EMDR)-by-time (T0 vs. T1) interaction effects.

Table 1. Clinical Data of Participants at T0 and at T1.

3. Conclusions

The present study examined the changes in the attachment state of mind, narrative coherence, and reflective function in a sample of AN patients after about a year of EMDR or CBT psychotherapy. The results presented, despite the small sample size, suggest that EMDR is a valuable effective treatment for ED and AN, in line with other clinical study [86]. Several sources starting from 1980 have reported a net correlation between ED and traumatic experiences. Research has been initially focused on the relation between ED and physical abuses and sexual harassment for the simple correspondence to a parental guidance failure. Recent studies showed that also emotional abuses, repetitive micro-traumatic relational experiences can result in further traumatic symptomatology.

A positive and secure attachment relation in children allows the definition of a self-image that deserves cares. It permits to rely on others in case of need, applying effective coping strategies. On the opposite, an insecure or disorganized attachment relation can result into a negative self-image.AN patients have developed poor strategies in regard to emotional management. This needs to be considered within a psychotherapeutic treatment, with an approach that should go beyond the simple symptomatic elements.

We hypnotize that EMDR method, in respect of other traditional approaches, results in a lower concern and less amount of weight-related thoughts related to body shape, with a consequent improvement on the emotional management and impulses of the patient. It has been suggested that individuals, after EMDR treatments, have lower confusion and apprehension in recognize and answer to emotions and impulses [76, 86]. These achievements

http://dx.doi.org/10.5772/65695

may contribute to increase the self-esteem and improve the social relations. We consider these preliminary results as a possible option in a therapeutic approachable to provide centrality to the "control" concept in its traditional frame, in its maintenance and possible resolution in a therapeutic framework.

EMDR seems to allow the elaboration of traumatic memories that characterize the AN patient's stories and to actively relate to disturbing memories, helping the resolution of the emotional blocks with a consequent elaboration of the first relations with the caregivers [87–89].

EMDR catalyzes a reconnection with body, emotions, and cognition along a continuum time span. It requires a coherent and smooth narration of the individual life story, without being overhang by negative feeling, such as anger, shame, and fear. These conclusions are supported by the increasing of Cohand RF scores on the AAI transcript of the patients who have participated in the present study.

3.1. Clinical implications

The control as a central aspect in ED has been established around the 1970 with the work of Marilyn Lawrence and Hilde Bruch. Between the 1980 and 2000, the progressive increment of the influence of cognitive-behavioral approach and, therefore, of the increased attempts to modify the ED directly on the symptomatic aspects without considering the traumatic remote sources of the disorders, had temporarily overtaken the study of the comprehension of the ED disorder and the treatment of its remote sources. The here employed protocol considers primarily the life story of the patients and their ability to elaborate and deal with emotions. With respect to traditional methods, a lower emphasis is given to the symptoms of early traumas. There are mainly four parts to consider in the application of EMDR protocol with AN patients.

A first point is to gather information on the previous and present life of the person, carefully analyzing resilience, risk, and maintenance disorder factors. The main focus in this phase is the evaluation of the attachment SoMs and the related risk factors, with a special attention to identify, within the patient's narration, eventual traumatic experiences that could have contributed to generate the AN behavior. A second step is to address and describe the time evolution of the disorder from its origin to the present, focusing on the context surrounding the patients right before the start of AN. It is also helpful, if applicable, to consider the stories of different forms of ED experienced by the patient and their relative treatments. A third part is related to the alimentation record of the family of the patient. From the nursing to the current alimentary habit, also questioning the parents ones. The latter investigation could provide a description of the meaning assigned to the food within the family by the parents and in the role of the food in the patient relation with the parents. The fourth and last part are related to the assessment of the control part, in terms of how it functions and how it protects the balance of personal self of the AN patient. A trust-based relation is necessary in people affected by AN. The patient has to feel to be an active part in the therapeutic process in order to not reiterate the impotence sensation that, in long term, could aggravate the control disorder of the patient. The security feeling allows a more effective exploration, by the patient, of his life story, with a focus on present and past aspects. It is essential, for the therapist, to listen and welcome all the different possible stories and perspectives to enable a complete narration by the patient. To obtain the trust from a patient, the therapist has to establish a link on the control aspect, defining its role in the resilience of the disorder. In order to induce in a patient the feeling of acceptance, it is necessary to discuss the consequences of the control and to describe its role and functions. It is absolutely required that the therapeutic does not judge the patient. Once a trust relation is established, more specific questions on the control and on its story can be posed with the focus to define the source, in time, of the disorder and on its role in protecting the patient. Furthermore, possible links with the parents or other relevant persons would be investigated. Via specific questions, it is possible to obtain a general view of the ensemble of factors that generated the AN. Allowing the expression of previously ignored feelings, re-elaborating them, and combining the different fragment, it is possible for AN patient to lose the stiff boundaries that they have constructed. Consequently, it will be possible to recognize the right to have needs, as nutrition, food, and relations.

3.2. Limitations and future directions

The present study has a clinical and exploration focus. Due to the low number of samples, it is not possible to satisfy the statistical requirement to represent a complete description of the overall population. Furthermore, a general quantitative description could fail to capture local and/or personal realities, defined by different life styles, society rules, and status quo. Hereby, clinical and methodological indications can provide significant indications and enable method enhancements. Further studies are needed to confirm and expand the present explorative work to obtain a larger clinical validation. A larger sampling would be auspicable to improve the statistical significance of the approach and the inclusion of additional elements that can enlarge the clinical efficacy of the method (e.g., the subjective perceptions of the caregivers' role during the treatments).

Author details

Maria Zaccagnino[1,2], Cristina Civilotti[3*], Martina Cussino[1,2], Chiara Callerame[1,2] and Isabel Fernandez[4]

*Address all correspondence to: cristina.civilotti@unito.it

1 University of Lugano, Lugano, Switzerland

2 EMDR Center for Eating Disorders, Milan, Italy

3 University of Turin, Turin, Italy

4 EMDR Italian Association, Varedo (MB), Italy

References

[1] Bruch H, editor. The golden cage: the enigma of anorexia nervosa. Cambridge: Harvard University Press; 1978.

[2] Jaffa, T., & McDermott, B. (Eds.). (2007). Eating disorders in children and adolescents. Cambridge University Press.

[3] Rosen DS. Eating disorders in children and young adolescents: etiology, classification, clinical features, and treatment. Adolescent Medicine Clinics. 2003; 14(1): 49.

[4] Kurz S, Van Dyck Z, Munsch, Munsch S, Hilbert A. Early-onset restrictive eating disturbances in primary school boys and girls. European Child and Adolescent Psychiatry. 2015; 24: 779–785.

[5] Russell GF. Anorexia nervosa through time. In: Szmukler G, Dare C, Treasure J, editors. Handbook of eating disorders: theory, treatment and research. Hoboken: John Wiley & Sons; 1995; p. 5–17.

[6] Mabe AG, Forney KJ, Keel PK. Do you "like" my photo? Facebook use maintains eating disorder risk. International Journal of Eating Disorders. 2014; 47(5): 516–523.

[7] Zennaro A, editor. The development of psychopathology: biological, environmental and relational factors. Boulogne, Italy: Il Mulino; 2011.

[8] Rieger E, Touyz SW, Swain T, Beumont PJ. Cross-cultural research on anorexia nervosa: assumptions regarding the role of body weight. International Journal of Eating Disorders. 2001; 29(2): 205–215.

[9] Garner DM, Garfinkel PE. Socio-cultural factors in the development of anorexia nervosa. Psychological Medicine. 1980; 10(4): 647–656.

[10] Stice E. Risk and maintenance factors for eating pathology: a meta-analytic review. Psychological Bulletin. 2002; 128(5): 825.

[11] Juaregui Lobera I, Bolaños Rios P, Garrido Casals O. Parenting styles and eating disorders. Journal of Psychiatric and Mental Health Nursing. 2011; 18: 728–735.

[12] Minuchin S, Rosman B, Baker L, editors. Psychosomatic families: Anorexia Nervosa in context. Cambridge: Harvard University Press; 1978.

[13] Jones DC, Vigfusdottir TH, Lee Y. Body image and the appearance culture among adolescent girls and boys an examination of friend conversations, peer criticism, appearance magazines, and the internalization of appearance ideals. Journal of Adolescent Research. 2004; 19(3): 323–339.

[14] Gorwood P, Bouvard M, Mouren-Simeoni MC, Kipman A, Ades J. Genetics and anorexia nervosa: a review of candidate genes. Psychiatric Genetics. 1998; 8(1): 1–12.

[15] Gorwood P, Kipman A, Foulon C. The human genetics of anorexia nervosa. European Journal of Pharmacology. 2003; 480(1): 163–170.

[16] Schmidt U, Treasure J. Anorexia nervosa: valued and visible. A cognitive-interpersonal maintenance model and its implications for research and practice. British Journal of Clinical Psychology. 2006; 45(3): 343–366.

[17] Rohde P, Stice E, Marti CN. Development and predictive effects of eating disorder risk factors during adolescence: implications for prevention efforts. International Journal of Eating Disorders. 2015; 48(2): 187–198.

[18] Ward A, Turnbull S, Steele M. Attachment in anorexia nervosa: a transgenerational perspective. Psychology and Psychotherapy. 2001; 74:497.

[19] Troisi A, Massaroni P, Cuzzolaro M. Early separation anxiety and adult attachment style in women with eating disorders. British Journal of Clinical Psychology. 2005; 44(1): 89–97.

[20] O'Kearney R. Attachment disruption in anorexia nervosa and bulimia nervosa: a review of theory and empirical research. International Journal of Eating Disorders. 1996; 20(2): 115–127.

[21] Tasca GA, Ritchie K, Zachariades F, Proulx G, Trinneer A, Balfour L, et al. Attachment insecurity mediates the relationship between childhood trauma and eating disorder psychopathology in a clinical sample: a structural equation model. Child Abuse and Neglect. 2013; 37(11): 926–933.

[22] Troisi A, Di Lorenzo G, Alcini S, Nanni RC, Di Pasquale C, Siracusano A. Body dissatisfaction in women with eating disorders: relationship to early separation anxiety and insecure attachment. Psychosomatic Medicine. 2006; 68(3): 449–453.

[23] Sharpe TM, Killen JD, Bryson SW, Shisslak CM, Estes LS, Gray N, et al. Attachment style and weight concerns in preadolescent and adolescent girls. International Journal of Eating Disorders. 1998; 23(1): 39–44.

[24] Delvecchio E, Di Riso D, Salcuni S, Lis A, George C. Anorexia and attachment: dysregulated defense and pathological mourning. Attachment Assessment in Treatments, Prevention and Intervention Programs. 2007; 52: 12–18.

[25] Mills P, Newman EF, Cossar J, Murray G. Emotional maltreatment and disordered eating in adolescents: testing the mediating role of emotion regulation. Child Abuse and Neglect. 2015;39: 39156–39166.

[26] Moulton SJ, Newman E, Power K, Swanson V, Day K. Childhood trauma and eating psychopathology: a mediating role for dissociation and emotion dysregulation? Child Abuse and Neglect. 2015;39: 39167–39174.

[27] Messman-Moore TL, Garrigus AS. The association of child abuse and eating disorder symptomatology: the importance of multiple forms of abuse and revictimization. Journal of Aggression, Maltreatment and Trauma. 2007; 14(3): 51–72.

[28] Ammaniti M, Lucarelli L, Cimino S, D'Olimpo F, Chatoor I. Maternal psychopathology and child risk factors in infantile anorexia. International Journal of Eating Disorders. 2010; 43(3): 233–240.

[29] Schore A. The human unconscious: the development of the right brain and its role in early emotional life. In Green V, editor. Emotional Developmental in Psychoanalysis, Attachment Theory, and Neuroscience. New York: Brunner-Routledge; 2003. p. 23–54.

[30] Schore A. Right brain affect regulation: an essential mechanism of development, trauma, dissociation, and psychotherapy. In Fosha D, Siegel D, Solomon M, editors. The healing power of emotion: affective neuroscience, development, and clinical practice. New York: Norton; 2009. 11 p. 112–144.

[31] Herman JL. Complex PTSD: a syndrome in survivors of prolonged and repeated trauma. Journal of Traumatic Stress. 1992; 5(3): 377–391.

[32] Shapiro F, editor. Eye movement desensitization and reprocessing: basic principles, protocols, and procedures. New York: Guilford, 2001.

[33] Van der Hart O, Nijenhuis ER, Steele K, editors. The haunted self: structural dissociation and the treatment of chronic traumatization. New York: WW Norton and Company; 2006.

[34] Liotti G, Farina B, editors. Traumatic Developments. Etiology, clinical and treatment of dissociative dimension. Milan, Italy: Raffaello Cortina; 2011.

[35] Van der Kolk B. Developmental trauma disorder: toward a rational diagnosis for children with complex trauma histories. Psychiatric Annals. 2005; 35: 401–408.

[36] American Psychiatric Association. Diagnostic and statistical manual of mental disorders (DSM-5®). Washington DC: American Psychiatric Pub; 2013.

[37] Liotti G. Trauma, dissociation, and disorganized attachment: three strands of a single braid. Psychotherapy: Theory, Research, Practice, Training. 2004; 41(4): 472.

[38] Felitti VJ, Anda RF, Nordenberg D, Williamson DF, Spitz AM, Edwards V, et al. Relationship of childhood abuse and household dysfunction to many of the leading causes of death in adults: the Adverse Childhood Experiences (ACE) Study. American Journal of Preventive Medicine. 1998; 14(4): 245–258.

[39] Dube SR, Felitti VJ, Rishi S. Moving beyond childhood adversity: associations between salutogenic factors and subjective well-being among adult survivors of trauma. In

Linden M, Rutkowski K, editors. Hurting memories and beneficial forgetting: posttraumatic stress disorders, biographical developments and social conflicts. London: Elsevier Insights, 2013. p. 139–149.

[40] Monteleone AM, Monteleone P, Serino I, Scognamiglio P, Genio M, Maj M. Childhood trauma and cortisol awakening response in symptomatic patients with anorexia nervosa and bulimia nervosa. International Journal of Eating Disorders. 2015; 48(6): 615–621.

[41] Monteleone AM, Monteleone P, Serino I, Amodio R, Monaco F, Maj M. Underweight subjects with anorexia nervosa have an enhanced salivary cortisol response not seen in weight restored subjects with anorexia nervosa. Psychoneuroendocrinology. 2016; 70: 118–121.

[42] Rhodes B, Kroger J. Parental bonding and separation-individuation difficulties among late adolescent eating disordered women. Child Psychiatry and Human Development. 1992; 22(4): 249–263.

[43] Latzer Y, Hochdorf Z, Bachar E, Canetti L. Attachment style and family functioning as discriminating factors in eating disorders. Contemporary Family Therapy. 2002; 24(4): 581–599.

[44] McKenzie-Mohr S, Lafrance S, editors. Women voicing resistance: discursive and narrative explorations. London: Routledge; 2014; p. 182–183.

[45] Kaye WH, Weltzin TE, Hsu LK, Bulik C, McConaha C, Sobkiewicz T. Patients with anorexia nervosa have elevated scores on the Yale-Brown obsessive-compulsive scale. International Journal of Eating Disorders. 1992; 12(1): 57–62.

[46] Bastiani AM, Rao R, Weltzin T, Kaye WH. Perfectionism in anorexia nervosa. International Journal of Eating Disorders. 1995; 17(2): 147–152.

[47] Sutandar-Pinnock K, Blake Woodside D, Carter JC, Olmsted MP, Kaplan AS. Perfectionism in anorexia nervosa: a6-24-month follow-up study. International Journal of Eating Disorders. 2003; 33(2): 225–229.

[48] Lawrence M. Anorexia nervosa—the control paradox. Women's Studies International Quarterly. 1979; 2(1): 93–101.

[49] Goossens L, Van Malderen E, Van Durme K, Braet C. Loss of control eating in adolescents: associations with adaptive and maladaptive emotion regulation strategies. Eating Behaviors. 2016; 22: 156–163.

[50] Titova OE, Hjorth OC, Schiöth HB, Brooks SJ. Anorexia nervosa is linked to reduced brain structure in reward and somatosensory regions: a meta-analysis of VBM studies. BMC Psychiatry. 2013; 13(1): 1.

[51] Lao-Kaim NP, Fonville L, Giampietro VP, Williams SC, Simmons A, Tchanturia K. Aberrant function of learning and cognitive control networks underlie inefficient

cognitive flexibility in anorexia nervosa: a cross-sectional fMRI study. PLoS One. 2015; 10(5) e0124027.

[52] Berzins L, editor. Dying to be thin: the prevention of eating disorders and the role of federal policy. Washington D.C.: American Psychological Association: Public Policy Office; 1997.

[53] Hay PJ, Touyz S, Sud R. Treatment for severe and enduring anorexia nervosa: a review. Australian and New Zealand Journal of Psychiatry. 2012; 46(12): 1136–1144.

[54] Watson HJ, Bulik CM. Update on the treatment of anorexia nervosa: review of clinical trials, practice guidelines and emerging interventions. Psychological Medicine. 2013; 43(12): 2477–2500.

[55] National Collaborating Centre for Mental Health. Eating disorders: core interventions in the treatment and management of anorexia nervosa, bulimia nervosa and related eating disorders. London: British Psychological Society and Royal College of Psychiatrists; 2004.

[56] Kreipe RE, Golden NH, Katzman DK, Fisher M, Rees J, Tonkin RS, et al. Eating disorders in adolescents. A position paper of the Society for Adolescent Medicine. Journal of Adolescent Health. 1995; 16: 476–479.

[57] Lock J, Agras WS, Bryson S, Kraemer HC. A comparison of short- and long-term family therapy for adolescent anorexia nervosa. Journal of the American Academy of Child and Adolescent Psychiatry. 2005; 44(6): 632–639.

[58] Knatz S, Murray SB, Matheson B, Boutelle KN, Rockwell R, Eisler I, et al. A brief, intensive application of multi-family-based treatment for eating disorders. Eating Disorders. 2015; 23(4): 315–324.

[59] Hay P. A systematic review of evidence for psychological treatments in eating disorders: 2005–2012. International Journal of Eating Disorders. 2013; 46(5): 462–469.

[60] Dare C, Eisler I, Russel G, Treasure JL, Dodge L. Psychological therapies for adults with anorexia nervosa: randomized controlled trial of out-patient treatments. British Journal of Psychiatry. 2001; 178: 216–221.

[61] Galsworthy-Francis L, Allan S. Cognitive behavioural therapy for anorexia nervosa: a systematic review. Clinical Psychology Review. 2014; 34(1): 54–72.

[62] Pike KM, Walsh BT, Vitousek K, Wilson GT, Bauer J. Cognitive behavior therapy in the posthospitalization treatment of anorexia nervosa. The American Journal of Psychiatry. 2003; 160: 2046–2049.

[63] Touyz S, Le Grange D, Lacey H, Hay P, Smith R, Maguire S, et al. Treating severe and enduring anorexia nervosa: a randomized control trial. European Psychiatry. 2015; 30: 357.

[64] Fairburn CG, editor. Cognitive behavior therapy for eating disorders: a comprehensive clinical guide. New York: Guilford Press; 2008.

[65] Murphy R, Straebler S, Cooper Z, Fairburn CG. Cognitive behavioral therapy for eating disorders. The Psychiatric Clinics of North American. 2010; 33(3): 611–627.

[66] Kass AE, Kolko RP, Wilfley DE. Psychological treatments for eating disorders. Current Opinion in Psychiatry. 2013; 26(6): 549–555.

[67] Byrne SM, Fursland A, Allen KL, Watson H. The effectiveness of enhanced cognitive behavioural therapy for eating disorders: an open trial. Behaviour Research and Therapy. 2011; 49(4): 219–226.

[68] Chassler L. Understanding anorexia nervosa and bulimia nervosa from an attachment perspective. Clinical Social Work Journal. 1997; 25(4): 407–423.

[69] Elgin J, Pritchard M. Adult attachment and disordered eating in undergraduate men and women. Journal of College Student Psychotherapy. 2006; 21(2): 25–40.

[70] Koskina N, Giovazolias T. The effect of attachment insecurity in the development of eating disturbances across gender: the role of body dissatisfaction. The Journal of Psychology. 2010; 144(5): 449–471.

[71] Fernandez I, Giovannozzi G. EMDR and Adaptive Information Processing. Psychotherapy as stimulation of the self-repairing psychological processes. Rivista di Psichiatria. 2012; 47(2): 4–7.

[72] Solomon R, Shapiro F. EMDR and the adaptive information processing model potential mechanisms of change. Journal of EMDR Practice and Research. 2008; 2(4): 315–325.

[73] Shapiro F, Solomon R, editors. Eye movement desensitization and reprocessing. Hoboken: John Wiley and Sons Inc.; 1995.

[74] Fernandez I, Maxfield L, Shapiro F. Eye movement desensitization and reprocessing (EMDR). In Giannantonio M, editor. Psicotraumatologia. Fondamenti e strumenti operativi. Milano: Centro Scientifico Editore; 2009.

[75] Pagani M, Di Lorenzo G, Verardo A, Nicolais G, Monaco L, Niolu C, et al. Neurobiological substrate of EMDR therapy. Rivista di psichiatria. 2012; 23 47(2): 16–18.

[76] Zaccagnino M, Cussino M, Callerame C, Civilotti C, Fernandez I. EMDR and CBT for Anorexic patients: a clinical comparative pilot. in preparation.

[77] Zaccagnino M. EMDR protocol for the management of dysfunctional eating behaviors in anorexia nervosa. In Luber M, editor. Eye movement desensitization and reprocessing (EMDR)scripted protocols and summary sheets: treating trauma, anxiety, and mood-related conditions. New York: Springer; in press.

[78] Copeley M, Forgash C, editors. Healing the heart of trauma and dissociation with EMDR and ego state therapy. New York: Springer Pub; 2008.

[79] George C, Kaplan M, Main M. Adult attachment interview. Unpublished manuscript. 1985.

[80] Garner DM. The eating disorder inventory-3. International Journal of Eating Disorders. 2004; 35: 478–479.

[81] Derogatis LR, Lazarus L. SCL-90-R, brief symptom inventory, and matching clinical rating scales. In Maruish M, editor. The use of psychological testing for treatment planning and outcome assessment. Hillsdale: Lawrence Erlbaum Associates, Inc.; 1994. p. 217–248.

[82] Gratz KL, Roemer L. Multidimensional assessment of emotion regulation and dysregulation: development, factor structure, and initial validation of the difficulties in emotion regulation scale. Journal of Psychopathology and Behavioral Assessment. 2004; 26: 41–54.

[83] Main M, Goldwyn R. Adult attachment interview scoring and classification manual–6th version. Unpublished manuscript. Berkeley: University of California; 1998.

[84] Main M, Goldwyn R, Hesse E. The Adult Attachment Interview: scoring and classification system. Version 7.1. Unpublished scoring manual. Department of Psychology. Berkeley, CA: University of California; 2002.

[85] Fonagy P, Target M, Steele H, Steele M, editors. Reflective-functioning manual, version 5.0, for application to adult attachment interviews. London: University College London; 1998.

[86] Bloomgarden A, Calogero RM. A randomized experimental test of the efficacy of EMDR treatment on negative body image in eating disorder inpatients. Eating Disorders: The Journal of Treatment and Prevention. 2008; 16(5): 418–427.

[87] Wesselmann D, Davidson M, Armstrong S, Schweitzer C, Bruckner D, Potter AE. EMDR as a treatment for improving attachment status in adults and children. Revue Européenne de Psychologie Appliquée/European Review of Applied Psychology. 2012; 62(4): 223–230.

[88] Zaccagnino M, Cussino M. EMDR and parenting: a clinical case. Journal of EMDR Practice and Research. 2013; 7: 154–166.

[89] Verardo A, Zaccagnino M, Lauretti G. Clinical applications in the context of attachment: the role of EMDR. Clinical applications in the context of attachment: the role of EMDR. Infanzia e Adolescenza. 2014; 13: 172–184

Chapter 11

The Body in Movement: A Clinical Approach

Michel Probst and Jolien Diedens

Additional information is available at the end of the chapter

http://dx.doi.org/10.5772/106289

Abstract

Physiotherapy or body-oriented therapy is often overlooked as an adjunctive treatment for patients with eating disorders (ED). However, the integration of physiotherapy is based on the physiotherapists' experience in both the body and the body in movement, two important issues integral to eating disorder pathology. From our clinical experience, physiotherapeutic techniques represent a potent clinical addition to available treatments. Patients with eating disorders have an intense fear of gaining weight and present a negative body experience. Excessive exercise and drive for activity or hyperactivity are considered to be a secondary symptom and are characterized by a voluntary increase in physical activity, a compulsive urge to move and by the dissociation of fatigue. Both characteristics are the two cornerstones for physiotherapy in children, adolescents, and adults in an inpatient or outpatient treatment. More concrete, the objectives for physiotherapy are (1) rebuilding of a realistic self-concept, (2) curbing hyperactivity, and (3) developing social skills. Physiotherapists have a wide array of skills that can be applied successfully in the treatment of anorexia nervosa (AN). The goal of this chapter is to present practical guidelines for physiotherapeutic management in eating disorder, more specific about mirror exercises, film images, and some additional individual or group exercises, recommendations based on more than 35 years of clinical experience.

Keywords: body image, physiotherapy, body-oriented therapy, mirror exercises, video confrontation

1. Introduction: body image and eating disorders

In the eating disorder pathology, body image disturbance is a central theme (see diagnostic criteria) [1] and distinguishes eating disorders from other psychological status that occasionally involve eating and weight abnormalities [2].

Bruch [3] was the first to recognize a group of three interrelated "perceptual and conceptual" disturbances in anorexia nervosa: (1) body image disturbances of delusional proportions;

(2) disturbance in perception or interoceptive disturbances such as an inability to accurately identify internal sensations such as hunger, satiety, or affective states; and (3) an overwhelming sense of personal ineffectiveness. The disturbance in body image of delusional proportions is described as follows: "the absence of concern about emaciation, even when advanced, and the vigor and stubbornness with which the often gruesome appearance is defended as normal and right and not too thin and as the only possible security against the dreaded fate of becoming illness" [2–4].

Since Bruch's description, a significant amount of literature on body image disturbances in eating disorders has been published over the last 50 years due to the relative new disorder and the demands of scientific evidence of the treatments. Her concept about body image is today integrated in the definition of body image proposed by Cash and Smolak [5] and which is today worldwide accepted.

Body image is a multidimensional concept with at least three aspects, including neurophysiologic, psychological, and behavioral. First, the neurophysiologic aspect refers to perceptual experiences as visual spatial, sensory judgments, physical sensations, body awareness, body recognition, physical appearance, and body size and shape. The psychological aspect refers to cognitive (thought process and thinking styles) and subjective experiences (feelings, emotions affect, and mood). A third behavioral component (avoidance and checking behavior) might actually be the result of neurophysiologic and psychological aspects [5–7].

The "perceptual aspect" refers to the degree to which the patient is not able to assess the own body size accurately. The most perplexing abnormality is the patient's apparent inability to recognize how thin the patient has become. In the literature, this phenomenon refers as a disturbed size awareness, that is, overestimation of some body parts (belly or thighs). Most of them recognize that they appear emaciated, but that further weight loss is a necessary condition to eliminate their protruding stomach. The cognitive and affective components of body image disturbance, without any obvious sign of perceptual mediators, refer to patients who react to their bodies with extreme forms of disparagement or occasionally aggrandizement for parts of their body. Patients with AN have a fear of ugliness and are forever concerned with their appearance, while denying the abnormalities of their starved bodies. In general, patients with ED perceive themselves as unrealistically big or fat and as out of proportion. They are proud of their emaciated bodies. The disturbed body experience is often expressed as a nonverbal message, a rejection of the body, a fear and a refusal to grow up. The behavioral component refers to the behavior as a consequence of the body image disturbance avoiding behavior such as mirrors, parties and activities, checking behavior, maladaptive physical activity, and excessive and compulsive (physical) activities [2, 4, 5, 7, 8].

Their experience with body weight and shape is distorted. Persons suffering from an ED evaluate their body in an unrealistic way. Even when underweight, they experience their body as normal or even too fat. They express a discrepancy between the way they see themselves and the way they see others. They are able to give an accurate estimate of another patient's body size while they do not realize, they look the same or even worse! They report inaccurate ideas about the consequences of food intake on their body structure. After a meal, they feel their stomach is "bulging" or their belly is "swelling." Most patients with ED nourish a negative

http://dx.doi.org/10.5772/106289

attitude toward their physical appearance. They are constantly focusing, criticizing, hiding, or fighting their body. The dissatisfaction applies to body parts that are not related to weight (wide hips, short height, short legs). Patients develop their own standards. They do not accept that the inner part of their thighs touch each other in stand. There is sometimes a similarity with people suffering from "imagined ugliness" or body dysmorphic disorder or from physical or sexual abuse. The problem is that weight loss does not increase their satisfaction and their confidence at all. They tremble at the thought of being touched and become anxious with physical closeness in general [2, 4, 5, 7, 8].

The theory of lenses illustrates clearly the conflict within body experience. The unbiased, objective, or neutral lens or "how does the person really look" indicates reality. The internal lens or "how does the person see himself" and the ideal lens or "how would the person like to look" refer to the (dis-) satisfaction and the discrepancy between thoughts and feelings and reality [7]. The external lens or "how do others see me" reflects the concern of the patient about how other persons think or perceive the patient. The external lens refers to (social) anxiety. The more the four lenses diverge, the more problematic the self-perception is. The core problem resides in the absence of self-esteem and the negative self-perception, which is expressed in the negative body image [4, 7–9].

Changing the way, patients with AN experience their bodies should be considered a priority in the treatment of this disorder. According to Bruch [3], a realistic self-concept and the acceptance of the body are necessary for recovery. Vandereycken et al. [10] claimed that one of the causes for the failure of some methods of treatment lies in the neglect of these aspects of therapy. Other authors [11–13] pointed to the negative prognostic value of a distorted body experience.

In this chapter, we want to review therapeutic interventions that specifically focus on improving the body experience of AN patients. Therefore, changing the way, patients with eating disorders experience their bodies should Be considered as a priority in the treatment of this disorder [3, 10–11].

Patients with eating disorder tend to acquire total control over their own body, both physically (weight, food, hunger, fatigue) and mentally (perfectionism, asceticism). The fear as losing control is translated into a huge fear of gaining weight, even with seriously underweight [14]. Therapies focusing on the treatment of eating disorders should aim to change these negative body experiences. [9].

2. Body-oriented therapy (BOT) and the role of physiotherapy

Although physiotherapy is often overlooked as an adjunctive treatment for patients with eating disorders, physiotherapy has a unique role to play in the treatment of eating disorders. Physiotherapists have a knowledge about both the body and the moving body, two important issues integral to eating disorder pathology. They can use physical interventions to help patients overcome their symptoms and to accept their changing body shape. From our clinical experience, physiotherapeutic techniques represent a potent clinical addition to available treatments of eating disorders. Since 1965, this physiotherapeutic approach is called in Belgium psychomotor therapy or body-oriented therapy, which is a specialty in physiotherapy [7, 9].

This specific approach includes exercises from physiotherapy and ideas of psychotherapy that focus on the body to improve psychic functioning. In this approach, patients are faced with primarily nonverbal experiences that can be discussed verbally later or elsewhere in treatment. This approach has been applied in clinical settings under different names and leaded by therapist with different education.

Literature [2, 7, 9, 10] suggested that BOT can influence the distorted body experience, the hyperactivity, and the fear of losing self-control [10]. Patients with eating disorders have an intense fear of gaining weight and present a negative body experience and a disturbed body perception (weight, circumference, and form). Excessive exercise and drive for activity or hyperactivity are considered to be a secondary symptom in the diagnostic of patients with eating disorders and are characterized by a voluntary increase in physical activity, a compulsive urge to move and by the dissociation of fatigue. These characteristics are the two cornerstones for physiotherapy in children, adolescents, and adults with eating disorders problem in an inpatient or outpatient treatment. Based on this previous study and on the specific behavior of eating disorders, three general objectives were formulated: (1) rebuilding a realistic self, (2) regulation of hyperactivity, impulses and tension, and (3) improvement of social interaction.

3. Treatment approaches

There are several ways to accomplish the above-mentioned objectives in physiotherapy. Group or individual therapy is possible. Physiotherapists have a wide array of skills that can be applied successfully in the treatment of patients with eating disorders. Different therapeutic interventions aimed at improving the body experience in patients with eating disorders can be used: postural training, relaxation training, mindfulness, tai chi and yoga, breathing exercises, physical activities, sensory awareness, and self-perception (mirror exercises and body awareness) (see **Figure 1**; **Table 1**) [2, 7, 9].

Not just doing exercise or performing activities are intrinsically therapeutic. The exercises are not only goals in themselves, but the patient's experience and inner perception play the central role. Movement is used as a therapeutic tool for stimulating the embodiment of the mind needing specific training and skills. The emphasis lies mainly on the acquisition of mental and physical proficiencies related to the body in motion and on supporting personal development to enrich the people in order to increase their independent functioning in society. The motor domain is employed as a gateway to ameliorate the social affective functioning of an individual. Within this approach, the physiotherapist creates a setting that favors the onset and the development of a process in the patient using their specific working methods in order to stimulate the patients to get in touch with their inner world [15].

By offering some wide range activities around the theme of " body in motion," patients are invited to come out of their comfort zone, to experience new things, thoughts (obsession, perfectionism, worrying), and many emotions (depressive feelings, fear, guilt, anger, stress, feelings of unease, estrangement, and dissatisfaction), and to get more in touch with their inner world. This allows them to gain a better insight into their own performance [2, 15].

http://dx.doi.org/10.5772/106289

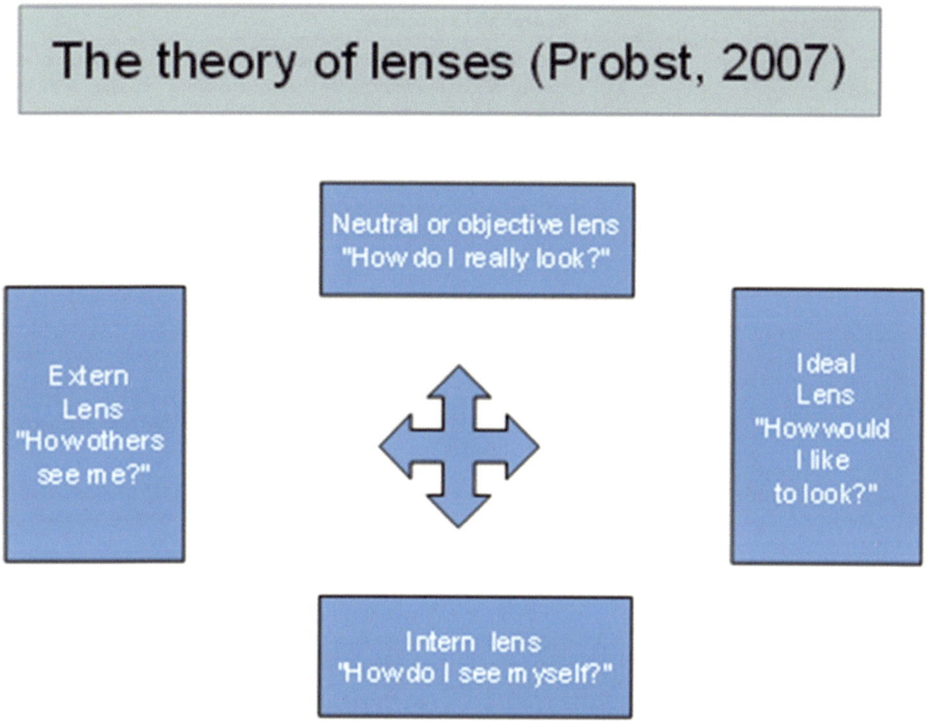

Figure 1. The theory of lenses.

The careful guidance and encouragement of the physiotherapist and the possibility to experience feelings in a safe environment allow the patient to develop behavior that he or she would not have developed otherwise. The underlying problems are not necessarily resolved, but the therapist tries improving his/her handling of problems. The patient shares his behavior, his feelings, and thoughts with the therapist and eventually with his peers. More emphasis is put on experiences, and how reactions to these experiences function as a dynamic power [15].

Throughout the physiotherapy intervention, an alternative frame of experiences can be made available. Experiencing that an alternative may exist will trigger new emotions and experiences, and a discrepancy between reality and the patient's perception of their reality will arise. The activities are aimed at learning, acquiring, training and/or practicing psychomotor, senso-motor, perceptual, cognitive, social, and emotional proficiencies. The following themes are taken into consideration: body and movement awareness, expressing and regulating emotions, augmenting the tolerance for frustration, refraining from impulsive behavior, improving the reality orientation, improving social interaction, learning to draw limits, strengthening self-confidence, improving body perception and self-perception, coping with emotionality, accepting responsibilities, dealing with fear of failure, developing self-reflection, exploring actual emotional and social life, and providing better insight into conscious inter- and intrapsychic conflicts [15].

It is obvious to present the patient a safe and structured framework, where everyone knows the rules and where the therapist is sufficiently informative about the therapeutic setting [2, 7, 9].

Physiotherapy intervention	Content and explanation
Postural exercises and postural awareness	A correct posture reduces physical symptoms, but also increases self-esteem; postural abnormality due to weakened muscles, which results in poor posture compensations (scoliosis, (]hyper-) kyphosis, lumbar (]hyper-) lordosis, scapula alata), and low back pain
Relaxation exercises	Relaxation reduces perceived stress and anxiety and the level of salivary cortisol. Relaxation techniques: progressive relaxation, autogenic training, yoga, mindfulness-oriented exercises, or biofeedback
Respiratory exercises	Respiratory exercises—especially those aimed at lowering respiration frequency, thereby amplifying abdominal respiration and lengthening expiration; the objective of breathing exercises is not simply to control respiration, but also to facilitate learning how to sense one's own body
Massage	The following forms of massage are used: relaxing and/or activating massage of the back and legs with or without instruments and passive mobilization of the limbs
Exercises targeting self-perception	Exercises targeting self-perception aim to amplify awareness of one's own body in its external appearance: mirror exercises, estimation techniques
Sensory awareness training	Sensory awareness training aims to discover the body through the senses in a nonthreatening manner. Awareness of touch Body boundary exploration, tactile awareness, body scanning ("trip around the body"), internal sensory exploration a "voyage into the body,"
Exercise, physical activity, sports, and games	Supervised exercise and physical activities such as fitness training resistance training, exercise, aerobics and callanetics, pilates, sports, and gymnastics

Table 1. Summary of therapy interventions.

The described picture of the body experience features highlights the perceptual, cognitive, affective, and behavioral aspects. It seems evident that the confrontation with their own body takes a crucial role in the treatment. Patients with eating disorders commonly criticize that they look fat viewing in the mirror [3, 6, 7]. The goal of this chapter is to present practical guidelines based on more than 35 years of clinical experience about two procedures namely the confrontation with mirrors and with life film images.

4. Mirror exercise

Mirrors play an important role in the life of the patient with eating disorders. Mirrors are to image what scales are to weight [16]. Some authors mention that the mirror is an illusion, one-half actual size. In fact, the size of one's reflection in a mirror is considerably smaller than one's real life body size [17]. Mirrors induce a self-centrality and show a greater awareness of one's own emotions and inner feelings. Mirrors have important effects. They make subjects more self-conscious, more critical, and more conforming. Mirror feedback can increase guilt, intensify self-dissatisfaction and affect mood, decrease the self-esteem, and increase conformity to the prevailing standard [16].

http://dx.doi.org/10.5772/106289

Scientific and clinical evidence provides some indication to address mirror exercise in the treatment of eating disorders. The aim of the mirror exercises is to target body experience concerns, to learn to use the mirror in a different way and to deal with the mirror and the associated emotions in a constructive way, to become aware of their own body, to start a habituation process about their own body. Mirrors are seen as a therapeutic ally. Mirrors could be helpful in forming a more stable integrated mental representation, they could break through the denying and could provoke an intense reality testing [2, 4, 9, 16–23].

The mechanisms responsible for mirroring are not known. Most likely mirroring is due to a combination of perceptual, affective, cognitive, and physiologic components of body perception. There is evidence that body exposure leads to a reduction of overestimation [23, 24], negative cognitions [16, 21, 25, 26], and feelings of fear, uncertainty, and sadness [22] as well as to the activation of the autonomic and endocrine system in the hypothalamus. Regular confrontation with the body leads to a habituation and refers to diminished dissatisfaction and a reduced anxiety toward the body. This adaptation process would lead to a more adequate behavior and in some cases even to feelings of success.

Mirror behavior refers to three behaviors: an appropriate mirror behavior, the mirror avoidance or refusing to look in mirrors, and the mirror checking, that is, constantly judging their body shape or body parts. It reveals a deep need to inspect and control the body and body changes in a vain pursuit of a perfect body (narcissistic feature). Checking behavior could be an expression of low self-esteem, anxiety, or addictive behavior [4].

The study of Jansen et al. [25] emphasizes another important issue. In contrary to noneating symptomatic subjects, eating symptomatic participants focused more on their own "ugly" body parts. When high symptomatic and noneating symptomatic subjects look to other bodies, the patterns are reversed. High symptomatic subjects focused their attention on the beautiful parts of other bodies. Normal controls concentrated on the ugly parts of the other bodies. The hypothesis is that a change in the processing of information might be needed for body exposure [25].

Mirrors are a useful tool for transforming body image when constructively combined with the power of visualization [16], with cognitive behavioral therapy (CBT) [21, 25] and with empirically supported CBT exposure therapy and mindfulness-based approaches [27]. Delinsky and Wilson [27] found that mirror exposure was effective in increasing body image satisfaction, reducing body image avoidance, and body checking. Jansen et al. [25] mentioned also that mirror exercises are very efficient if they are combined with cognitive restructuring. Hilbert et al. [28] state that mirror exposure may be useful for improving the awareness of body-related cognitive errors as negative bias, unrealistic standards, and dichotomous thinking.

4.1. Recommendations for mirror exercise based on our clinical practice

Different ways are available to accomplish mirror exercises. Some basic recommendations are proposed based on our clinical experience. Offering a safe framework with respect for the privacy is fundamental. Before starting, detail information concerning the procedure and the expectations is explained and patient's attitude toward the mirror is collected. The therapist possesses a gradation of possibilities. In the rule, the exercise (see addendum) takes about 30 min including an end-discussion and can be done in-group (with respect for everyone's privacy) or individually. Patients are invited to do the exercise in underwear. The therapist emphasizes the patient's responsibility during the exercise. The therapist looks to another way and refrains as much as possible from comments during the discussion. The frequency of the mirror exercise (i.e., twice a week) at several times (i.e., during the morning and in the afternoon; before and after the meals) develops a certain habituation effect.

In the first phase, the exercises are performed under the supervision of a therapist. In a latter phase, the patient can exercise alone or with a partner. In that phase, it is recommended to keep a mirror diary in which the frequency, the duration, the degree of fear before and after the exercise, and the feelings during the exercises are noted in order to improve the motivation. Using a hand mirror, body lotion, and background music are helpful tools [4].

The proposed mirror exercise consists of different steps. The first instruction is to look, to observe, and to describe, here and now, in a neutral, objective, respectful, mild, and curious manner their own body in the mirror. This instruction highlights that the purpose is not to criticize their own body or to compare with other bodies, but to increase their familiarity with one's own body. The patient stands in front of the mirror and learn to feel that he/she has the control over the body and not the negative feelings. The comparison between the mental picture and the image in the mirror is exercised by closing and after 30 s by opening the eyes. Later, the attention is aimed on possible changes and on patient's body parts that are attractive. Another instruction is to deal with different questions such as "who am I," "who do I think I am," "what do I do during my mirror exercises," "what are my wishes for the future," and "who do I want to be." At the end, the therapist invites the patient to congratulate him/herself [4].

From our clinical experience, there is a great support to implement mirror exercises in the treatment of eating disorder patients. Regular mirror confrontation together with a cognitive behavioral approach can lead to a decrease in body avoidance, checking, and dissatisfaction. After a time, the patients experience feelings of success and higher emotional responses than with other exercises. In our setting, mirror exercises are combined with a body-oriented therapy that also proposes other body-oriented exercises and within a multidimensional cognitive behavioral framework. The therapist must remain alert for possible negative impact of body exposure on the self-perception, such as negative fixations and a changing mood. A preceding interview and a debriefing after the mirror exercises could prevent these negative features [2, 4].

Patients in our inpatient treatment program retrospectively reported greatly valuing the mirror exercises that are incorporated into the body image treatment [2, 4, 9, 20]. Some AN and BN patients state that mirror exercises are one of the most important ingredients of our treatment program [4, 20]. These clinical impressions are supported by other authors [21–28].

5. Confrontation with film images

The use of film images (or video-recording) in the rehabilitation of patients with eating disorders is Not so common. However, since the idea launched by Yager et al. [29], the use of film

http://dx.doi.org/10.5772/106289

images was included in the eating disorder program. The method has been applied systematically for several years in a greatly modified form of Yager's method [29]. The approach consists of making standardized film recordings of the patient at the start of the treatment and on discharge. The patient is dressed in bikini/underwear because clothes or bathing suits would hide parts of the body which are important for persons with eating disorders. The recording lasts about 10 min. General shots of the complete body in frontal, back, and profile positions in addition to close-ups of parts of the body are taken. In the psychomotor sessions during the first week of the treatment, the pictures are shown to the patient and to the group the patient belongs to. The week before discharge, the patient is confronted both with the admission and the final recording. After viewing the recordings, the patient is invite to express his/her thoughts and feelings. Then, the fellow patients in the group have the opportunity to express their feelings as well and ask questions. On discharge, the two recordings are compared. The therapist refrains from giving comment but notes the responses [30, 31].

This procedure has even if it seems unusual a lot of important advantages for the patients. The patients look to and evaluate the complete body as it is perceived by others. Therefore, patients Can not pretend that they did not know how they looked like, even if image fades fast in time. This is unquestionably the most important positive aspect. This procedure could also be used to affect the body perception in a therapeutic sense. The patient's perception of her condition usually improves and disease denial decreases [30, 31].

The clinical experience with more than 1300 patients has increasingly strengthened the impression that the reactions to the recording provide very important information for the therapy. The reactions can be cluster into following reactions of indifference, surprise, confusion, uncertainty and fear, dissatisfaction, disgust, denial, shame, insight, and satisfaction.

Viewing the pictures in a group offers also an advantage. Watching other patient's recordings (heteroconfrontation) is just as important as self-confrontation. The combination of self-confrontation and group confrontation can increase the motivation and enable correction of the body perception and facilitates the development of a realistic positive body image [31]. No negative fundamental side-effects were experienced with this confrontation. Of course, the therapist must carefully offer a safety framework where the patients are informed about what, when, where, and how prior to the session. When the procedure is integrated in a multidisciplinary therapeutic setting, the theoretical risks of fear, reduced self-esteem, and a deterioration of the symptoms can be dealt with [30, 31].

6. Additional exercises (individual/group)

6.1. The estimation of shapes by a rope

The goal of this exercise is to observe patients' reactions during the different exercises and to confront the patient little by little with their wrong ideas concerning their own body. The patient receives one rope of 120 cm. This rope is always lying on the floor. Participants are asked to estimate/to guess the size of some shapes; for example, estimation means that you try to make an appropriate judgment without measuring. More concrete: What do you think about the size of the proposed object? What will be the approximate size?

When all the questions are clarified, the therapist can start the exercise. The exercise consists of different tasks:

- Estimate the circumference of a neutral object for instance the base of a trash bin or a bottle, by using the rope.
- Estimate the girth/outline of your body at the level of the belly button, above spina iliaca anterior superior (waist). How do you estimate the size of your waist?
- Estimate the girth/outline of the body of the therapist at the same level.
- Estimate your ideal girth/outline at the same level.
- Measure your girth/outline of your body and place it on the floor.

The results are an illustration of how patients think and feel. After each task, the therapist compares the result of the estimation with the real measurement. It is advisable not to focus on the result but more on the message that is expressed by the estimation.

6.1.1. Guidelines for the therapist

In the rule, most of the patients are able to make more or less an appropriate estimation of neutral objects. It is the task of therapist to judge whether the estimation lies within the normal range. In exceptional situations, the therapist is confronted with a deviant estimation, mostly depending of the level of familiarity with the chosen object. The general conclusion of this first introduction exercise is that in general there is nothing wrong with our eyes and with our perception.

In the second task, all the patients will overestimate their size. It is important that therapist and patient(s) discuss the estimation. After the estimation, the therapist can verify whether the estimation corresponds with the real size. Therefore, the patient is standing and the therapist shows the estimated size on the body of the patient, afterward the therapist shows the real (measured) size. In all cases, the patient will overestimate their own size, sometimes even two times the real size. The conclusion is that the estimation of our own size is not objective, but it is influenced by our thoughts and feelings. It is acceptable that they are unsatisfied with their own body because they have an unrealistic idea about their own size.

In the third task, the patient will be confronted with the fact that they are unable to estimate their own body size, but in the rule, they are able to estimate the size of somebody else. This is for the patient an important finding. The message of this exercise is that you have to be more open for what others (parents, group members, friends, relatives, partner, etc.) say. The message of the second and third task is that patients have to be very careful to believe their own thoughts and feelings in regard of their body.

The fourth task is an additional, not required, task. The patient will be confronted with the fact that in most of the cases, the ideal image is larger than the real image. This can provoke some emotional reactions. It is shocking to see the large difference between the shape of the body that they have in their minds and their actual body.

http://dx.doi.org/10.5772/106289

The last task is the most important one. The patient can measure their own size in standing position and make the real size on the floor. As therapist, it is important to observe the verbal and nonverbal reactions. This exercise provokes high emotional reactions. Some of the patients do not like to look to that size. Others do not believe that this is reality and measure again, sometimes five times. Some of them are confused, and others deny or minimize the results of the exercise.

The whole exercise is not a goal in itself; it is just a means to provoke some reactions and to discuss these reactions. Therefore, it is important to underline that after each task, patients are able to discuss, to express their thoughts and feelings, and to give comments. During the evaluation at the end of session, the exercise can be evaluated. The reactions represent the attitude of the patient about his/her body. The ideas elaborated during the rope exercise can be used during the mirror exercises.

6.2. A letter to your body or body part

The idea of writing a letter to your body originates in the narrative therapy. It is a very concrete task, where feelings and thoughts are expressed. The person is asked to write a letter from their own point of view. This process should promote empathy, understanding others, and flexibility. Writing letters allows that those who are involved can reflect on the problem in question without falling into communication. The process of writing is the most important. Afterward, everyone has the freedom to share the letters with the therapist and/or peers. It is important to explore what the exercise did with them. Writing can be a first step toward more depth and that is exactly what therapy is all about.

In this guided imagery exercises, the person is asked to write a letter to the body or to a loaded or unloaded body part. This is done in the same way as one would write a letter to a relative or friend. In a later phase, the same person will be asked to reread the letter and formulate a response from the body (or body part) addressed to the sender. Two examples from a 21-year-old patient with bulimia nervosa and from a 17-year-old patient with anorexia nervosa illustrate this exercise (see Boxes 1 and 2).

6.3. The exercise "middle point"

This is a group exercise. Patients are sitting close to each other in a circle. The therapist asks whether they feel comfortable. The awareness of feeling comfortable is being explored. After this exploration, the therapist explains the exercise: The patients are invited one by one to come in the middle of the group during 60 s without talking. It is the creativity of the patient to fill in the minute. The therapist observes the patients and gives the patient after each attempt the possibility to express their own experiences and feelings; the group members are also allowed to ask questions.

The focus of the exercise lies in "how to cope with stress, with low self-esteem, with attention (to be in the middle point), with the idea that others are looking (see and be seen).

Body awareness, communication, and relational aspects are other important items. Patients are invited and not obliged to execute the exercise. Even if some patients do not take the opportunity to perform the exercise, they will be confronted with a lot of emotions. The execution of the exercise is free; there is nothing wrong or good. Most of the time it shows how a patient thinks and feels. The focus lies on the exploration of the awareness of oneself in relation to others.

Dearest Belly

When I look at my body, you are the part that I hate the most. I don't know why you're so important in my life. You decide who I am and how I feel. It's just like you encourage me every day, and after every meal, to vomit. I sometimes think you're so fat! Why can't you just stay thin? I hate to be confronted with you day after day. Because I hate you so, you obstruct a part of my healing. Why do I have the feeling that everything I eat is stored in my belly? There is not an hour that goes by without thinking of you. I don't want this anymore. I want to go on, whether or not you want to help me out. I won't let you live my life, but from now on I take matters into my own hands. I was a happy woman and I still have everything to be that happy woman again. You can't take that away from me. You're a part of me that will always be difficult for me, but gradually I will try to accept you. Give me some time and I really hope that we can be buddies for life in the future. What do you think?

Love Bianca.

Dear Bianca,

Why do you worry so much about your belly? I'm just a body part, just like any other. I don't want you to worry about me. Everyone has a belly. It's normal that your stomach isn't very tight and you have a full feeling after your meals. A belly has its own shape, but that is typically female. You should be happy that you look so beautiful. Accept me as I am and you'll see that I won't change so much. Instead of beating or pinching me, try to give me some extra attention sometimes by rubbing me with a body lotion. I really like.

As you write in your letter, you were once a very happy woman. You can still be that. Do not worry about how you want me to be, but accept me as I am. Once you stop worrying about me, we can be good friends. I would love to see you happy again in the near future. Didn't I hear you talking to your boyfriend about getting babies? I'd be honored to feel your baby inside me. Think about that. If you want children, you have to let go and accept me as I am!

I know you can, and that you will soon be the happy girl who you were before. We continue working on our friendship.

Greetings

Your Belly

Box 1. Letter from a 21-year-old patient Bianca with bulimia nervosa.

At the end of the session, the link between the exercise within a therapeutic session and the outside world needs to be underlined and elaborated. There a lot of alternatives possible. The

http://dx.doi.org/10.5772/106289

Dear Belly,

Just before I was anorexic, you were still very common. I could walk around in bikini in the summer without any problem.

But 2 years ago everything became quite different. I didn't expose you, I didn't dare to walk around anymore. But still I did it and others started to gaze at me. I was proud of this, because you were skinny and they were thick. You are a very important body part for me, because you decide how I feel for the rest of the day. Sometimes you seem thicker and that scares me. Sometimes you seem skinny and that still makes me proud. I'm not going to lie about that. Ideally I would keep you as you are now. You give me some kind of security, a feeling that I'm worth it.

When I look at the future, I'm scared. I'm afraid of what will happen if I need to gain weight and you will return "normal?" I don't want to be normal. I want to be different from the others, I want to stand out from the others. And you help me with this. I don't want to give up on you. Not yet … now. But I realize that I'll have to, I want to continue. But then I have to give up on you and I have seen you like my god recent years. What now? I don't know anymore. It's all so confusing. Who should I listen to? The angel or the devil? The eternal dilemma: I think white or black. It would better be … gray.

But the essential thing is that I do not know how to deal with this situation. At the moment I'm not sure, but one thing is certain, I would like to be proud and happy …

So I think that I should taper the obsessive attention that I give you. Quietly, and it will not be easy. I realize that it will be hard, because it is similar to rehabilitation from drugs or alcohol. A dangerous addiction that is difficult to combat. I hope I can go on and can accept you in the end as you will be.

Big Kiss,

Sonia.

Dearest Sonia,

Since about 2 years I've been one of the most important things in your life. You've done me a lot of deficit by eating less. I often longed to eat, but that you did not give me. I know you're proud of me because I'm flat but that is a wrong idea. You'd better gain some weight and be happier than to stay lean and be unhappy. Yet I know it won't be easy for you. I will never say that. But think of all the people who believe in you and want to help you. You have cheated on them for years and yet they continue to support you. Isn't that more important to you than me, a body part? You say you want to be different from the others. Realize that you are unique because of who you are and not for what you do. Keep on fighting.

Big hug,

Your Belly

Box 2. Letter from a 17-year-old patient Sonia with anorexia nervosa.

therapist can manipulate the height (sitting on the floor or on a chair or in a standing position) or the distance between the participants.

6.4. The labyrinth

The labyrinth is a sail divided in 100 equal squares. The players have to follow an unknown route mapped in advance by the therapist. This route departs from one side and will revert to the other side. The route can take any form. The rules can be adapted to the players but need to be explained before the start. During the execution of the exercise, the therapist can make an appointment with the players not to speak, write, and establish codes, neither on the field nor outside. Only one person can be present simultaneously in the labyrinth. The therapist gives after each step the message "just go on" or "wrong step." Each player can make two wrong steps. After two wrong steps, the player needs to go back the way out. Another player takes the place till he makes two wrong steps. The game is over when all group members reach the other side. Different adaptations are possible in function of the group composition.

This exercise tests memory, demands attention, and develops a problem-solving strategy. Before and during the game, the patients could be confronted with anxiety, with fear to fail, with pressure. During the exercise, other group members are observing the person trying to find the way out. How does the person cope with seen and be seen? How does one feel when one has a black out in the middle of the labyrinth? Depending on the rules, It is also a good exercise in communication. This exercise has not only a cognitive, or emotional aspect but also a symbolic dimension that can be discussed during the evaluation. Life is a labyrinth, sometimes one has to take risks. It is much more difficult to take decisions when one is in the middle of the problem than when one look from outside to the problem. Sometimes to solve a problem one need to accept help, together it is easier to face problems. Listen to others is necessary. Persons have to believe in themselves. If one does it alone, one will make the same mistake.

7. Epilogue

The literature about the recovering process in eating disorders assesses rarely the patient's opinion and experience. However, the exploration of patients' subjective remarks and experiences of the patients with this approach can provide important indications. Therefore, the patients were interviewed at discharge [2, 4, 20, 32, 33]. One of the topics was "Do patients with eating disorders benefit from physiotherapy?"

¨"I just want to add that psychomotor therapy has helped me a lot."

¨"I want to thank the psychomotor therapist for his help. He taught me a lot. He often had to exhort me, but he made me look at myself in a different manner."

¨"I think psychomotor therapy was not always fun. The tasks were always difficult, but I learned a lot by executing them."

""It doesn't affect me having to say goodbye. Through psychomotor therapy the psychomotor therapist made me feel more confident and now I dare a lot more. I thank him for his patience and the interest he showed in me."

"For me psychomotor therapy was often a difficult and confronting therapy, but it did help me a lot to get where I am now…"

"I have the feeling that the psychomotor therapy helped me on the way of a complete acceptance of myself…"

"Sometimes the nature of the tasks we had to carry out surprised me but afterwards I always thought I had learned a lot."

""I find it difficult to linger over myself. But psychomotor therapy helped me in this. I feel I can be less resistant to change."

""The psychomotor therapy was not the easiest therapy for me but the psychomotor therapist helped me through it. There were even moments when I could enjoy it. My body is no longer a necessary evil but a team-mate I have to take into account…"

These statements are in the line of earlier research [32] but need to be interpreted scrupulously. What is the value of these statements? How sustainable are they? They were collected by interview upon discharge, expressed in the presence of the therapist and are perhaps influenced by the "hello-good-bye effect."

These qualitative remarks completed with more objective evaluations and observations, and remarks by other team members give some indications about the value of psychomotor therapy for certain patients. At least, a final remark with respect to the changes in body experience after treatment has to be made. When we compare our results 1 year after admission with the data of normal subjects, we see that eating disorder patients still have a more negative body experience. But can one expect body experience to change so quickly and is it realistic to expect "normalization" anyway? How many eating disorder patients will not retain a special relationship to their bodies throughout their lives? [2, 4, 7, 32, 34, 35].

At least, a final remark with respect to the changes in body experience after treatment has to be made. The comparison of the results of 1-year follow-up with the data of nonclinical subjects revealed that eating disorder patients still have a more negative body experience. Is it realistic to expect a "normalization?" The development of body experience is a process. Can such a change be supposed so quickly? The most of patients with eating disorder will throughout their lives retain a special relationship to their bodies [2, 4, 7, 32, 34, 35].

BOT is perceived as an effective form of therapy as patients encounter improvements in self-awareness, both physically and mentally. A closer contact with the own body, a more positive body experience, insight in a disturbed body image and distorted way of thinking, and improved self-esteem arise as a result of BOT and contribute to the process of accepting the own body. The role of the therapist, the presence of peers, one's own motivation and openness, and the time aspect are considered as key elements of BOT. These results should be targeted in future studies with larger sample sizes.

Appendix: Mindful mirror exposure

Welcome at this mirror exposure. I invite you to stand in front of the mirror and to prepare yourself for this mirror exposure.

Besides that, I invite you to participate in this exercise while wearing only your underwear. The reason for this, our clothes hide our most important body parts.

The intention of this exposure is to look at your own body in a mild, curious, non-judging way. But most of all, to look at your body in a respectful way. The goal is to become more familiar with your own body.

So try to look in a neutral and objective way at yourself in the mirror. It is not the aim to criticize yourself, nor to compare, but above all to look at your body.

Watch your posture. During the mirror exercise you can move or touch yourself. Try to pay attention to your posture and take a proud posture: Stand straight up, knees stretched, shoulders slightly to the back, head up and a smile on your face. Do you notice any difference?

Because you probably will be distracted to some specific parts of your body. We will systematically run over the different body parts journey around the body).

We will start with:

The head and the face

- Look at your hair specifically take a look at the color, length,..., of your hair
- Look at your forehead, eyebrows. Pull your eyebrows up or frown and feel the tension in your forehead
- Look at your eyes with eyelashes, eyelids, color of your eyes, and your appearance
- Look at your nose including nose bridge, nostrils, and naris
- Look at your mouth: lips, teeth, and corners of your mouth
- Look at your chin, cheekbones
- Look at your cheeks, are they little bit pale or are they rose-tinted?
- Look at your ears with your earlobes and auricles.

Now look at the global image of your head and face.

Further we look at the neck muscles. If you turn your head to the left and the right, you can feel the tension in those muscles of your neck.

Further down are the clavicles, with behind the shoulder muscles. When you move your shoulders forward, you accentuate your collarbones. When you shrug, you feel the tension in your shoulder muscles.

Then focus on your right shoulder, right upper arm with, among other things, at the front side of your arm the biceps (arm bender) and backside of your arm the triceps (arm extensor).

http://dx.doi.org/10.5772/106289

I invite you to bend and stretch the muscles in your upper arm.

Relax your arm now and feel the relaxation, and notice especially the difference between tension and relaxation.

Focus your attention now at:

- Elbow joint
- Forearm
- Wrist and hand
- The back of your hand
- The hand palm and five fingers starting with the thumb, forefinger, middle finger, ring finger, and little finger. Every finger has three little bones except the thumb that only has two of them. Note that all of the fingers are different
- When you move your finger, you can see the tendons of the finger extensors
- Now we will turn our hand and focus our attention toward the palm of the hand and the thumb thenar. The thenar is a collection of muscles that make the specific movements of the thumb possible. I invite you to make a fist and feel the tension in your hand. Relax your hand now and feel the relaxation
- Notice especially the difference between tension and relaxation

Then look at your whole right arm.

It goes without saying that what we have did at the right side we will also do for our left side.

So focus at your left shoulder, left upper arm with the biceps or triceps. I invite you to bend and stretch the muscles in your upper arm.

Relax your arm now and feel the relaxation, and notice especially the difference between the tension and relaxation.

If you recognize you are distracted by body parts which concern you, I invite you to get your concentration back and to follow again. Focus now at your sternum. Together with your ribs it forms your thorax. The thorax protects some vital organs, such as your heart and two lungs. By deep breathing in and out, you notice a change in the size of your chest. I invite you to breathe in and out deeply and perceive this change.

On top of your ribs you see your pectoral muscles and on top of them you have your both breasts.

Beneath your breast area you find your abdominal area with abdominal muscles, umbilicus and at both sides the loin.

Notice that your belly goes parallel up and down with your breathing.

May I ask you to put both hands on your abdomen and examine how your hands move along parallel with your breathing.

How do you feel this?

How do you experience this?

Then focus on the right hip and the gluteal muscles, of which we have three. Namely: the biggest, the middle one and the smallest gluteal muscle. Those muscles ensure that you can stand on one leg. I invite you to lift you left leg once to feel the tension in your right buttock. Relax your back and feel the difference between tension and relaxation.

So, we will focus now at the right upper leg with at the front side the quadriceps (knee extensors) and at the rear side the hamstrings.

If you pull your knee back, you can feel the tension in your knee extensors. Relax and feel the difference between tension and relaxation. Lower is the right knee, with the patella at the front and at the back of the knee the popliteal.

Then we have the right lower leg with your shin-bone and splint-bone and your calf muscles that ends in your Achilles tendon. The calf muscles ensure that you can stand on the tips of your toes. I invite you to go to stand once on your toes and feel the tension in your lower legs. Lower your heel and stand with your whole feet at the ground.

- Notice the difference between tension and relaxation.

We also come to the right ankle, heel, foot, dorsum of foot, toes and phalanges, but which are small.

If you hang your toes, you can observe the tendons of your toe extensors.

It goes without saying that what we have at the right, we also have at the left: the left hip with the gluteal muscles, of which we have three. Namely the biggest, middle and small gluteal muscle. Those muscles make sure that you can stand on one leg. I invite you once you lift right leg to feel the tension in your left buttock. Relax your back and feel the difference between tension and relaxation.

So, we will focus now at the right upper leg with at the front side the quadriceps (knee extensors) and at the rear side the hamstrings. If you pull your knee back, you can feel the tension in your knee extensors. Relax and feel the difference between tension and relaxation.

Lower is the right knee, with the patella at the front and at the back of the knee the popliteal.

Then we have the left lower leg with your shin-bone and splint-bone and your calf muscles that ends in your Achilles tendon. The calf muscles ensure that you can stand on the tips of your toes. I invite you to go to stand once on your toes and feel the tension in your lower legs.

Lower your heel and stand with your whole feet at the ground.

Notice the difference between tension and relaxation.

Now we also come to the left ankle, heel, foot, dorsum of foot, toes and phalanges, but which are small.

http://dx.doi.org/10.5772/106289

If you hang your toes, you can observe the tendons of your toe extensors.

And so we come to the end of the journey around our body.

Now we look back to our body at all. In a gentle, curious, not-judgmental but especially respectful way. Once again mind your proud posture.

Look to the whole image of your body

- Turn 90° to the right and look at your body in profile (10–15 s)
- Turn again 90° to the right and look over your shoulders to the backside of your body
- Turn 90° to the right and look at your body in profile
- Turn 90° to the right: frontal
- Turn for one last time 90° to the right, and now you're standing again in front of the mirror.

I invite you to close your eyes and make a mental image of your body as you saw just now in the mirror. So try to make a mental picture of your body. This is not an easy task and it requires some effort.

(After 15–20 s)

Open your eyes and see or your mental image corresponds with the image you see in the mirror. What are similarities? What are the differences?

Close your eyes again and try again to make a mental image of your body. Open your eyes and check or your mental image corresponds with your mirror image.

Look back at your whole body and try to answer the following three questions.

- Who am I? Or who do I think am?
- What am I doing? Am I honest towards myself if I reply on this? Do I not make a fool of myself?
- Where do I want to go? Who I would like to be? Where do I stand for?

Try to search for one positive element of your body. It does not have to be a big part of your body; it can be just a little detail. Also try to motivate why you experience it as positive. Try to find another element then the last time/times when you did mirror exercises.

Look back at your whole body and see or something has been changed since your last mirror exposure.

At the end of the mirror exercises it is important to congratulate yourself for the courage and effort that was needed to successfully complete the exercise or to convince yourself that you are worth it. By standing straight up, look deeply into your own eyes and say loud and with conviction: "I'm worth it."

With this final sentence we finish the mirror exercise. I invite you to dress up again. Than together we can exchange views.

Author details

Michel Probst* and Jolien Diedens

*Address all correspondence to: michel.probst@kuleuven.be

Department of Rehabilitation Sciences and Physiotherapy at the Catholic University of Leuven, KU Leuven, Belgium

References

[1] American Psychiatric Association. Diagnostic and statistical manual of mental disorders. (DSM-V), 5th ed. Washington, DC: APA Press, 2011.

[2] Probst M. Body experience in eating disorders: research and therapy. European Bulletin of Adapted Physical Activity [Internet]. Eufapa.upol.cz. 2006 [cited 24 June 2016]. Available from: http://www.eufapa.upol.cz

[3] Bruch H. Perceptual and conceptual disturbances in anorexia nervosa. Psychological Medicine. 1962;24:187–194.

[4] Probst M, Pieters G, Vancampfort D, Vanderlinden J. Body experience and mirror behaviour in female eating disorders patients and non-clinical subjects. Psihologijske Teme [Psychological Topics]. 2008;17(2):335–348.

[5] Cash T, Smolak L. Body image. A handbook of science, practice and prevention. New York: Guilford, 2011.

[6] Cash JT. What do you see when you look in the mirror? Helping yourself to a positive body image. New York: Bantam Books, 1995.

[7] Probst M, Majeweski M, Albertsen M, Catalan-Matamoros D, Danielsen M, De Herdt A et al. Physiotherapy for patients with anorexia nervosa. Advances in Eating Disorders. 2013;1(3):224–238.

[8] Probst M. Handboek eetstoornissen [Handbook eating disorders]. Utrecht: De Tijdstroom; 2008.

[9] Probst M, Coppenolle H, Vandereycken W. Body experience in anorexia nervosa patients: an overview of therapeutic approaches. Eating Disorders. 1995;3(2):145–157.

[10] Vandereycken W, Depreitere L, Probst M. Body-oriented therapy for anorexia nervosa patients. American Journal of Psychotherapy. 1987; 41: 252–259.

[11] Danielsen M, Rø Ø. Changes in body image during inpatient treatment for eating disorders predict outcome. Eating Disorders. 2012;20(4):261–275.

[12] Keel P, Dorer D, Franko D, Jackson S, Herzog D. Postremission predictors of relapse in women with eating disorders. American Journal of Psychiatry. 2005;162(12):2263–2268.

[13] Exterkate CC, Vriesendorp P, De Jong C. Body attitudes in patients with eating disorders at presentation and completion of intensive outpatient day treatment. Eating Behaviors. 2009;10:16–21. dx.doi.org/10.1016/j.eatbeh.2008.10.002.

[14] Probst M, Goris M, Vandereycken W, VanCoppenolle H. Body composition of anorexia nervosa patients assessed by underwater weighing and skinfold-thickness measurements before and after weight gain. The American Journal of Clinical Nutrition. 2001;73:190–197.

[15] Probst M, Knapen J, Poot G, Vancampfort D. Psychomotor therapy and psychiatry: what's in a name? The Open Complementary Medicine Journal. 2010;2(1):105–113.

[16] Freedman RJ. Body love (updated edition). New York: Harper & Row, 2003.

[17] Shafran R, Fairburn C, Robinson P, Lask B. Body checking and its avoidance in eating disorders. International Journal of Eating Disorders. 2003;35(1):93–101.

[18] Cash TF, Pruzinsky T. (Eds.) Body images: development, deviance, and change (pp. 51–79). NY: Guilford, 1990.

[19] Cash TF. What do you see when you look in the mirror?: Helping yourself to a positive body image. New York: Bantam Books, 1995.

[20] Probst M. Spiegels en lichaamsbeleving bij vrouwelijke patiënten met eetstoornissen versus niet klinische subjecten [Mirrors and body experience in female patients with eating disorders versus non-clinical subject]. In: Simons J. (Eds.), Actuele themata uit de psychomotorische therapie: jaarboek (pp. 99–118). Leuven: Acco, 2005.

[21] Key A, George C, Beattie D, Stammers K, Lacey H, Waller G. Body image treatment within an inpatient program for anorexia nervosa: the role of mirror exposure in the desensitization process. International Journal of Eating Disorders. 2002;31(2):185–190.

[22] Tuschen-Caffier B, Vögele C, Bracht S, Hilbert A. Psychological responses to body shape exposure in patients with bulimia nervosa. Behaviour Research and Therapy. 2003;41(5):573–586.

[23] Farrell C, Shafran R, Fairburn C. Body size estimation: testing a new mirror-based assessment method. International Journal of Eating Disorders. 2003;34(1):162–171.

[24] Vocks S, Legenbauer T, Wächter A, Wucherer M, Kosfelder J. What happens in the course of body exposure? Emotional, cognitive, and physiological reactions to mirror confrontation in eating disorders. Journal of Psychosomatic Research. 2007;62(2):231–239.

[25] Jansen A, Nederkoorn C, Mulkens S. Selective visual attention for ugly and beautiful body parts in eating disorders. Behaviour Research and Therapy. 2005;43(2):183–196.

[26] Mountford V, Haase A, Waller G. Body checking in the eating disorders: associations between cognitions and behaviors. International Journal of Eating Disorders. 2006;39(8):708–715.

[27] Delinsky S, Wilson T. Mirror exposure for body image disturbance. International Journal of Eating Disorders. 2004;35:449.

[28] Hilbert A, Tuschen-Caffier B, Vögele C. Effects of prolonged and repeated body image exposure in binge-eating disorder. Journal of Psychosomatic Research. 2002;52(3):137–144.

[29] Yager J, Rudnick FD, Metzner RJ. Anorexia nervosa: a current perspective and some new directions. Psychiatric research in practice: biobehavioral themes (pp. 131–150). New York: Grune and Stratton; 1981.

[30] Probst M, Vandereycken W, Van Coppenolle H. L'image du corps et l'anorexie mentale. L'emploi de la confrontation par vidéo dans la th rapie psychomotrice [Body image and anorexia nervosa. The use of video-confrontation in psychomotor therapy]. Acta Psychiatrica Belgica. 1988;88:117–126.

[31] Probst M, Van Coppenolle, H, Vandereycken, W. The use of videoconfrontion in the treatment of patients with eating disorders. In: Vermeer A, Bosscher R, Broadhead G. (Eds.), Movement therapy across the life-span (pp. 116–122). Amsterdam: VU University Press, 1997.

[32] Probst M. Onderzoek in de psychomotorische therapie: de perceptie van de psychomotorische therapie door patiënten met eetstoornissen [Perception of psychomotor therapy in patients with eating disorders]. In: Simons J. (Eds.), Actuele themata uit de psychomotorische therapie (pp. 133–151). Leuven: Acco, 2007.

[33] Machado G, Ferreira M. Physiotherapy improves eating disorders and quality of life in bulimia and anorexia nervosa. British Journal of Sports Medicine. 2014;48(20):1519–1520.

[34] Geerdens C, Vanderlinden J, Pieters G, De Herdt A, Probst M. Missing data in long-term follow-up of patients with eating disorders using the body attitude test. European Eating Disorders Review. 2012;21(3):224–229.

[35] Probst M, Vandereycken W, Van Coppenolle H, Pieters G. Body experience in eating disorders before and after treatment: a follow-up study. European Psychiatry. 1999;14(6):333–340.

Section 5

Other Topics

Communication Challenges Within Eating Disorders: What People Say and What Individuals Hear

Martha Peaslee Levine

Additional information is available at the end of the chapter

http://dx.doi.org/10.5772/65305

Abstract

Communication challenges are apparent in many different ways when working with individuals who struggle with eating disorders. These issues can include the influence of parenting styles to society's weight messages to comments by professionals as they interact with those struggling with eating disorders. Other challenges come from the skewed interpretations that individuals with eating disorders can place on messages that they receive. This chapter examines the literature on many of these issues, highlights challenges with clinical examples, and proposes potential tools to ameliorate some of the impact of these issues on communication.

Keywords: communication, eating disorders, anorexia nervosa, bulimia nervosa, binge-eating disorder, parenting, negative comments, media images, teasing

1. Introduction

Communication requires the exchange of ideas, which means that there is a communicator and a receiver. We need to consider communication as it relates to eating disorders from both sides. What is being said? And what is being heard? There are times that these two aspects are very different. For example, when a person tells another, "You look so healthy!" Most of us would accept this as a compliment. Individuals with anorexia nervosa often hear this exact comment as "You've gained weight". They hear and interpret comments through a specific filter that can distort messages. Yet there are times that messages communicated to individuals are heard just the way that they were meant, and it is the comment itself that is the issue. Such an example would include when a client of mine, who was finally recovering from her eating disorder and was doing well in college was criticized by her family for not having a job. This comment, clearly, meant that she was not meeting expectations. That is how it was heard.

This inability to please others, even when she was working so hard to recover and complete school started her back on the path of restricting and purging.

Other expectations are communicated by society through implied standards. Even the DSM 5 recognizes these messages when it defines certain risk factors: "Historical and cross-cultural variability in the prevalence of anorexia nervosa supports its association with cultures and settings in which thinness is valued" ([1], p. 342). "Internalization of a thin body ideal has been found to increase risk for developing weight concerns, which in turn increase risk for the development of bulimia nervosa" ([1], p. 348). These values are often communicated through the media, which can have a significant effect on individuals.

This chapter will examine communication challenges through a review of the literature and examples from clinical experience. In the end, recommendations to help improve communication will be offered. The eating disorders addressed in this chapter are defined by the DSM 5 and include anorexia nervosa, restrictive eating leading to a significantly low body weight with an intense fear of gaining weight; bulimia nervosa, recurrent episodes of binge eating and subsequent compensatory behaviour in an attempt to prevent weight gain; binge-eating disorder, recurrent episodes of binge eating, such that one eats until uncomfortably full, binges even when not hungry, eats this quantity of food alone because of embarrassment and feeling distressed or guilty after the binge, and finally unspecified eating disorder, which includes behaviour similar to the above categories but in which the symptoms do not meet all of the qualifications [1].

While the effects of different interpersonal interactions will be split out and examined separately, it is important to recognize that these influences work together to create an atmosphere that fuels the eating disorder. Many authors describe the "tripartite model of influence" with the primary core sources affecting body dissatisfaction being parents, peers, and the media [2, 3]. Attempts to understand these various factors have been made with the development of the CIMEC (Questionnaire of Influences on Body Shape Model), which measures the influence of different sociocultural influences [4].

2. Intrapersonal factors

While there are many challenges with the messages communicated via the media, society, family members, and peers, there are additional challenges related to how individuals with eating disorders perceive these messages. Individuals struggling with eating disorders when compared to asymptomatic controls are more likely to identify hostile intent in a series of social vignettes [5]. Adolescent girls were provided with social dilemmas, such as not being invited to a best friend's birthday party. The control group described that they would talk with the friend or made positive assumptions, such as it must have been assumed that she would come. Individuals struggling with eating disorders, however, rarely picked the option of talking with the friend and brought negative assumptions to the interaction, such as assuming that the friend had only been pretending to like her. They most often picked avoidant coping strategies, including eating disorder symptom uses [5].

http://dx.doi.org/10.5772/65305

Those with anorexia nervosa (AN) and bulimia nervosa (BN) have a higher tendency to use suppression strategies to handle negative emotions as compared to healthy controls who use reappraisal strategies [6]. Individuals with eating disorders suppress the hurt rather than trying to reframe a situation or challenge their assumptions. With BN, avoidant coping strategies are more apparent when the individual is struggling with depression [7].

There is additional evidence that individuals with eating disorders are on high alert for threats. In a computer-driven test, women with a high level of bulimic symptoms were significantly more likely to identify a threatening word when it was present and less aware of it being absent, which suggested a bias towards always expecting a threat to be present [8]. Individuals with anorexia nervosa (AN) often think the worst when considering how others see them, and these experiences then negatively affect their body image, such that they feel themselves fat and believe others see them as ugly or disgusting [9]. One can see the challenge these negative perceptions and expectations have in interpersonal interactions.

Other studies have demonstrated engrained reactions that differ for individuals struggling with eating disorders (ED) as compared with healthy controls. For example, using a lexical decision task, individuals at risk of eating disorders were found to react more quickly to fat-related words than to words unrelated to fat; healthy controls had the opposite pattern [10]. In another study when compared with controls, eating disorder patients were quicker to identify body-related information and more distracted by food information [11]. At-risk individuals appear triggered by these types of words, which then affect how they attend to words and concepts in conversational settings. In addition, clients have described that if they restrict in a social setting then much of their focus is on food or body comparisons. They are not only primed for this focus, but also their ED behaviours fuel it.

Interpersonal interactions also rely on nonverbal communication. So while individuals with eating disorders may be overly attending to certain words, distracted by others, and reading negative meanings into many situations, what happens in the face-to-face contact with others? Individuals struggling with AN have less facial expression in response to positive and negative emotional stimuli and tend to look away while watching a negative film clip as if trying to avoid negative feelings [12, 13]. In particular, individuals with AN have less intense and shorter in duration spontaneous smiles as compared to individuals with BN and healthy controls within these settings [14]. This reduced expression of positive affect can maintain a pattern of social avoidance seen in individuals with AN [14]. Individuals with AN also have more difficulty imitating facial expressions of emotions [15]. They can appear distant and uninterested. Individuals with eating disorders, especially AN, have deficits in their own emotional awareness [16]. This challenge in expressing their own emotions can lead to a tendency to provide vague or over-generalized answers to questions about their emotional state [17]. One client described that she does not really know how she feels so she cannot put it into words. This has led to interpersonal conflicts with her spouse who wants to know how she is feeling and how he can help improve her mood.

Individuals with eating disorders also struggle in the opposite direction, that of being able to accurately interpret another person's emotional expression [16]. Individuals with high levels of eating pathology have a challenge in recognizing subtle expressions of emotion and have a tendency to misidentify more intense emotions, reading fear as anger and anger as sadness [18]. As Ref. [19] describes, "Thus, if the experience of anger, disgust and rejection are usually linked to each other in people with AN, it may be that faces portraying disgust were experienced by people with AN as rejecting and thus were interpreted as 'angry'" (p. 40). This can relate to the previously described interpersonal situations and the tendency of individuals with eating disorders to interpret others' interactions in a negative light and see them as rejecting. Another study demonstrated that individuals with AN, especially those with strong obsessive-compulsive symptoms, had difficulty in recognizing sad facial affect [20]. Difficulties in these emotional spheres can have huge impacts on individuals with eating disorders as they work to make interpersonal connections. Helping individuals understand their misinterpretation of facial cues and the link to feelings of rejection may be very important in the treatment of individuals with AN [19].

In addition, anger and, at times, sadness are seen as toxic and a danger both for the individual and the others involved [21]. According to Ref. [21], "The analysis highlighted how people with anorexia often did not regard themselves as entitled to be an 'emotional' human being, or that being 'emotional' would lead to rejection from significant others" (p. 298). In the clinic setting, family members often provide this message to individuals struggling with eating disorders. Even as a brother was criticizing his sister and she was trying to defend herself, he told her to not get mad. In other situations, clients have been told by family members that they are "just too sensitive". These comments take away the power of these women to be able to react to criticism. It relieves the attacker of responsibility and hands it to the individual who is struggling with the eating disorder. It essentially says, "This is not related to what I said, this is all you. You are just too sensitive". This leads us into examining aspects of interpersonal interactions with family and peers.

3. Interpersonal factors: parents

Individuals with eating disorders, especially those struggling with anorexia nervosa, can misinterpret situations and emotions. However, are there times that interpersonal interactions could be fuelling the eating disorders? Overall, the majority of adolescents report valuing their parents' opinions and believe their parents care about them. Yet those adolescents who perceived a poor level of parental communication and caring were at a high risk of developing unhealthy weight-control behaviours, especially if they felt that their mother cared very little or not at all [22]. Ref. [23] used a projective test to examine family dynamics and found that patients with eating disorders expressed more discord within the family picture and described, in particular, cold and loveless relationships in the family, in which they did not feel validated. While perceptions may not always be the reality, within a group of adolescents those with binge-eating disorder (BED), as compared to controls, had higher levels of perceived maternal criticism and lower levels of perceived warmth [24]. Ref. [25] identified that, "Whether overt or perceived, negative verbal communications appear stronger predictors of eating disorders than those that are indirect in nature such as family conflict" (p. 209). Weight-teasing by family members has been found to be most strongly and most consistently correlated with problematic weight issues [26]. Individuals who have more eating disorder characteristics often describe feeling less comfortable discussing their problems with their parents, feel that issues are not taken seriously and often feel lectured at rather than finding a collaborative stance [27].

Families in which the daughter is struggling with AN perceive their family functioning as significantly worse than matched controls and the daughters perceive the family functioning in a much worse light than the rest of the family [28, 29]. The most frequent parenting style in families where a child struggles with an eating disorder is low in care and high in control [30]. They do not feel cared for but feel as if they do not have any control or the ability to navigate the family situation. Individuals struggling with eating disorders who have a more positive perception of their family functioning generally had a more positive outcome, irrespective of the severity of their symptoms [29].

In one study, daughters and mothers of control families seemed to share similar views of family communication, but daughters with eating disorders often did not have a shared perception with either parent about the family's communication. This left them isolated and potentially participated in maintaining the eating disorder [28]. Evidence suggests that this difference in the daughter's perception is related to her distrust of people in general and to her feelings of inadequacy [31]. She feels isolated and not understood. Individuals who consider their mothers "neglectful" in the first 16 years of their lives often demonstrate a higher drive for thinness and more body dissatisfaction [30]. They may be trying to understand why their mothers are so withdrawn from them and are trying to find ways, through the messages of society, to make themselves into individuals who are loveable. When individuals experience neglectful parenting, they have lower self-esteem [30]. In clinic interactions, some of the young woman often describe a feeling of isolation in the family and relate that their eating disorder is the only thing that they can count on.

For individuals struggling with bulimia nervosa (BN), three family variables appear to be involved, including negative comments related to appearance, external control of food intake, and rules related to family mealtime [32]. Often family meals have been seen as positive and protective, but it depends on how the meals proceed. One client whom I worked with described that when she was growing up, her parents would not speak to each other but would argue through her. She was the conduit for all conversation and disagreement during the family meal. Afterwards, she would go to her room and binge and purge to try to relieve herself of this negativity. This clinical example reflects research findings that document a link between negative family food-related experiences and disordered eating [33]. Families who have poor problem-solving skills can spur increased bulimic symptoms because individuals need to relieve feelings of distress and frustration in that immediate point in time when a problem is being mulled over but not solved [34], whereas individuals who restrict often experience excessive cohesiveness in the family. This sense of over-control is a more global experience and not a discrete episode related to solving a problem. The response to this style of parenting typically leads to more restrictive behaviours because that is the only thing they can control [34].

While we will examine the effect of the media and peer interactions, it appears that parental comments have the largest impact on young adults and the development of body dissatisfaction and eating disorders. Females can be influenced not only by negative comments, but also by positive comments, when the focus still fuels the pressure to stay thin; in males, only negative comments have been related to body dissatisfaction [35]. In addition, in females, eating disorder patients have lower self-esteem as compared to controls and are very sensitive to both positive and negative remarks, such that just one comment can have a significant effect [36]. Dissatisfaction with appearance, lack of regular meals and poor communication with parents increase the likelihood of eating disorder symptoms in both girls and boys [37].

An additional challenge within parent-child relationships is in families where communication between the father and child emphasizes conformity and sets very high standards, which are often unachievable [38]. This spurs self-perfectionism and can make the individual vulnerable to media and society standards, because of the message to conform and achieve. "Those fathers with a communication and conflict resolution style that promotes collaboration/compromise and therefore autonomy in their children help to minimize the risk of the child having significant problems around eating" ([39], p. 60).

A recent example in my program was a father whose daughter had just returned from an extended stay in a residential eating disorders program. She describes that her first morning backs that she was peeling a grapefruit because that is how they ate it at the program. Her father said, "Why are you eating it like that? Don't normal people cut their grapefruit in half?" This is a small example but it had a huge effect on her. She felt criticized, felt "not normal", and a failure despite trying to comply with the meal plan that she had been discharged on. While knowing this father, I do know that he cares deeply about his daughter. But controlling and critical comments can set a standard that seems unreachable and may end up leading to individuals not pursuing their goals since they feel that no matter what they do, they are going to fail anyway.

One challenge within the father-daughter relationship is that daughters want connection/closeness, but fathers often value separateness and independence in their children and so remain distant [40]. These male/female emotional distinctions can get played out within dysfunctional families. There is often a tendency to avoid conflict so communication is stunted. Girls may be aware of the underlying emotional tone but feel powerless to change it; boys, less concerned with family interactions, find support outside the family as they seek their independence [40]. This can leave daughters more vulnerable.

Daughters often model their mothers' relationships to food. This can be a significant issue if mothers have had their own challenges with food and body image. Ref. [41] identified modelling between mothers and daughters in their emotional responses to food and correlations between their eating disorder symptom scores. While daughters mimicking their mothers' eating behaviours may be important, parental comments on the daughter's weight and appearance have a stronger effect than modelling behaviour, such as dieting [42]. This stays true even as women move on into adulthood. The level of concern that adult women have about their weight and their overall body dissatisfaction is often related to comments that they remember their parents making to them when they were young girls [43]. The comments were weight-related or criticism of their appearance.

http://dx.doi.org/10.5772/65305

So how can parents help their children who may be overweight or obese? This is clearly a current societal challenge. The evidence suggests that the focus should be on healthy eating rather than focusing on weight or size. Even for non-overweight adolescents, having one parent engage in weight conversations was triggering, such that the prevalence of dieting went from 15.6% when neither parent engaged in weight conversations to 35.2% when one parent engaged in this talk and 37.1% when both parents engaged in this focus [44]. This is an important consideration because adolescents who report dieting end up experiencing (after 5 years) weight gain, becoming overweight and developing disordered eating [45]. Ref. [46] showed that in recollections of family meal times, comments about appearance/weight control and emphasis on mother's weight were significantly more present in women who were overweight as compared to those who were underweight. He suggests that "…emphasis on mother's weight may be the single most destructive factor mis-shaping a young girl's bodily self-esteem…" (p. 43).

Clinically, it is a challenge when mothers struggle with their own relationships with food and their body image. In working with clients, many describe their mothers' focus on calories or the nonfat nature of a food item, and they find this triggering. Unfortunately, many of these food-related discussions and observations are so engrained in our culture that women may not even realize that are making these comments. Mothers will also body check in front of their daughters, ask whether a certain pair of jeans makes them look fat, and other experiences, which can sometimes be seen as "bonding" but in fact can be extremely triggering to the daughter who may be struggling with her own issues.

This is further escalated if the mother has a clear eating disorder whether it has been diagnosed and treated or not. Often the untreated eating disordered behaviours can be extremely challenging. Daughters find it hard to comply with their meal plan when their mothers are only eating plain lettuce or not even sitting down to eat. Some mothers of patients in our program modelled that they do not eat when they are feeling stressed and often engaged in exercise with their daughters who were being treated in an intensive day program. These mixed messages communicate an ambivalence related to the eating disorder and recovery. How can the daughter value her complete nature and inner talents, when ongoing discussions focus on weight, diets and appearance? Many times, these interactions occur without the mother even being aware of the negative messages. For mothers who have clearly documented eating disorders, there are other ongoing struggles. They worry about being a negative role model, and they want to shield the child from an awareness of symptom use, but this becomes impossible, and in the end, many children end up as caregivers for their parents [47]. Mothers with eating disorders may, in particular, have more difficulty interacting with their daughters around food than their sons, with increased monitoring and food restriction and more appearance-related comments [48]. Difficulties in social communication have been observed in children at a high-risk of an eating disorder, particularly if they were exposed to a mother who experienced bingeing with or without purging behaviours [49]. Their findings suggested a possible shared liability for eating disorders, social anxiety and autism spectrum disorders and raised the possibility that maladaptive eating could result from social difficulties in these individuals [49].

Often certain shared traits in the family precede the eating disorder and can fuel symptom use. These traits run in family, such as anxiety and compulsivity. Family members clearly become anxious when their family member is sick and that anxiety can make the individual more anxious, which can escalate symptom use, and this can fuel the cycle [50]. Overly analytic family members who focus on detail and continually try to argue the individual out of their eating disorder can often strengthen the symptoms because the patients have the chance to rehearse and state their beliefs over and over such they become even more entrenched [50]. These tendencies can have other effects. In one couple, the husband had the need to think through the pros and cons of every decision in a very compulsive way. He would then ask his wife for her opinion of the options. No matter what she answered, he provided the cons of her choice such that she always worried that she had made a mistake. She felt like she was never right and felt inadequate, and this escalated her restricting behaviour.

In addition to the difficulties within family dynamics that might be present prior to the eating disorder, there are challenges that can affect the family once the eating disorder develops, which can cause continual strain for the family and can exacerbate the eating disorder symptoms. Approximately, one-third of caregivers working with children struggling with eating disorders had moderate to severe levels of psychological distress, including depression and anxiety [51]. A review demonstrated consistent findings of psychological distress, expressed emotion, and accommodating and enabling behaviours in caregivers for people with eating disorders [52]. This can become understandable when we consider the stress that families can be under as they work to provide care to their loved one with an eating disorder. This burden can increase as the years of illness increase, and this can impact the caregivers' functioning, such that accommodating behaviours are more frequent, remains the longer the illness [52]. This is understandable if we consider that compromises with the eating disorder might be made as the individual becomes more ill, having them eat anything may be better than trying to engage them in the family meal. In addition, caregivers in the family can get worn down as the day-to-day arguments over meals and exercise continue. In most families, mothers spend 2–5 times as that of fathers in caregiving tasks [51]. In these interactions, mothers have demonstrated more accommodating behaviours, which are often used to decrease distress or anger in their child who is struggling with an eating disorder [51]. However, these accommodating behaviours lead to poorer social aptitude for individuals struggling with AN [51]. This can lead to more social isolation and an ongoing cycle of challenges.

4. Interpersonal factors: peers

Many clients describe that they were teased about weight-related issues during middle and high school either by family members or their peers. Ref. [53] found that among overweight children, three times as many as compared to non-overweight children were teased, and this teasing occurred more frequently, lasted for years, was more emotionally upsetting and was associated with bulimic behaviours. This predicted lower confidence in physical appearance and a tendency to isolate and participate in sedentary activities because the over-weight children were not avoiding just one bully, they were avoiding an entire peer group that teased them [53]. There is a clear association between teasing and body dissatisfaction and disordered eating [54].

http://dx.doi.org/10.5772/65305

Outside of teasing, the prevalence of "fat talk" (conversations pertaining to comments about appearance, dieting, and the need to lose weight) can also be an issue just as we saw with communication between mothers and daughters. College students both with and without an eating disorder discuss people's shape and appearance, but those with an eating disorder engage in more fat talk and are more attuned to and preoccupied with eating and body image [55]. Fat talk is a way that the thin ideal is transmitted between individuals and can affect social connections, such that those who do not comply with this type of talk can be viewed more negatively [56]. Ref. [57] found that fat talk is common among young women and is associated with body dissatisfaction, body checking, negative affect and eating disorder behaviours; this is particularly true if individuals engage in the "fat talk" as opposed to just overhearing it. Body talk can also affect men, not only related to eating disorder behaviour but also the extreme drive for muscularity; however, in conversations with friends, men do express body satisfaction, a topic that is a rarity within women's conversations [58]. It appears that there is a weaker association between fat talk and disordered eating in men as compared to women and in older individuals as compared to those who are younger [59]. The higher association between fat talk and eating disorders in women may be related to the fact that these messages reinforce broad societal messages related to women's appearance [59].

There are also issues related to dieting and weight loss advice that is affected by an individual's appearance. For young women athletes, individuals with higher a BMI received less anti-dieting advice than those with lower BMI, even though both groups had the same level of disordered eating symptoms [60]. This pattern has been present for non-athletes as well and has been seen in comments by healthcare providers, at times. There is often a focus on weight loss when individuals are overweight to obese and not an exploration of how this goal is being accomplished. Individuals may be using dysfunctional eating disorder behaviours, but this is not often confirmed until there is a physical evidence of low weight or other physical issues.

5. Interpersonal factors: online experiences

Individuals with eating disorders can have challenges with interpersonal connections. Some of this can be related to issues that have already been discussed. For example, they have a tendency to interpret interactions through a self-critical lens that often has them withdraw from these situations. Many of our cultural interactions revolve around food, which can be extremely challenging for individuals who struggle with eating disorders. In addition, many clients describe that their eating disorder makes them feel isolated. Often when they come into treatment they find a community. This can be supportive or can keep them stuck in their eating disorder because by recovering, they lose part of their identity and support.

Individuals sometimes turn to online groups to find a support system. Members of online forum groups perceive less support from others in their lives as compared with age-matched peers and describe receiving better support overall and specifically related to their eating concerns through the group conversations [61]. Communication within these forums can be helpful, providing advice of how to get help, or they can support the eating disorder behaviours. This is especially true related to online groups that function around disordered eating.

Ref. [62] evaluated online discussion groups related to general psychiatric issues, abuse or a forum for eating disorders. All of the forums provided users with constructive/positive responses to posts, which could be seen as encouraging social support. However "destructive" posts and topic threads, which encouraged negative behaviours, were more than twice as common in the eating disorder group as compared with the other two forums. In the thin focused culture that we live in, no one tends to encourage staying depressed or being abused, but positive feedback can be provided to encourage individuals to try and get thin.

This is evident in online discussion groups that are pro-ana (pro-anorexia nervosa) or pro-mia (pro-bulimia nervosa) and encourage eating disorder behaviour. Social support is most frequently communicated among pro-ana bloggers, which leads to intense friendships and bonds that can have both positive (encouraging seeking treatment) and negative effects (comments that encourage further weight loss) [63]. Interviews with pro-ana group participants demonstrated that each individual had significant evidence of disordered eating and had joined the group specifically to gather advice about weight loss and support for their symptom use [64]. While Ref. [65] found that groups that form a recovery focus can offer individuals much needed support, Ref. [61] describes that in addition to support, forums encourage eating disorder behaviours. Although pro-recovery activity has been found on Facebook, they attract fewer users than pro-anorexia groups [66]. Pro-ED websites do not necessarily imply "anti-recovery", but users who come for information about seeking treatment may instead find validation of their eating disorder identities and tips about how to continue their symptoms use and hide it from others [67].

Individuals who receive extremely negative comments to their Facebook statuses experience higher shape, weight and eating concerns. These individuals often have a negative feedback seeking style that promotes critical comments, and this, in turn, increases their restrained eating [68]. How individuals ask for feedback can affect what is said, and their further negative interpretation of these comments can escalate the damaging effect.

6. Interpersonal factors: media

Messages from the media can influence eating disorders in a number of ways. First is the overall presentation of society's "thin ideal" and unrealistic expectations, especially with the mixed messages about the indulgence on food yet with the need to still conform to a certain svelte appearance. "Whereas the ideal female has become progressively thinner over the last 30 years, the male ideal has become increasingly dense and muscular" ([69], p. 298). Media images of the "thin ideal" can have an immediate effect on women's moods such that they feel angrier and more depressed after examining just 20 images; women who are more dissatisfied with their bodies or have feelings of ineffectiveness or interpersonal distrust are more vulnerable to these effects [70]. These images of unattainable thinness can influence some women to eat more, perhaps related to feeling one's status as worse in a culture of thinness and exacerbating negative effect and lowered self-esteem [71]. In addition, magazine articles often focus on diet and weight loss and can contribute to negative weight control behaviours to help women meet their thin ideal [72]. Restricting calories and taking diet pills appear to be influenced by reading fashion magazines [73]. The emphasis of the magazines of self-improvement is typically in the realm of physical beautification [73]. These are just some of the skewed messages that are being communicated.

Second is how the media portrays eating disorders since these messages can influence individuals as they consider pursing help. Ref. [74] found that magazine articles tended to focus on unusually thin sufferers of eating disorders with a disproportionate focus on anorexia nervosa, such that readers can get the erroneous view that someone who is overweight cannot have an eating disorder. This concern seems to be merited as many times normal weight individuals who struggle with bulimia report that others have made comments to them that they do not look like they have an eating disorder. The articles often provide a superficial presentation of eating disorders, so that readers do not get a sense of the complex emotional issues that underlie eating disorders and the complex path for recovery [74]. Articles about eating disorders are typically placed in the entertainment-related sections, so are seen as "soft" news stories [75]. In addition "...profiles of individuals with EDs also understated the complexity of causes and outcomes associated with anorexia and bulimia and overstated the likelihood of an easy recovery" ([75], p. 48). These messages can be exceptionally hard for sufferers and their families. The messages communicated by the media are often that eating disorders are not that serious and can be easily overcome. When perfectionistic young women struggle with recovery, they view these messages as criticisms of themselves—they are not strong enough to recover—and families are lulled into expectations that this illness will be easy to treat. Since the response to individuals with AN is often, "Just eat!" one can see the pervasive harm of these superficial messages.

7. Interpersonal factors: healthcare professionals

While healthcare professionals should be more aware of the potentially negative effects of their comments and the health risk of eating disorders, this does not always seem to be the case. Clients have returned from referrals for bone scans to assess the possibility of osteoporosis and describe that the technician said, "I wish I could have anorexia for just a little while". Doctors have not listened to the concerns of patients and families related to weight loss. There is such a focus on obesity that losing weight is not seen as a significant concern. This can delay necessary treatment for individuals and lead to a greater risk of complications. Ref. [76] quoted one patient who was being seen for binge-eating disorder (BED) as being told by her paediatrician *"to do my push-away exercise, meaning push food away"* (p. 58). Patients describe needing a safe environment where they can talk about their issues and a competent understanding of the illnesses by their providers. Often if providers do not have a good understanding of eating disorders, they minimize the problem [77]. This can affect the individual's pursuit of treatment and level of shame. In addition, often individuals are not seeking treatment on their own but are being pushed to discuss treatment at the encouragement of someone else, and this can lead to intense anxiety over losing control of the eating and their life [77]. Practitioners need to be aware of this anxiety and engage individuals in the session so they can express their goals, their concerns and what steps they are willing to take.

Even in a field that should have compassionate professionals, when assessing BED, psychiatrists recommended that patients employ willpower to break the symptom use and often phrased questions in ways that patients felt judged. Despite patients wanting to explore factors that they felt were driving the binges, such as negative emotions, the psychiatrists often did not explore those areas, focusing instead on type of food eaten, amount, etc. [78]. A word cloud provided a stark visual as to how the psychiatrists and patients each viewed BED, with the psychiatrists focused on symptoms such as binge, weight, ever vomit, how much weigh as compared to the patients whose top words included depressed, stress, anxiety, sweet [78]. The word clouds highlighted the most frequent terms introduced by either the psychiatrist or the patient during their sessions. With such remarkable differences in viewpoints, one can see where communication might falter in these encounters.

Professionals need to be aware of not only what they say, but also of their body language. If they appear not engaged, bored and dismissive of the problem or violate the patient's safe space, individuals who are already ambivalent about seeking treatment may flee from an uncomfortable interaction and not pursue potential treatment. Attention to tone of voice, body language, etc. can help "...alleviate the patient's feelings of loneliness and make her feel safe and listened to" ([77] p. 220). When staff from a inpatient children's hospital were surveyed, nurses had more sympathy towards the ED patients than the paediatric residents (58.1 vs. 37.5%), but only 12.5% of the nurses felt rewarded caring for their ED patients and only 6.3 % of the residents [79]. This level of frustration has the potential to be transmitted to the patients and their families, which can affect their decision about whether to pursue or continue with medical care.

All frontline practitioners, including dentists, should increase their competence related to eating disorders. Dental fear is higher among women with ED as opposed to the general population, which can impact dental visits, even though purging can lead to dental erosion [80]. Ref. [81] offers an extremely useful sample dialogue to help approach patients about a possible eating disorder when dental signs are discovered. These guidelines can help other practitioners. They emphasize making certain there is enough time to discuss the issue, enough privacy, to start slowly with the observations that have been made and listen to the patient's thoughts as to what might be causing the damage, if they do not offer information suggest possible causes of the damage, explore the patients' relationship with food, body image and eating, and then offer referrals for help with the eating issue as indicated. The suggested dialogue in this article offers a comprehensive view of eating disorders and a compassionate approach that could be employed by all health professionals.

8. Recommendations

Considering this information are there guidelines that can improve overall communication with individuals who struggle with eating disorders?

A. We need to understand that eating disorders are not only isolating for the individual, but also often for the family as well as they try to cope with the rules and expectations that

http://dx.doi.org/10.5772/65305

the eating disorder demands. Working with the patient and family to help them engage in food-related events will be important. However, it may be necessary for the clinician to help broker some of these experiences. Dining out can be hard for individuals with an eating disorder, but the meal can be planned ahead of time and a positive family interaction can occur. Yet taking the individual to a buffet may be so overwhelming that it can lead to a retreat from that experience back into the safety of the eating disorder. Families often do not understand how stressful everyday food events can be for someone struggling with an eating disorder. The extent of this challenge may need to be communicated by the healthcare professional.

B. Family messages can unintentionally be provided that keep the symptoms in place [82]. One set of parents who were considering divorce told the staff and daughter that they were going to stay together until she was well. What incentive did she have to get better? Once she was well, her family would dissolve. Another patient described that her family was very involved and caring when she was sick, but then as she got well, they disappeared from her life because they were no longer worried about her health. The only way to keep them close and involved was by staying ill. Practitioners may need to decipher these messages.

C. Families need help understanding the way that some of their behaviours reinforce the eating disorder so they can find alternatives. For example, do they incorporate all the eating disorder rules into the family just to keep peace? If either parent's behaviour is accommodating or enabling the eating disorder that will adversely affect recovery [83]. Are there ever negative consequences for the eating disorder behaviours or does mom just clean up vomit from the bathroom and not confront the issue? Families will need help with small steps that can help shift the dynamics within the family. They will need to working together, making small changes, such as working on more positive communication, openly and calmly discussing issues rather than avoiding the topic of symptom use, and working together against the eating disorder. In one couple in which the girlfriend was over-exercising, we had to help support the boyfriend to not feel obligated to go on long hikes with her. He was trying to keep her happy but was fuelling the eating disorder thoughts. Another individual's boyfriend would often buy her binge food so that she would not steal it, would not get angry, and sometimes as a reward for doing well in her recovery. This is a very mixed message.

D. Families need information to help them understand eating disorders. Understanding the biological risk factors can help decrease some of the shame, blame and guilt. Understanding how their loved ones who struggle with an eating disorder process messages and struggle with perfectionism may help in interactions. Carers often describe that they want more information, practical advice and guidance [84]. Psychoeducation can help lower distress and create a more understanding perspective [85].

E. We need to help parents as caregivers and focus on decreasing overprotection so their children can feel a sense of control in their lives [30]. With this comes the need to assist families to improve open communication and skilled conflict resolution. One aspect of this is for family members to listen to each other and not to interrupt so that everyone has an opportunity to express their needs and opinions in a supportive atmosphere. Sometimes a "talking stick" or other object can be helpful. The person holding the stick gets to speak and cannot be interrupted.

F. We need to help those struggling with eating disorders to become more assertive. A basic formula for expressing one's self is "When you..., I feel..., because..." ([86], p. 145). If someone dismisses the individual's feelings, they can say "'That may be so...' (You are neither agreeing nor disagreeing with them.)...'...But I want you to know how your behaviour affects me'"([86], p. 147). This pattern of expressing one's self may need to be repeated before others will start to listen. The individual struggling with an eating disorder needs to be able to express their opinions without the use of their symptoms.

G. Teaching families some of the tools that we as physicians should be using, such as summarizing what you think the other person has said. It is through these conversations, "So if I understand you, you feel..." that misinterpretations and assumptions can be clarified and corrected.

H. Work to help families feel empowered because many family members may struggle with their own sense of low self-esteem [30]. Low self-esteem can cause individuals to use unfavourable comparison strategies, that is, that their daughter is sicker than others [87]. This can increase maternal stress and affect the family's overall level of functioning. The child is seen in the sick role rather than as one able to recover. A recent clinic example included a mother who the daughter perceived as distant and neglectful. The mother spoke highly of a girl she knew who recovered from her eating disorder and was doing so well. Yet the daughter felt that the mother never acknowledged her own struggles. This comparison led to the daughter feeling like she needed to get sicker in order to get her mother's attention. We need to help strengthen connections within families and work to help each member understand the hidden messages that words and actions convey.

I. Help families understand that they need to engage in self-care behaviours so that they do not experience caregiver burnout. One way to discuss this is that family members need to be role models for healthy coping so that their children can learn from them [88]. Physicians need to help communicate these messages so that families take care of themselves. They need permission, and they need to understand that unless they care for themselves, they will not be able to help their child recover [88].

J. Understand that the eating disorder can become such an engrained part of Individuals' identities that they become fearful of whom they will be without the illness. As described in [89], p. 863, "The recovery process brought losses because in rejecting the illness, they were also rejecting a major part of their identity". This concept is important so that friends, family and healthcare professionals can help individuals reconnect with interests prior to the eating disorder, help them discover new interests or work to understand what led to the illness—what function it serves—so that they can replace that function in a healthier way.

K. Strong feelings of guilt and shame related to the eating disorder may make it difficult for individuals to ask for help and support with their recovery [89]. Families and caregivers need

http://dx.doi.org/10.5772/65305

to understand that a lack of communication does not mean that their loved one does not need their help. They may be fearful of being seen as a burden. In addition, there are times that individuals struggling with an eating disorder will feel when not being asked questions about the illness is an indication that the caregiver is no longer worried about them [90].

L. At times, patients have difficulty expressing themselves. They do not really know how they feel or they fear expressing their opinions. Sometimes they communicate through their eating disorder. One patient told me that when the family was struggling with an issue, she let her body speak for her. When she increased her restricting, she was trying to let her family know her feelings. As described by a parent "…The unspoken words are more important than the spoken word" ([91], p. 423). The individual struggling with an eating disorder may put a good face on how things are going and say that everything is all right. If there is evidence to the opposite, do not ignore it!

M. Physicians and other healthcare providers need to be more sensitive to issues of eating disorders and the potential effects of their comments. If a healthcare provider suspects an eating disorder, they need to ask about body concerns and eating habits in a compassionate style. Their assumptions and comments can have lasting effects.

N. Improved education should also include school nurses, teachers and coaches. Often early signs of eating disorders can present in these different environments. Adults need to be able to recognize the warning signs and be able to initiate discussions in a compassionate and well-educated manner.

O. While there may be family communication issues, which may suggest the need for family therapy, family members should not be made to feel guilty about the eating disorder. The goal should be for the family to align with and help the individual tackle the eating disorder.

P. As parents or providers, if one is interacting with a child or young adult who may need to lose weight, the focus needs to be on health and not on dieting. Weight-related teasing only hurts the individual's self-esteem. Dieting only starts the individual on a futile cycle. When parents engage in weight-related conversations, they increase the risk that their children will diet, use unhealthy weight-control practices or binge-eat [44]. Capitalize focus instead on pursuing a range of fun activities!

Q. We need to teach children to practice media literacy (and practice it ourselves). This can help blunt the impact of the messages that bombard us on a daily basis. We need to remember how images are created and photoshopped so that when we compete with the model in a magazine, we recognize that we are trying to match a fantasy.

R. Families should also consider environmental cues, how many fashion magazines do they have in the house? What shows are they watching? What messages are being promoted? Consider the messages that are being provided—"unlike the media, parents are able to deliberately adapt their communication with their children" ([35], p. 148).

S. We need to work with parents both of our patients and parents in general to examine the messages that they are providing to their children. A home environment needs to nurture positive feelings about one's body and one's self.

9. Conclusion

We live in a world that is focused on a thin ideal. The messages that we receive from the media can influence people's overall self-esteem and be especially triggering for individuals who are at risk for eating disorders. It is important that we practice media literacy and that we treat ourselves and others with compassion. Weight-related comments and teasing can escalate the risk of disordered eating. Families and professionals should instead focus on health and providing support. Excessive expectations can lead to perfectionism and disordered eating as a way to comply with unreachable goals. Within interpersonal interactions, all individuals, especially those struggling with eating disorders, need to be encouraged to express their opinions. If they are not allowed or encouraged to use their words, they will use their bodies and symptoms to let people know something is wrong. We need to be aware of what we say and what those who struggle with eating disorders hear. Let's work to ensure that there are positive messages filled with compassion and care.

Author details

Martha Peaslee Levine

Address all correspondence to: mlevine1@hmc.psu.edu

Departments for Pediatrics, Psychiatry and Humanities, Penn State College of Medicine, Hershey, PA, USA

References

[1] American Psychiatric Association (2013). Diagnostic and Statistical Manual of Mental Disorders, Fifth Edition. Arlington, VA, American Psychiatric Association.

[2] Hardit, S.K. & Hannum, J.W. (2012). Attachment, the tripartite influence model, and the development of body dissatisfaction. *Body Image, 9*, 469–475.

[3] van den Berg, P., Thompson, J.K., Obremski-Brandon, K & Coovert, M. (2002). The tripartite influence model of body image and eating disturbance: a covariance structure modelling investigation testing the mediational role of appearance comparison. *Journal of Psychosomatic Research, 53*, 1007–1020.

[4] Toro, J., Salamero, M., & Martinez, E. (1994). Assessment of sociocultural influences on the aesthetic body shape model in anorexia nervosa. *Acta Psychiatrica Scandinavica, 89*, 147–151.

[5] McFillin, R.K, Cahn, S.C., Burks, V.S., Levine, M.P., Lane-Loney, S., & Levine, R.L. (2012). Social information-processing and coping in adolescent females diagnosed with an eating disorder: toward a greater understanding of control. *Eating Disorders, 20*, 42–59. doi:10.1080/10640266.2012.635565

[6] Davies, H., Swan, N., Schmidt, U., & Tchanturia, K. (2011). An experimental investigation of verbal expression of emotion in anorexia and bulimia nervosa. *European Eating Disorders Review, 20*, 476–483.

[7] Tobin, D.L. & Griffing, A.S. (1995). Coping and depression in bulimia nervosa. *International Journal of Eating Disorders, 18*(4), 359–363.

[8] Waller, G., Quinton, S., & Watson, D. (1995). Processing of threat-related information by women with bulimic eating attitudes. *International Journal of Eating Disorders, 18*(2), 189–193.

[9] Espeset, E.M.S., Gulliksen, K.S., Nordbø, R.H.S., Skårderud, F., & Holte, A. (2012). Fluctuations of body images in anorexia nervosa: patients' perception of contextual triggers. *Clinical Psychology and Psychotherapy, 19*, 518–530.

[10] Ferraro, F.R., Andres, M., Stromberg, L., & Kristjanson, J. (2003). Processing fat-related information in individuals at risk for developing an eating disorder. *The Journal of Psychology, 137*(5), 467–475.

[11] Smeets, E., Roefs, A., van Furth, E., & Jansen, A. (2008). Attentional bias for body and food in eating disorders: Increased distraction, speeded detection, or both? *Behaviour Research, 46*, 229–238. doi:10.1016/j.brat.2007.12.003

[12] Davies, H., Schmidt, U., Stahl, D., & Tchanturia, K. (2011). Evoked facial emotional expression and emotional experience in people with anorexia nervosa. *International Journal of Eating Disorders, 44*(6), 531–539.

[13] Rhind, C., Mandy, W., Treasure, J., & Tchanturia, K. (2014). An exploratory study of evoked facial affect in adolescent females with anorexia nervosa. *Psychiatry Research, 220*, 711–715.

[14] Dapelo, M.M., Hart, S., Hale, C., Morris, R., & Lynch, T.R. (2015). Facial expression of positive emotions in individuals with eating disorders. *Psychiatry Research, 230*, 70–77.

[15] Dapelo, M.M., Bodas, S., Morris, R., & Tchanturia, K. (2016). Deliberately generated and imitated facial expressions of emotions in people with eating disorders. *Journal of Affective Disorders, 191*, 1–7.

[16] Jänsch, C., Harmer, C., & Cooper, M.J. (2009). Emotional processing in women with anorexia nervosa and in healthy volunteers. *Eating Behaviors, 10*, 184–191.

[17] Oldershaw, A., Hambrook, D., Stachl, D., Tchanturia, K., Treasure, J., & Schmidt, U. (2011). The socio-emotional processing stream in anorexia nervosa. *Neuroscience and Biobehavioral Reviews, 35*, 970–988.

[18] Ridout, N., Wallis, D.J., Autwal, Y., & Sellis, J. (2012). The influence of emotional intensity on facial emotion recognition in disordered eating. *Appetite, 59*, 181–186.

[19] Dapelo, M.M., Surguladze, S., Morris, R., & Tchanturia, K. (2016). Emotion recognition in blended facial expressions in women with anorexia nervosa. *European Eating Disorders Review, 24*, 34–42.

[20] Castro, L., Davies, H., Hale, L., Surguladze, S., & Tchanturia, K. (2010). Facial affect recognition in anorexia nervosa: is obsessionality a missing piece of the puzzle? *Australian and New Zealand Journal of Psychiatry, 44*, 1118–1125.

[21] Fox, J.R.E. (2009). A qualititative exploration of the perception of emotions in anorexia nervosa: a basic emotion and developmental perspective. *Clinical Psychologyand Psychotherapy, 16*, 276–302.

[22] Ackard, D.M., Neumark-Sztainer, D., Story, M., & Perry, C. (2006). Parent–child connectedness and behavioural and emotional health among adolescents. *American Journal of Preventive Medicine, 30*(1), 59–66.

[23] Ciccolo, E.B.F. (2008). Exploring experience of family relations by patients with anorexia nervosa and bulimia nervosa using a projective family test. *Psychological Reports, 103*, 231–242.

[24] Schmidt, R., Tetzlaff, A., & Hilbert, A. (2015). Perceived expressed emotion in adolescents with binge-eating disorder. *Journal of Abnormal Child Psychology, 43*, 1369–1377.

[25] Hanna, A.C. & Bond, M.J. (2006). Relationships between family conflict, perceived maternal verbal messages, and daughters' disturbed eating symptomatology. *Appetite, 47*, 205–211.

[26] Neumark-Sztainer, D., Bauer, K.W., Friend, S., Hannan, P.J., Story, M., & Berge, J.M. (2010). Family weight talk and dieting: How much do they matter for body dissatisfaction and disordered eating behaviors in adolescent girls? *Journal of Adolescent Health, 47*(3), 270–276.

[27] Larson, B.J. (1991). Relationship of family communication patterns to Eating Disorder Inventory scores in adolescent girls. *Journal of the American Dietetic Association, 91*, 1065–1067.

[28] Emanuelli, F., Ostuzzi, R., Cuzzolaro, M., Baggio, F., Lask, B., & Waller, G. (2004). Family functioning in adolescent anorexia nervosa: a comparison of family members' perceptions. *Eating and Weight Disorders, 9*, 1–6.

[29] Holtom-Viesel, A. & Allan, S. (2014). A systematic review of the literature on family functioning across all eating disorder diagnoses in comparison to control families. *Clinical Psychology Review, 34*, 29–43.

[30] Jáuregui Lobera, I., Bolaños Ríos, P., & Garrido Casals, O. (2011). Parenting styles and eating disorders. *Journal of Paychiatric and Mental Health Nursing, 18*, 728–735.

[31] Dancyger, I., Fornari, V., & Sunday, S. (2006). What may underlie differing perceptions of family functioning between mothers and their adolescent daughters with eating disorders? *International Journal of Adolescent Medicine and Health, 18*(2), 281–286.

[32] Crowther, J.H., Kichler, J.C., Sherwood, N.E., & Kuhnert, M.E. (2002). The role of familial factors in bulimia nervosa. *Eating Disorders, 10*(2), 141–151.

[33] Kluck, A.S. (2008). Family factors in the development of disordered eating: Integrating dynamic and behavioural explanations. *Eating Behaviors, 9*, 471–483.

[34] Waller, G. (1994). Bulimic women's perceptions of interaction within their families. *Psychological Reports, 74*, 27–32.

[35] Rodgers, R.F., Paxton, S.J., & Chabrol, H. (2009). Effects of parental comments on body dissatisfaction and eating disturbance in young adults: a sociocultural model. *Body Image, 6*, 171–177.

[36] Vanderlinden, J., Kamphuis, J.H., Slagmolen, C., Wigboldus, D., Pieter, G., & Probst, M. (2009). Be kind to your eating disorder patients: the impact of positive and negative feedback on the explicit and implicit self-esteem of female patients with eating disorders. *Eating and Weight Disorders, 14*, e237–e242.

[37] Hautala, L.A., Junnila, J., Helenius, H., Väänänen, A., Liuksila, P., Räihä, H., Välimäki, M., & Saarijärvi, S. (2008). Towards understanding gender differences in disordered eating among adolescents. *Journal of Clinical Nursing, 17*, 1803–1813.

[38] Miller-Day, M. & Marks, J.D. (2006). Perceptions of parental communication orientation, perfectionism, and disordered eating behaviors of sons and daughters. *Health Communication, 19*(2), 153–163.

[39] Gale, C.J., Cluett, E.R., & Laver-Bradbury, C. (2013). A review of the father-child relationship in the development and maintenance of adolescent anorexia and bulimia nervosa. *Issues in Comprehensive Pediatric Nursing, 36*(1–2), 48–69.

[40] Maine, M. (2004). Father Hunger: Fathers, Daughters, and the Pursuit of Thinness. Carlsbad, CA, Gürze Books.

[41] Lewis, S., Katsikitis, M., & Mulgrew, K. (2015). Like mother, like daughter? An examination of the emotive responses to food. *Journal of Health Psychology, 20*(6), 828–838.

[42] Bardone-Cone, A.M., Harney, M.B., & Sayen, L. (2011). Perceptions of parental attitudes toward body and eating: associations with body image among black and white college women. *Body Image, 8*, 186–189.

[43] Wansink, B., Latimer, L.A. & Pope, L. Eat Weight Disord (2016). doi:10.1007/s40519-016-0292-6

[44] Berge, J.M., MacLehose, R., Loth, K.A., Eisenberg, M., Bucchianeri, M.M., & Neumark-Sztainer, D. (2013). Parent conversations about healthful eating and weight, associations with adolescent disordered eating behaviors. *JAMA Pediatrics, 167*(8), 746–753.

[45] Neumark-Sztainer, D., Wall, M., Guo, J., Story, M., Haines, J., & Eisenberg, M. (2006). Obesity, disordered eating, and eating disorders in a longitudinal study of adolescents: How do dieters fare 5 years later? *Journal of the American Dietetic Association, 106*, 559–568.

[46] Worobey, J. (2002). Early family mealtime experiences and eating attitudes in normal weight, underweight and overweight females. *Eating and Weight Disorders, 7*, 39–44.

[47] Tuval-Mashiach, R., Ram, A., Shapiro, T., Shenhave, S., & Gur, E. (2013). Negotiating maternal identity: Mothers with eating disorders discuss their coping. *Eating Disorders, 21*(1), 35–52.

[48] Sadeh-Sharvit, S., Levy-Shiff, R., Feldman, T., Ram, A., Gur, E., Zubery, E., Steiner, E., Latzer, Y., & Lock, J.D. (2015). Child feeding perceptions among mothers with eating disorders. *Appetite, 95*, 67–73.

[49] Kothari, R., Barona, M., Treasure, J., & Micali, N. (2015). Social cognition in children at familial high-risk of developing an eating disorder. *Frontiers in Behavioral Neuroscience, 9*(208). doi:10.3389/fnbeh.2015.00208

[50] Treasure, J., Sepulveda, A.R., MacDonald, P., Whitaker, W., Lopez, C., Zabala, M., Kyriacou, O., & Todd, G. (2008). The assessment of the family of people with eating disorders. *European Eating Disorders Review, 16*, 247–255.

[51] Rhind, C., Salerno, L., Hibbs, R., Micali, N., Schmidt, U., Gowers, S., Macdonald, P., Goddard, E., Todd, G., Tchanturia, K., Lo Coco, G., & Treasure, J. (2016). The objective and subjective caregiving burden and caregiving behaviours of parents of adolescents with anorexia nervosa. *European Eating Disorders Review*. 24(4), 310–319

[52] Anastasiadou, D., Medina-Pradas, C., Sepulveda, A.R., & Treasure, J. (2014). A systematic review of family caregiving in eating disorders. *Eating Behaviors, 15*, 464–477.

[53] Hayden-Wade, H.A., Stein, R.I., Ghaderi, A., Saelens, B.E., Zabinski, M.F., & Wilfley, D.E.(2005). Prevalence, characteristics, and correlates of teasing experiences among overweight children vs. non-overweight peers. *Obesity Research, 13*(8), 1381–1392.

[54] Menzel, J.E., Schaefer, L.M., Burke, N.L., Mayher, L.L., Brannick, M.T., & Thompson, J.K. (2010). Appearance-related teasing, body dissatisfaction, and disordered eating: a meta-analysis. *Body Image, 7*, 261–270.

[55] Ousley, L., Cordero, E.D., & White, S. (2008). Fat talk among college students: How undergraduates communicate regarding food and body weight, shape & appearance. *Eating Disorders, 16*, 73–84.

[56] Cruwys, T., Leverington, C.T., & Sheldon, A.M. (2016). An experimental investigation of the consequences and social functions of fat talk in friendship groups. *International Journal of Eating Disorders, 49*, 84–91.

[57] Jones, M.D., Crowther, J.H., & Ciesla, J.A. (2014). A naturalistic study of fat talk and its behavioural and affective consequences. *Body Image, 11*, 337–345.

[58] Engeln, R., Sladek, M.R., & Waldron, H. (2013). Body talk among college men: content, correlates, and effects. *Body Image, 10*, 300–308.

[59] Tzoneva, M., Forney, K.J., & Keel, P.K. (2015). The influence of gender and age on the association between "Fat-Talk" and disordered eating: an examination in men and women from their 20s to their 50s. *Eating Disorders, 23*(5), 439–454.

[60] Kroshus, E., Kubzansky, L., Goldman, R., & Austin, S.B. (2015). Anti-dieting advice from teammates: a pilot study of the experience of female collegiate cross country runners. *Eating Disorders, 23*, 31–44.

[61] Ransom, D.C., La Guardia, J.G., Woody, E.Z., & Boyd, J.L. (2010). Interpersonal interactions on online forums addressing eating concerns. *International Journal of Eating Disorders, 43*, 161–170.

[62] Johnsen, J.K., Rosenvinge, J.H., & Gammon, D. (2002). Online group interaction and mental health: an analysis of three online discussion forums. *Scandinavian Journal of Psychology, 43*, 445–449.

[63] Tong, S.T., Heinemann-LaFave, D., Jeon, J., Kolodziej-Smith, R., & Warshay, N. (2013). The use of pro-ana blogs for online social support. *Eating Disorders, 21*(5), 408–422.

[64] Rodgers, R.F., Skowron, S., & Chabrol, H. (2011). Disordered eating and group membership among members of a pro-anorexia online community. *European Eating Disorders Review, 20*, 9–12.

[65] Wesemann, D. & Grunwald, M. (2008). Online discussion groups for bulimia nervosa: an inductive approach to internet-based communication between patients. *International Journal of Eating Disorders, 41*, 527–534.

[66] Teufel, M., Hofer, E., Junne, F., Sauer, H., Zipfel, S., & Giel, K.E. (2013). A comparative anaylsis of anorexia nervosa groups on Facebook. *Eating and Weight Disorders, 18*, 413–420.

[67] Rouleau, C.R. & von Ranson, K.M. (2011). Potential risks of pro-eating disorder websites. *Clinical Psychology Review, 31*, 525 531.

[68] Hummel, A.C. & Smith, A.R. (2015). Ask and you shall receive: desire and receipt of feedback via Facebook predicts disordered eating concerns. *International Journal of Eating Disorders, 48*, 436–442.

[69] Borzekowski, D.L.G & Bayer, A.M. (2005). Body image and media use among adolescents. *Adolescent Medicine Clinics, 16*(2), 289–313.

[70] Pinhas, L., Toner, B.B., Ali, A., Garfinkel, P.E., & Stuckless, N. (1999). The effects of the ideal of female beauty on mood and body satisfaction. *International Journal of Eating Disorders, 25*, 223–226.

[71] Polivy, J. & Pliner, P. (2015). "She got more than me". Social comparison and the social context of eating. *Appetite, 86*, 88–95.

[72] Utter, J., Neumark-Sztainer, D., Wall, M., & Story, M. (2003). Reading magazine articles about dieting and associated weight control behaviors among adolescents. *Journal of Adolescent Health, 32*, 78–82.

[73] Thomsen, S.R., Weber, M.M., & Brown, L.B. (2002). The relationship between reading beauty and fashion magazines and the use of pathogenic dieting methods among adolescent females. *Adolescence, 37*(145), 1–18.

[74] Inch, R. & Merali, N. (2006). A content analysis of popular magazine articles on eating disorders. *Eating Disorders, 14*(2), 109–120.

[75] O'Hara, S.K. & Smith, K.C. (2007). Presentation of eating disorders in the news media: what are the implications for patient diagnosis and treatment? *Patient Education and Counseling, 68*, 43–51.

[76] Herman, B.K., Safikhani, S., Hengerer, D., Atkins, Jr., N., Kim, A., Cassidy, D., Babcock, T., Agus, S., Lenderking, W.R. (2014). The patient experience with DSM-5 defined binge eating disorder: characteristics, barriers to treatment, and implications for primary care physicians. *Postgraduate Medicine, 126*(5), 52–63.

[77] Gulliksen, K.S., Nordbø, R. H.S., Espeset, E.M.S., Skårderud, F., & Holte, A. (2015). The process of help-seeking in anorexia nervosa: patients' perspective of first contact with health services. *Eating Disorders, 23*, 206–222.

[78] Kornstein, S.G., Keck,Jr., P.E., Herman, B.K., Puhl, R.M., Wilfley, D.E., & DiMarco, I.D. (2015). Communication between physicians and patients with suspected or diagnosed binge eating disorder. *Postgraduate Medicine, 127*(7), 661–670.

[79] Raveneau, G., Feinstein, R., Rosen, L.M., & Fisher, M. (2014). Attitudes and knowledge levels of nurses and residents caring for adolescents with an eating disorder. *International Journal of Adolescent Medicine and Health, 26*(1), 131–136.

[80] Willumsen, T. & Graugaard, P.K. (2005). Dental fear, regularity of dental attendance and subjective evaluation of dental erosion in women with eating disorders. *European Journal of Oral Sciences, 113*, 297–302.

[81] Burkhart, N., Roberts, M., Alexander, M., & Dodds, A. (2005). Communicating effectively with patients suspected of having bulimia nervosa. *Journal of the American Dental Association, 136*, 1130–1137.

[82] Lemmon, C.R. & Josephson, A.M. (2001). Family therapy for eating disorders. *Child and Adolescent Clinics of North America, 10*(3), 519–542.

[83] Salerno, L., Rhind, C., Hibbs, R., Micali, N., Schmidt, U., Gowers, S., Macdonald, P., Goddard, E., Todd, G., Coco, G.L, Treasure, J. (2016). An examination of the impact of care giving styles (accommodation and skilful communication and support) on the one year outcome of adolescent anorexia nervosa: testing the assumptions of the cognitive interpersonal model in anorexia nervosa. *Journal of Affective Disorders, 191*, 230–236.

[84] Winn, S., Perkins, S., Murray, J., Murphy, R., & Schmidt, U. (2004). A qualitative study of the experience of caring for a person with bulimia nervosa. Part 2: Carers' needs and experiences of services and other support. *International Journal of Eating Disorders, 36*, 269–279.

[85] Uehara, T., Kawashima, Y., Goto, M., Tasaki, S., & Someya, T. (2001). Psychoeducation for the families of patients with eating disorders and changes in expressed emotion: a preliminary study. *Comprehensive Psychiatry, 42*(2), 132–138.

http://dx.doi.org/10.5772/65305

[86] Johnston, A. (1996). Eating in the Light of the Moon. Carlsbad, CA, Gürze Books.

[87] Jáuregui Lobera, I., Garrido, O., Santiago Fernández, M.J., & Álvarez Bautista, E. (2010). Social comparison as a coping strategy among caregivers of eating disorder patients. *Journal of Psychiatric and Mental Health Nursing, 17*, 775–782.

[88] Patel, S., Shafer, A., Brown, J., Bulik, C., & Zucker, N. (2014). Parents of children with eating disorders: developing theory-based health communication messages to promote caregiver well-being. *Journal of Health Communication, 19*, 593–608.

[89] Lindgren, B-M., Enmark, A., Bohman, A., & Lundström, M. (2015). A qualitative study of young women's experiences of recovery from bulimia nervosa. *The Journal of Advanced Nursing*, 71(4), 860–869.

[90] Papathomas, A., Smith, B., & Lavallee, D. (2015). Family experiences of living with an eating disorder: a narrative analysis. *Journal of Health Psychology, 20*(3), 313–325.

[91] Cohn, L. (2005). Parents' voices: what they say is important in the treatment and recovery process. *Eating Disorders, 13*(4), 419–428.